Adult Telephone Triage Guidelines

(Age 18 Years +)

A 5-Tier Approach
to Triaging Symptom Urgency

Sheila Wheeler

TeleTriage Systems Publishers

NOTICE TO THE READER

The authors and publisher have made every effort to provide accurate information. However, they are not responsible for errors, omissions, or for any outcomes related to the use of the contents of this book and take no responsibility for the use of the products and procedures described.

To the best of our knowledge, the dispositions in this book reflect safe practice; nevertheless, they cannot be considered absolute and universal recommendations. The authors and publisher disclaim any responsibility for any adverse effects resulting from any suggested home treatment, or from any undetected errors related to readers' misunderstanding of the text.

TeleTriage Systems Publishers
44 Madrone Avenue
San Anselmo, CA 94960
415.453.8382
teletriage@gmail.com

For information and permissions, write Sheila Wheeler, TeleTriage Systems Publishers, 44 Madrone Ave, San Anselmo, CA 94960

Printed in the United States of America

Library of Congress Cataloging in Publication Data

Wheeler, Sheila Q.

Adult Telephone Triage Guidelines - Age 18 + Years
Includes bibliographical references and index

ISBN 0-9883212-0-3 ISBN 978-0-9883212-0-5

1. Adult emergencies 2. Triage (Medicine) 3. Telephone in medicine 4. Medical protocols.
(DNLM: 1. Triage - nurse's instruction 2. Triage- handbook 3. Adult Nursing- methods- handbooks. 4. Telemedicine. 5 Telephone. 6 Clinical protocols in Adults

*Dedicated to telenurses throughout the world
and to the future of telephone triage
and telehealth.*

PROTOCOL DIRECTORY

User's Guide & Operating Standards

Master Guideline

Abdomen Problem:

1. (Upper & Generalized): Pain w or w/o Trauma

2. (Lower): Pain w or w/o Trauma
   Abdomen Problem Supplemental Information

Abuse:

Abuse 1 (Sexual) Reporting Tree

Abuse 1 (Sexual) Supplemental Information

Abuse 2 (Physical) Supplemental Information

Back Problem (Upper & Lower): Pain w or w/o Trauma

Back Problem Supplemental Information

Behavioral Problem Supplemental Information (School-Age Children manual; Infants and Children manual)

Bites (Skin Problem 1):

1. (Human/Animal): Human; Cat; Dog; Bat; Horse; Squirrel; Skunk; Raccoon; Fox

2. Snake; Jellyfish; Sea Urchin; Stingray

3. Bee Stings, Yellow Jacket, Hornet, Wasp; Spiders, Scorpions; Fleas; Ticks

   Bites (Skin Problem 1) Supplemental Information

Bowel Problem:

1. Diarrhea (Severe/Moderate/Mild); Bloody Stool

2. Constipation; Stool Color Change
   Bowel Problem Supplemental Information

Breast Problem: (Adults manual; School-Age Children manual) • See Women's Health section

1. Female (Non Pregnant, Non Postpartum): Pain w or w/o Trauma; Discharge; Lump;
   Lesions

2. Male: Pain w or w/o Trauma; Discharge; Lump; Lesions
   Breast Problem (Male/Female) Supplemental Information

Breastfeeding Problem: Pain w or w/o Fever; Sore Nipples; Painful Breasts • See Women's Health section

Breastfeeding Initial Assessment Questions

Breastfeeding Problem Supplemental Information

Burn (Skin Problem 2):

1. Thermal; Chemical; Electrical
2. Radiation (Sunburn)
   Bum (Skin Problem 2) Supplemental Information

Chest Pain: Pain w or w/o Trauma

Chest Pain Supplemental Information

Cold Exposure: Hypothermia; Frostbite

Cold Exposure Supplemental Information

Confusion: Sudden; Chronic

Confusion Supplemental Information

Dizziness: W or w/o Trauma

Fainting

Dizziness; Fainting Supplemental Information

Ear:

1. Pain w Trauma; FB; Hearing Loss; Ringing; Earlobe Trauma

2. Pain w/o Trauma; Discharge; Congestion; Earlobe Swelling
   Ear Supplemental Information

Emotional Problem: (Adult manual; School-Age Children manual)

1. Suicide in Progress; Threat; Ideation
   Suicide Supplemental Information

2. Panic; Depression; Anxiety; Agitation; Aggression; Withdrawal; Hallucination
   Emotional Problem Supplemental Information

Extremities:

Upper: Pain w or w/o Trauma; Swelling; Lacerations; Fractures

Lower 1: Pain w Trauma; Swelling; Lacerations; Fractures

Lower 2: Pain w/o Trauma; Swelling; Weakness/Non Use; Limp

Extremities (Upper & Lower) Supplemental Information

Eye:

1. Pain w Trauma; Bum; FB; Vision Changes; Blood In

2. Pain w/o Trauma; Photophobia; Blood In; Discharge; Swelling; Vision Changes
   Eye Supplemental Information

Face/Jaw: Pain w or w/o Trauma; Swelling; Weakness

Face/Jaw Supplemental Information

Fever: Fever w Assoc. Symptoms

Fever Supplemental Information

Temperature Taking Instructions Supplemental Information

Head Problem:

1. Pain; Laceration; Level of Consciousness Change w Trauma

2. Pain; Level of Consciousness Change w/o Trauma
   Head Problem Supplemental Information

Heat Exposure: Heat Stroke; Heat Exhaustion; Heat Cramps

    Heat Exposure Supplemental Information

Joint Problem (Upper & Lower): Pain w or w/o Trauma; Swelling (Shoulder, Elbow, Wrist, Hip, Knee, Ankle); Limp (See also Extremities, Upper/Lower)

    Joint Problem Supplemental Information

Lip/Mouth; Teeth/Gums; Tongue: Pain w or w/o Trauma; Swelling; Laceration; Lesions

    Lip/Mouth; Teeth/Gums; Tongue Supplemental Information

Neck Problem: Pain w or w/o Trauma; Swelling; Lumps

    Neck Problem Supplemental Information

Newborn Concerns Supplemental Information (Infants and Children manual)

Nose/Sinus Problem: Pain w or w/o Trauma; FB; Bleeding; Discharge; Congestion

    Nose/Sinus Problem Supplemental Information

Penile/Scrotal/Testicle Problem: Trauma; FB; Pain; Discharge; Lumps; Lesions

    Penile/Scrotal/Testicle Problem Supplemental Information

    Penile Problem: STD Supplemental Information

Postpartum Problem (Adults manual; School-Age Children manual) • See Women's Health section: Leg Pain; Painful Urination; Incisional Pain; Fever; Bleeding; SOB; Diarrhea; N/V; Abd. Pain

    Postpartum Concerns Supplemental Information

    Postpartum Emotional Problem Supplemental Information

Pregnancy Problems: (Adults manual; School-Age Children manual) • See Women's Health section

    High Risk Pregnancy Initial Assessment Questions

1. Labor; Abdominal Pain; Vaginal Discharge; Vaginal Bleeding

2. Trauma; Headache; Chest Pain; < Fetal Movement; N/V; Swelling; Burning on Urination; Itching
   Pregnancy Concerns Supplemental Information

Rectal Problem: Pain w or w/o Trauma; FB; Bleeding; Itching; Discharge; Lesion

    Rectal Problem Supplemental Information

Respiratory Problem:

1. Breathing Problem/Cough: Respiratory Distress; Choking; SOB; Stridor: w or w/o Trauma

2. Throat: Choking; FB/Trauma; Pain; Bum: Chemical/Thermal
   Respiratory Problem Supplemental Information

Seizures: W or w/o Trauma

Shock: Distributive; Cardiogenic; Hypovolemic

Skin Problem:

Bites: See Bites (Skin Problem 1)

Bum: See Bum (Skin Problem 2)

3. Discoloration: Bruise; Yellow; All Color Changes
   Skin Problem 3 (Discoloration) Supplemental Information

4. Laceration/Wound: Amputations; Major & Minor Lacerations; Abrasions; Puncture
   Wounds
   Skin Problem 4 (Laceration/Wound) Supplemental Information

5. Lesion/Lump/Swelling: W or w/o Trauma
   Skin Problem 5 (Lesion/Lump/Swelling) Supplemental Information

6. Rashes; Childhood Rashes: W or w/o Itching
   Skin Problem 6 (Rashes; Childhood Rashes) Supplemental Information

Substance Abuse: (Adults manual; School-Age Children manual)

Substance Abuse Supplemental Information

Urinary Problem: Pain w or w/o Trauma; Frequency; Urgency; Discharge; Output/Color

Changes; Blood in

Urinary Problem Supplemental Information

Vaginal Bleeding (Non-Pregnant) • See Women's Health section: Abnormal Bleeding: Painful, Irregular, Excessive;

Absence of Menses

Vaginal Bleeding (Non-Pregnant) Supplemental Information

Vaginal Problem (Non-Pregnant) • See Women's Health section: FB; Trauma; Discharge; Pain; Lesion; Itching; STD

Exposure
OB/GYN Procedures

Vaginal Problem: STD Supplemental Information Vomiting/

Nausea: w or w/o Diarrhea; Headache; Abdominal Pain

Vomiting/Nausea Supplemental Information
Questions\

Women's Health

ACKNOWLEDGMENTS

To my friends and family for their belief in me, their moral support,
sense of humor, perspective and words of wisdom.

My deepest gratitude goes to my husband Richard, and my children, Joe and Kate
for their love, patience and encouragement
as I worked incessantly on this project.

A special thanks to Jeff Clawson, MD, and Vimla Patel, PhD,
for pioneering work that influenced this manual.

And many thanks to all Task Force members—
expert nurse reviewers and physicians-
who took pains to make this an excellent product.

Finally, a special thanks to Elsa Tsutaoka, MD
for her excellent and painstaking work as contributing author,
and to Cindy Lamendola, RN, NP,
for her invaluable contributions as expert reviewer.

PREFACE

These protocols were originally launched in 1994 for two health care facilities - one, a large county hospital, and the other, a small community clinic. Both facilities served low-income, high-risk, low-literacy patients.

This manual was developed by nurses and reviewed by physicians. As editor in chief, I hired, trained and managed a task force of over 30 nurses and physicians with expertise in geriatrics, pediatrics, emergency medicine, women's health, crisis intervention and other subspecialties. A smaller panel of physicians reviewed the final product. Over the ensuing years, the protocols were revised and updated annually. I continued to utilize expert nurses and physicians throughout that process. Two different electronic versions were developed.

In the development process, the task force consulted all pertinent "gold standard" references as well as existing protocols. With a template, the nursing process, and a unique approach to the "search feature"—site based protocols— firmly in mind, we set about to build a better mousetrap. We discarded designs that were not user-friendly and titling systems that were confusing. We beefed up the User's Guide and endeavored to integrate everything nurses would want in this manual-documentation form, abbreviations, a glossary and a repository of home treatment instructions. The process was highly collaborative and took over two years for the initial volumes.

The challenge was to create a user-friendly triage tool for nurses that facilitated communications and instruction for the patient. It quickly became clear that we would need to "pretranslate" the content to the fifth to eighth grade literacy levels, so nurses would be spared that task when communicating with low-literacy clients. This concept originated with the work of Jeff Clawson, MD, pioneer in protocols for emergency medical dispatchers.

The original manual was a three-volume, age-based product, addressing the unique needs of infants/preschool and school-age children and adults. The problem-solving design is based on research on a pattern recognition model preformed by Vimla Patel, PhD., an expert in medical decision making who performed research on how nurses make telephone triage decisions in real life. The unique design is a synthesis of both algorithm and case-based reasoning which mimics the brain's natural problem solving by utilizing context and a symptom recognition/matching strategy.

The new edition has been reviewed, revised and updated. A four-in-one product, it is a working reference tool with a comprehensive User's Guide, Standards Manual and CD ROM training program. Finally, research related to medical error, decision support and critical thinking has been included and related to telephone triage practice.

Nurses wishing to obtain telephone triage Continuing Education may visit www.teletriage.com, to take a course on Protocol Competency, or a range of other telephone triage CE courses.

TASK FORCE MEMBERS
2009 Contributing Authors/Reviewers

CONTRIBUTING AUTHOR
Elsa Tsutaoka, MD
Primary Care Physician
Southeast Health Center, San Francisco
Assistant Clinical Professor
University of California
San Francisco, California

REVIEWER
Cindy Lamendola, MSN, ANP
Nurse Practitioner, Clinical Research Coordinator
Stanford University School of Medicine
Stanford, California

PAST Contributing Authors/Reviewers

Laura Wachter Alexander, RN, BSN, IBCLC
Lactation Consultant and Prenatal Instructor
California Pacific Medical Center
San Francisco, California

Stacy Bischoff,RN,NP
Women's Health Care Nurse Practitioner
ATM A Group
San Rafael, California

Patricia A. Crane, MSN, RNC, NP
Forensic Nurse Consultant
Sexual Assault Nurse Examiner
San Jose, California

Jeff Howell, RN, CEN
Private Practitioner
Emergency Department
California Pacific Medical Center
San Francisco, California

Russ J. Kino, MD
Director
Emergency Services
Saint John's Hospital and Health Center
Santa Monica, California

Joan Marks, BSN, NP
Private Practice
Greenbrae, California

Eve R. Meyer, MSW, MSHA
Executive Director
San Francisco Suicide Prevention
San Francisco, California

Suellen Miller, RN, CNM, MHA, PhD
University of California Berkeley School of Public Health
Berkeley, California

Robert H. Pantell, MD
Chief
General Pediatrics Division
Professor of Pediatrics
University of California, San Francisco
San Francisco, California

Edwin Cary Pigman, MD
Assistant Professor
Department of Emergency Medicine
George Washington University Medical Center,
Washington, DC

Adrienne Plasse, CNM, MPH
Clinical Instructor
Marin County Women's Health Care-
   San Rafael
University of California
San Francisco, California

Deborah Quilter
Author, Consultant
Beyond Ergonomics
New York, New York

Elizabeth San Luis, MSN, PNP
Ambulatory Care Center
University of California Medical Center
San Francisco, California

Sally Thresher, MSN, NP
Clinical Nurse Specialist
San Francisco Youth Guidance Center
San Francisco, California

Susan Valeriote, RN, CPNP, MS
Pediatric Nurse Practitioner
San Francisco, California

Task Force Members

Donna M. Vincent, RN, BSN, MA
Telehealth Consultant
Emerald Hills, California

Lindsay Wheeler, DC
Chiropractic Practice
Berkeley, California

Sheila Wheeler, RN, MS
President
Tele Triage Systems
San Anselmo, California

Introduction to New Edition

The 2017 edition includes new research that supports the ongoing use of checklists (Gawande, 2009; Wachter 2015), prevention of root causes of error (Joint Commission), using a systems approach (Institute of Medicine), AAACN Practice Standards and Position Papers by the American College of Emergency Physicians and the Emergency Nurses Association.

New content includes: 5-Tier Triage Flow Chart for Telephone Triage, Standard Guideline, QA Audit, Standards and research on safety, root causes of error, and Five-Tier Triage. (IOM, 2011, IOM, Joint Commission, 2011, Donabedian, 2003, Patel, 1996, AAACN, 2012, ACEP & ENA, 2015).

Please note: This book was produced by scanning an earlier version. Imperfections in the format generated by the scanning process may be apparent. Also note: while the approach we have used since 1995 is bolstered by current research, symptom descriptions and supplemental home treatment information was last revised in 2009 and 2005 for the Adult and Pediatric versions respectively. Always have the medical director review any guidelines prior to implementation.

Customize this manual by placing pages in a binder with tabs for use as a base set. Add your facilities' preferences on colored sheets at the end of each guideline. "Growing your own" paper guidelines from scratch may take years to accomplish, may be more expensive than expected, and may not produce high quality results. Paper-based guidelines are economical; electronic algorithms can be extremely costly.

Structure and Process the guideline design is grounded in Medical Traditions of pattern recognition and is further supported by new safety trends, research and professional standards. This edition builds and expands upon previous editions in the following areas:

1. Nursing Process
2. Checklist (Gawande, 2009)
3. Avoidance of Root causes of error (Joint Commission)
4. 5-Tier Triage (ACEP & ENA (2015), Manchester Triage Group (2015))
5. AAACN Standards *(2011)*
6. QA Audit (2017)

NEW CONTENT 2017

"Triage represents a grey area between medicine and nursing, where medical diagnoses are not essential in order to make a decision about the appropriate interventions, and where the dimension of *urgency* become the primary focus of the reasoning process."(Lephrohon, Patel, 1995)

Like the Merck Manual, these guidelines are a reference. They have been "field tested" without incidence of errors, omissions or lawsuits since publication in 1995. In this edition, the five-tier triage approach has been refined and updated per standards set forth by the Manchester Triage Group, ACEP and ENA with improved Nomenclature (descriptions, definitions, examples) for clarity. Revisions to these guidelines include updated and enhanced design elements listed below:

- *Introduction & Afterword*
- o *Telephone Triage Flow Chart*
- o *Adult and Pediatric Master Guideline with Standards*
- o *QA Audit of Performance Standards based on AAACN standards*
- o Telephone Triage Position Papers: ACEP & ENA
- o *Call Center and Performance Standards*

PLEASE NOTE:
- Before using, please review carefully three major sections: Users Guide, Individual Guidelines and Appendices.
- *Due to the limitations in the production of the revised guidelines, we were unable to add page numbers.*
- Please refer to the Table of Contents to locate a given Guideline – listed alphabetically.
- The Appendices follow the Vomiting/Nausea Guideline and contains useful resources: i.e.Patient Brochure, QA Audit, 14-page Director of Hotlines and Websites for Support Groups. Please read the Afterword and CE course information as well.
- There will be occasional guideline formatting variability, due to changes in formats from the original design.
- Directory of Hotlines and Websites for Support Groups has not been revised, but it is a useful resource for web searches on a wide range of topics.
- *Clinical content* was revised per list below:
    i. *Adult: 2009*
    ii. *School-Age: 2005*
    iii. *Infant-Child: 2003*

Guideline Uses

These age-based guidelines integrate telephone triage Structure and Process for safe, timely telephone triage (appropriate outcomes) useable in several ways:

- *Multi-purpose* -- suitable for *both* telephone- *and* face-to-face on-site triage (in office, ED, health center or clinic settings)
- *Paper References* as a standalone reference or adjunct to electronic guidelines.

The Master Guideline contains general descriptions of a range of conditions with 5-Tier Triage time frames and access sites for timely dispositions. It can serve as a:

- Contingency policy or *"Fall Back"* for the "out of protocol experience" -- when no guideline seems to fit the patient symptoms.
- Pre-emptive policy or *"Go-to"* guideline *before* selecting a specific guideline
- The Master Guideline may be also viewed as an orientation tool for new practitioners to review current Policies and Procedures of your facility.

Please note: **Design and methodology** described in the Afterword section at the end of the manual. Please read this section, and the User's Guide before using the guidelines.

Customize the guidelines, by placing them in a binder with Alphabetical Tabs (45). Add your own facilities' policies, procedures and additional guidelines on colored paper after each tab.

Resources

- **For Telehealth Update CE Course,** please see the last pages of this manual
- **Preceptor Workbook with Answer key** (200-page) please see last pages of this manual

USER'S GUIDE AND OPERATING STANDARDS

▶ **Notice to the User**

- Medical Approval: The protocols should be reviewed and approved by the Medical Director prior to implementation.

- User Qualifications: These guidelines were designed to be used by experienced RNs with formal training in telephone triage.

- Training Program: For optimal results and optimal risk management, Sheila Wheeler provides a comprehensive on-site or home study training program in Practice and Protocol Competency.

   For more information about home study programs, conferences, consultation, content licensing, medical call center referral, medical-legal services, please visit: www.teletriage.com.

▶ **About Telephone Triage**

What Does Research Reveal about RN Decision Making?

Telephone triage—the safe, effective, appropriate disposition of health-related problems by RNs—always involves "decision making under conditions of uncertainty and urgency" (Lephrohon and Patel 1995). It involves "Uncertainty" because decisions are often made based on partial or inaccurate information; "urgency" because calls must be processed within a brief time frame—usually 6-10 min average. In new research, telephone triage has been compared to the work of air traffic controllers, EMDs, and firefighters—all high-stake activities. Vimla Patel, PhD, described how a group of RNs working in an emergency department setting made "real world" decisions in telephone triage. She discovered that these nurses used pattern recognition, rules of thumb, and context as major strategies to make decisions.

How Does This Research Relate to These Protocols?

The research on nurse decision making by Patel (Lephrohon and Patel 1995) and other experts has important implications for protocol design and for these Protocols in particular. The strategies of pat-tern recognition, rules of thumb, and context have been incorporated into all elements of this system—training, Protocols, and forms. The goal of this design is to mimic how the brain naturally solves problems in "real world" situations.

   Because patients are complex and symptom presentations often ill-structured, novel, variable, and unique, one needs a system that is correspondingly complex yet flexible, attuned to symptoms' nuances and subtleties while at the same time providing firm support for decision making. Protocols based on a pattern-recognition approach have these qualities. Furthermore, because telephone triage is a high-stakes activity, a well-integrated *system* is needed to manage the uncertainty and urgency. That system (an inter-dependent group of items forming a whole and serving a common purpose) should be operated by a pro-fessional. Thus, the designers of these Protocols intend them to be used by RNs with decision-making experience.

If Protocols Are Well-Developed and Comprehensive, Why Must RNs Manage the Calls?

While Protocols are an important component of the telephone triage system, the bottom line is the expe-rienced, well-trained RN. Current standards of practice stress the use of the RN. Protocols alone cannot guarantee safe practice.

Don't Protocols Take the Place of Training?

This is an area of confusion and controversy. Managers should be aware of the risks of relying on Pro-tocols to take the place of formal instruction. Overreliance on the tool can lead to mistriage. Training in the principles and skills of history taking, communications, assessment, disposition, and decision mak-ing is the foundation, followed by an orientation to the Protocols. Potential problems and misunder-standings can be averted through instruction in the correct and safe operation of the Protocols and documentation form. It will also address "protocol bias" that develops when RNs who have been using one type of protocol must become acquainted with a new one.

In order to determine the right disposition, the nurse must go through a decision-making process, the task being to create context or build a picture or pattern. Linked to this concept is that of "drilling down" to excavate the information. The process, then, is to ask *enough* of the *right questions,* in the *right way* to elicit *enough* of the *right data,* and to choose the *right Protocol(s)* and *right disposition.* This process will be outlined in detail in the pages that follow. The first step often begins with a cursory or global approach.

▶ Assessment Strategies

A Global Approach

How Many Questions Must I Ask?

How far the RN must "drill down" to finally reach a decision is uniquely determined by the acuity of symptoms and the patient presenting them. Some problems require more in-depth questioning and RNs will pursue data collection to different degrees—sometimes referred to as "skimming" or "sleuthing." There are times to do both. For example, in the case of chest pain, most nurses quickly elicit the large chunks of information "skimming" before making a decision. In other cases, such as vague abdominal pain, the RN may spend more time and gather larger quantities of detailed information—"sleuthing." Problems arise when some protocol designs (or professionals) treat problems superficially and fail to drill down far enough. These protocols are designed to enable the RN to drill down as far as the instance requires—yet allow for quick skimming as well. The four acronyms summarized below (SAVED, SCHOLAR, PAMPER, and ADL) are described in detail in *Telephone Triage: Theory, Practice and Protocol Development* (Wheeler 1993).

How Can I Quickly Assess and Prioritize Problems?

The telephone triage process usually begins with a broad, global assessment. Most nurses quickly build a picture through gathering information about the patient's age, gender, chief complaint, literacy or language level, emotional state (determined via the words, tone, pacing of voice), and sometimes previous medical history. This key contextual information can quickly identify high-risk patients or situations. This process, while appearing superficial, yields key chunks of information and may take as little as 60 sec.

Broad categories of high-risk patients and symptoms are signified by the acronym "SAVED" standing for: *severe, strange,* or *suspicious symptoms, age, veracity* problems, *emotional* distress, *debilitation,* and *distance.* These "red flags" are loaded with information. Identifying high-risk status aids in prioritizing and helps to "defend" dispositions, facilitating decisions regarding upgrading and disposition time frames. Red flags help all practitioners to function more effectively. Listed below are examples of each category:

Severe, Strange, or Suspicious Symptoms

Patel (Lephrohon and Patel 1995) notes that "it is easier to identify an emergency than to rule one out." Severe pain ("9 on a scale of 10"), severe bleeding (spurting, bright red), or severe trauma (falls from a height of over 15 ft) are conditions that the average layperson could identify as urgent.

Strange symptoms include ill-structured, vague, atypical, or unusual presentations, symptoms that only astute professionals might recognize as urgent. Falling into this category are sudden, unexpected, or new symptoms, recurrent symptoms, or a marked change in the patient's condition.

Suspicious symptoms include the "big six": head, abdomen, chest, respiratory, dizziness, and "flu." These symptoms always require thorough investigation by a professional, primarily because they are often associated with underdiagnosed conditions such as ectopic pregnancy, MI, or appendicitis—all serious diagnoses. Suspicious symptoms also apply to any situation where the nurse has a "gut feeling" or a "hunch about a problem." If the nurse is uncomfortable with the Protocol disposition, he or she may upgrade a problem or bring the patient in sooner. When red flags of suspicion are raised, nurses are encouraged to use their intuition.

Age

Age is one of the most important pieces of data obtained. The very young, the very old, and women of child-bearing age are always considered high-risk patients. Premature infants and those under 3 mo are typically considered at highest risk. The "frail elderly"—anyone over 75 yr of age, suffering from multiple or chronic diseases, functional disability, or psychosocial problems—must always be treated with extreme care. The childbearing years, always a high-risk period, now extend from age 11 into the 60s! In regard to chest pain, the latest research demonstrates that women over age 50 have the same risks of cardiac disease as men over age 35.

Veracity

Veracity refers to the ability to reproduce the facts of the situation accurately. Obstacles to data-gathering arise whenever there are second-party calls, low-literacy callers, language barriers, extremely young or very inexperienced mothers, or a caretaker unfamiliar with the patient.

Emotional Status (Caretaker and/or Patient)

Nurses can pick up many cues through careful attention to the words as well as the tone and pacing of the caller's voice. There may be hysteria or denial or inappropriate affect in parent or caretaker with a history of psychiatric problems or substance abuse. Anxiety is always a red flag. Frequent calls in a short period of time can be an indicator of both caller anxiety and problem acuity.

Debilitation

In general, debilitation refers to chronic illness. Chronic illness may include but is not limited to the following:

- All Populations: AIDS, asthma, diabetes, sickle cell, low-income homeless
- Frail Elderly: Cardiac problems, COPD, dementia
- All Immunocompromised: Lack of adequate immunizations, chemotherapy, HIV, splenectomy, steroid therapy/chronic, transplants, nephrotic syndrome
- Pediatric Populations: Congenital heart disease, cystic fibrosis, spina bifida, hydrocephalus, prematurity with secondary complications

Distance

Distance can become an important factor when (1) the parent/caretaker is calling from a remote location several hours from hospital; (2) in an urgent situation, the patient is unable to arrive by car within 1 hr owing to traffic or lack of available car; and (3) the patient must take public transportation that is sporadic or nonexistent after certain hours at night. Ail of these situations heighten the need for reliable, prompt, safe transportation.

After performing a global assessment, the nurse may quickly discover an emergent situation, abbreviating the assessment process and necessitating paramedic transport. However, in most cases, the call requires more sleuthing.

History Taking: Assessing the Problem and Patient

What Is the Key Information to Elicit about the Chief Complaint?

To elicit key information about most symptoms (SCHOLAR), ask the following questions:

Symptoms and associated symptoms

Characteristics

History of complaint in past

Onset of symptoms

Location of symptoms

Aggravating factors

Relieving factors

What Is the Key Information to Elicit about the Patient?

Sometimes getting a brief patient history is helpful. This "snapshot" provides additional context, sometimes necessary to make the correct decision. The acronym "PAMPER" is summarized below:

- Pregnancy/breastfeeding
- Allergies
- Medications
- Previous chronic illness
- Emotional stress
- Recent injury, illness, ingestion

How Does One Assess Elderly or Poor Historians?

With, some elderly, and poor historians, it is difficult to get adequate information for two major reasons: (1) the patient is a poor historian and/or (2) the patient has vague or ill-structured symptoms. In both cases, the acronyms SCHOLAR and PAMPER may not be applicable. Use activities of daily living (ADL) to elicit and compare the client's current state with their baseline state. With children and the elderly especially, these indicators of current health or illness may help paint the clearest picture, when symptoms are often vague, ill-structured, or absent. *Marked changes* in any of these indicators can be a red flag:

- *INTAKE*
- Eating
- Drinking
- *OUTPUT*
- Elimination (urine, BM, emesis)
- *ACTIVITY*
- Work/play/daily routine
- Sleep pattern
- Appearance
- Skin color
- Mood

The above lists may be duplicated and hung on the wall by the phone for quick reference. Complete descriptions of each of the acronyms may be found in *Telephone Triage: Theory, Practice and Protocol Development* (Wheeler 1993) (available at www.teletriage.coml.

▶ Decision-Making Strategies

Rules of Thumb for Age-Based Populations

Rules of Thumb is another strategy that forms the foundation for managing calls from high-risk groups. These strategies are derived from years of experience and often operate at an intuitive level. Several of the rules of thumb below are based on ACEP policies as well. The examples below are divided into those that apply to all ages followed by age-based rules specific to adult, adolescent, and child populations.

AH Ages

All severe pain should be seen urgently.

Trauma: Always be alert to unwitnessed accidents and to mechanism of injury (major trauma: MV A, falls > 15 ft, blunt trauma). Assess and investigate completely. Caretakers' assessments may be faulty or they may focus on a problem that is minor (e.g., avulsed tooth) and miss a more serious one (e.g., head injury).

Several calls in a short period of time (several hours) without ability to describe seriousness of patient's symptoms may be an indicator of acuity.

Beware of the developing disease: what starts out as vague abdominal pain with low-grade fever may, over several hours or days, develop into appendicitis.

Self-limiting symptoms existing > 1 wk but not becoming markedly worse can be treated at home with optimal appointment in 24+ hr.

Age is a major factor in many Rules of Thumb. In fact, age alone (and especially extremes of age) can markedly influence the level of risk—owing to certain illnesses as well as greater vulnerability because of communication barriers or dependency on caretakers, as illustrated below:

Adolescent Populations

Assess all children with unexplained symptoms for possible unintentional or purposeful ingestion/exposure to toxins, inhalants, street or prescription drugs.

Teenagers are especially vulnerable to depression and suicide (and rarely, homicide) because of several factors: easy access to alcohol and drugs, increased sexual activity, complex societal demands, negative role models, and increased family disruptions. The precipitating factor is usually a loss—betrayal of a trust, romantic breakup, failure in school or sports, move to a new neighborhood, peer pressures, conflict regarding dependence and independence, poverty, unwanted pregnancy, sexual problems, peer- or media-emphasized suicide, treatment for mental illness, and/or any legal problems.

Elderly Populations

Symptoms in the elderly may be atypical, silent, or late (e.g., the patient may feel fatigue as only symptom of pneumonia).

Assess all elderly patients for dehydration status (as appropriate).

Elderly populations are at greater risk for hypothermia and hyperthermia.

Assess all elderly with unexplained symptoms for adverse drug reaction (ADRs), "chemical restraints," or possible ingestion—intentional or accidental. Exposures may be caused by toxins, alcohol, or overmedication with prescription or OTC medications.

The elderly are at risk for ADRs. The greater the number of drugs the patient uses, the greater the incidence of ADRs. As the number of daily doses increases, compliance decreases.

Elderly patients may be poor or forgetful historians. Err on the side of caution.

▶ Protocol Design Features

Design Philosophy

These protocols are unique in both organization and content. The authors included everything that advice nurses might want in a triage and advice tool, and tried to avoid too many "bells and whistles." If the nurse thoroughly understands the design, it will not only enhance his/her practice but also expedite calls. The goal is to create a tool that is neither overly simplistic nor treat problems superficially, and yet not so complicated that it proves too cumbersome to use. The Protocols are simple enough to be user-friendly and yet comprehensive enough to provide constant support for the decision maker.

Decision Support versus Decision Making

According to one definition, computer systems may be one of two types: decision making or decision support. *Decision-making* systems are expert systems that allow an unqualified person to "make a decision that is beyond his/her level of training and experience." On the other hand, *decision-support* systems are expert systems that remind an experienced decision maker of options or issues to consider that she/he once knew but may have forgotten. These protocols are based on a *decision-support* approach.

Quick Reference

In the style of *The Merck Manual,* these Protocols are designed to be a "quick reference." However, that is where the similarities end. This manual is a working tool—to be consulted constantly rather than infrequently. Unlike *The Merck Manual,* the disease descriptions contained herein are highly distilled, organized by acuity level, and contain disposition, home treatment, referral, and teaching sections.

Symptoms Patterns

Each Protocol presents an array of descriptions of commonly encountered conditions or diseases—"classic pictures." In order to be most useful to the user, these descriptions are comprehensive rather than minimalistic. They are often described as a progression, from beginning symptoms to "full-blown" condition.

The rationale for this is the rule of thumb to "beware the developing disease." This information can be passed on to patients when instructing them about symptoms to watch for as indicators of worsening conditions.

Concise but Complete

According to some experts, patients call with a limited number of problems. The authors found that about 50 protocols cover 95% of all callers' problems. Since each protocol includes about 20 possible diagnoses, the 45-50 Protocols in this manual address over 1000 possible conditions.

Anatomical Site-Based Titles

The Protocols match "real world" wording and presentation as much as possible; patients usually describe symptoms in relation to location or site on the body. For example, "1 have—a *headache,*" "—a swollen *ankle,* " "—an *eye* discharge," "— an earache." In addition, the anatomical site-based approach is very visual. Starting with the location of the problem on the body (e.g., Eye Problem) is a major chunk of context and makes sense in a pattern-matching approach. The next step would be to narrow it down further (or flesh it out more) to the particulars (e.g., Eye Problem: trauma, discharge, blood in, vision difficulties, pain, etc.).

While an anatomical site-based approach might resemble a "systems approach" (Urinary to GU; Abdomen to GI; Chest to Cardiology), it is different. Rely on the caller's description of the site and symptoms at first.

With a strict symptom-based approach, difficulties arise when people (Protocol designers and/or nurse and patient) can't agree on the best words to use for symptoms (e.g., "ear ringing" or *"ringing* in ears"; "*belching*" or *"gas"; "hives"* or *"rash"; "stomach* ache," *"pain* in stomach," or "abdominal pain"). Using a variety of lay terms for symptoms, even when listed alphabetically, predictably results in confusing, time-consuming searches for the nurse.

Unique Features

Age-Based Protocols and Content

Protocols such as Breastfeeding, Bums, Bites, and others apply to all ages. Within all Protocols, you will also find certain age-specific information. Thus, age is listed when it has significant bearing on a certain disease or condition.

Women's Health Section

Women's Health Protocols are now in a separate section.

Key Assessment Tools

The Master Protocol and Pain Assessment provide unique support when no Protocol applies, and to elicit more detail about pain, respectively . They are meant to be consulted frequently . Pain is a common presenting symptom; monitoring and measuring pain—the fifth vital sign—is now a standard.

Community Alert

This is a new feature, designed to enhance RN sensitivity and awareness of the influence of community-based events (such as Super Bowl Sunday) and environmental factors (heat waves and cold snaps) that can increase the incidence of problems such as domestic violence and heat-and cold-related illness, respectively. Telephone triage nurses and call centers, often the first point of contact, have the capability to serve as "early warning systems," to notify providers and local EDs, when call volume related to these problems increases.

Content

Most Protocols are written in conversational, "cook-book" style, and in lay language at fifth- to eighth-grade level. This feature facilitates communication with all callers, especially low-literacy callers. The information is intended to be read to the patient as needed. This saves time by eliminating the extra step of translating symptom descriptions and instructions for home treatment, first aid, or self-assessment from college level to fifth-grade level language.

Protocol Length

The original goal was to develop the Protocols to one page in length. However, many Protocols are divided into two parts (e.g., Ear Problem 1, Ear Problem 2). As a general rule, Protocols with "1" in the title (e.g., Ear Problem 1) include trauma, whereas those with "2" in the title do not. If there is no number in the title, there is only one Protocol, and all symptoms, including trauma and nonacute, will be in that Protocol. Most Protocols have an accompanying Supplemental Information which must be consulted when using the Protocol. In some cases (as with Menopause) there is a Supplemental Information but no Protocol chart.

Initial Assessment Questions (IAQs)

Breastfeeding and Pregnancy Problems have Initial Assessment Questions. This section must be consulted prior to using the Protocol, in order to identify or rule out risk factors, as well as Toxicity or Dehydration in the infants of mothers calling with breastfeeding problems.

Flexible Disposition Time Frames

All Protocols have three standard disposition time frames (Emergent, Urgent, and Acute/Nonacute). These time frames overlap slightly and are intended as flexible limits within which the RN can operate. The site of the patient visit may vary according to what is accessible. For example, lack of access to office visits on weekends, holidays, and after hours means the patient who needs a same-day appointment must be seen in the ED or Urgent Care.

Format Variations: Atypical Format

Some Protocols do not follow the standard format and are atypical. The Abuse 1 (Sexual) Reporting Tree is atypical and the only example of its kind. Fainting, Seizures, and Shock Protocols include First Aid as well as causes and descriptions for RN reference.

Diagnosis "Lumping"

In an effort to be consistent in descriptions of medical problems, the Task Force tried to keep each complex of symptoms for a particular diagnosis separate. However, in many cases symptom complexes are so similar that the diagnoses are "lumped" together. In these cases, the disposition was usually upgraded to the higher level of acuity—to err on the side of caution.

Recurring Standard Topics

While there are specific Protocols for Abuse and Fever, these topics are also standard items found in nearly every Protocol. There is no specific Protocol for Ingestion, however. Ingestion may go undetected. Therefore, it too is found in Supplemental Information, in the section entitled "Drug Side Effect". Ingestion also appears on the Documentation Form under "Recent Ingestion" as reminder to explore unexplained symptoms in adults, adolescents or elderly clients.

"Problems" and "Concerns"

Throughout the Protocols, "Problems" and "Concerns" have been differentiated: Problems are defined as acute symptoms and are covered in the triage chart. Concerns are defined as nonacute symptoms or informational issues, covered in the Supplemental Information sections as in Birth Control and Menopause, Pregnancy and Postpartum Concerns.

Abuse 1: Sexual

The Abuse Reporting Tree is in an algorithmic format unlike any other Protocol. This algorithm or decision tree takes the place of the Protocol. Establish first if there is major trauma or if assailant is nearby. When major trauma is ruled out, the next priority is to preserve evidence. See Instructions for Preserving Evidence in the Supplemental Information section. Abuse 2: Physical covers adult and teen domestic violence, and elder abuse.

Bowel Problem

Bowel Problem is primarily concerned with symptoms related to bowel movements—diarrhea, constipation, etc.

Breastfeeding Problem

Breastfeeding Problem has IAQs. Please refer to IAQs prior to using the Protocol. Since there are *two* patients involved in the Breastfeeding Problem, assess *both* the mother and infant. (See also Postpartum Emotional Problem.)

Confusion

Confusion in adults and children is always a serious symptom. In the elderly especially, remain alert to the possibility of accidental or intentional overdose, overmedication (chemical restraints) or polypharmacy. With adolescents, suspect accidental ingestion as well as intentional ingestion (suicide attempt) in teen and young adult population.

Fever

Fever is atypical because in order to follow the standard format and to keep it a manageable length, it was necessary to "punt" to other Protocols.

Rectal Problem

Rectal problem only addresses problems of the rectum: Pain with or without trauma, foreign body, bleeding in very small amounts, itching, and lesions. Diarrhea/constipation are covered under Bowel Problem. An exception to the rule is the reference to "large amount of rectal bleeding," which is covered.

▶ A Tour of Protocol Elements

Detailed descriptions correspond to examples in the sample Protocol on the following pages.

Item	Description/Purpose
1. Title and Subtitle	Subtitles indicate key symptoms in Protocol left-hand column.
2. Key Symptoms Assessment	Symptoms presented by patient must match one of these words in order to move into center column questions (Acuity Level).
3. Symptom Patterns/Associated Symptoms	[Preceded by *plus* (+).] If patient describes one symptom (usually very severe) or more (several lesser symptoms) that match the symptom patterns move, to the disposition box in the right-hand column, and follow the instructions.
4. Considerations/Diagnoses	[Possible diagnoses in *parentheses* ()•] *The advice nurse must never document or verbalize to the caller the diagnosis found within the parentheses; they are for the RN's information and reference only.*
5. Disposition/Advice	The Disposition/Advice column is composed of two parts: the Disposition and the Protocol Advice; always advise the patient of the disposition—when and where to come for treatment; the site of care may vary depending upon the hour and day of the call. For some acute problems when care within 8-24 hr is not feasible, after hours, patients may need to be seen in the ED. Please see Disposition Options for details of how to use this section.
6. Cross-References	(If applicable, at the end of the Protocol, in the Assessment column). This section is designed to provide users with other possible Protocol choices; specific cross-references are also found throughout the Protocol in parentheses.
7. Arrows	The Disposition/Advice section may include other directives, First Aid instructions, or self-assessment to perform immediately; each of these items is linked to a specific complex of symptoms by an arrow; *arrows* indicate actions for the RN to take: directives for pt. self-assessment, First Aid directives, or referral to ED.
8. Self-Assessment (SA)	In Disposition/Advice section designated as *SA*.
9. First Aid Directives	(Designated as *First Aid* in Disposition/Advice section).
10. Specific Referrals	Specific referrals to Suicide Prevention, Poison Center, and instructions to *COME TO ED NOW!*
11. Supplemental Information (SI)	On a separate sheet, this section includes Home Treatment Instructions; Tutorial Information for the nurse as well as information and home treatment instructions for the patient.
12. Home Treatment References	*Always consult the Home Treatment* (Home lx SI, Appendix A) when directed by the Protocol. This section may be developed in-house; see Appendix A for examples. Home Treatment may be found in the specific Protocol or in Appendix A.

SAMPLE PROTOCOL: BURNS
Skin Problem: Burns 1
Electrical; Thermal; Chemical

ASSESSMENT	ACUITY LEVEL	DISPOSITION/ADVICE
Key Questions	**Emergent Symptom Patterns**	**EDOmin-1 hr**
All electrical burns	+ ± Chest pain, palpitations, > heart rate, fainting, Hx of lightning strike? (cardiac dysrhythmia) —	- - ▶ All electrical burns have potential for progressive injury; may be worse than it looks! Seconds count
All thermal burns	--▶	See Burns SI, First Aid
Burn w decreased consciousness	/+ Weak, dizzy, cold/mottled/pale skin, blue lips/nail beds, rapid/shallow breathing, unresponsive, loss of consciousness? (shock) (See Shock)	Y SA: Estimate using one palm of *victim's* hand (not including fingers) = 1%
Burn w respiratory I symptoms	+ Hoarseness, cough, wheezing, SOB, singed/black nares, facial bum, smoke inhalation, black sputum? (inhalation injury)	
Burn (deep)	+ White, dark, charred appearance, loss of skin, regardless of size? (3rd degree)	
Burn (over 9%)	+ Red, mottled, blisters, extreme pain? (2nd degree, major)	
Burn of finger(s) (circumferential)	Unable to remove rings? (> risk circ.)	
Facial/neck burn? (retinal, inhalation burn)		
All chemical burns (Including eyes)	...............................- - ....▶	All chemical burns have potential for progressive injury; may be worse than it looks! Seconds count!

Key Questions	**Urgent Symptom Patterns**	**ED/UCC/Office 1 -8 hr•**
Burn (circumferential)	+ Face/neck/hands/feet/arms/legs/perineum/anyjoint? (circ. obstruction) ------------------------------------»—	See Burns SI, First Aid
Burn w blisters	+ Red, mottled, extreme pain, 5%-9%? (2nd degree) - -<	See Burns SI, First Aid

Key Questions	Acute/Nonacute Symptom Patterns	FA 8+ hr ± Home Tx ©
Burn Hx	+ Foul smelling, purulent discharge, > swelling, > streaks and pain, fever? (infection)------- —— ------------▶	Check tetanus status See Burns SI, First Aid
Burn (moderate)	+ Tetanus immunization > 10 yr? (> risk infection) + Red, blisters, pain 1%-5%? (2nd degree)	

Burn (minor)	+ Reddened, mild, swelling, moderate pain, no blisters?
	   (1st degree)
	+ Red, mottled, blisters, pain, < the size of one
	   hand (1%)? (2nd degree)	

Cross-Reference ©
Abuse

SKIN PROBLEM: BURNS 2
Sunburn

ASSESSMENT	ACUITY LEVEL	DISPOSITION/ADVICE
Key Questions	Emergent Symptom Patterns	ED 0 min-1 hr
Sunburn w < consciousness	+ Fever (high), sev. fatigue, confusion, fainting, hot, dry red skin, rapid shallow breathing? (See Heat Exposure)	
Key Questions	Urgent Symptom Patterns	ED/UCC/Office 1-8 hr
Sunburn	+ Eye pain, photophobia, < vision? (retinal involvement) + Extensive, deep sunburn, fever, pain (sev. to mod.), dehydration Sx, generalized swelling of burned area? (sun poisoning)	
Red, mottled, blisters	+ > 5%, Extreme pain? (2nd degree)	
Sunburn Hx	+ Foul smelling, purulent discharge, worsening swelling or pain, streaks, fever? (infection)	
Key Questions	Acute/Nonacute Symptoms Patterns	FA 8+ hr± Home Tx
Sunburn w blisters	+ Red, mottled, tender, covering 5% of body? (> risk infection)	
Open blisters	± Discharge ± fever? (> risk infection)	
Sunburn	+ Pain/tenderness, deeply pigmented skin types? (1st degree) + Red, mild swelling, moderate pain, no blisters? (1st degree)	
Cross-References Abuse	Heat Exposure	

SKIN PROBLEM: BURNS
Supplemental Information

Quick Reference: ▶ First Aid   ▶ Burn Assessment (Rule of Nines)

Thermal Burn   ▶ Burn Care

Chemical Burn   ▶ Blister Care

▶ First Aid

Thermal Burn

SA: Estimate using one palm of *victim's* hand (not including fingers) = 1%.

   If clothing sticks to skin, do not remove clothing! Immerse burned area for no more than 3 min in cool tap water.

   If clothing does not stick to skin, remove it.

- If > 5%, do not immerse. Cover with clean wet sheet + plastic wrap.

- If < 5%, immerse immediately in cool tap water x 10 min.

   Do not put butter, oil, or creams on burn!
   Do not put ice on burn: could lead to > skin damage, > shock.

- For transport: Wrap burn in clean plastic wrap to keep warm, clean, and reduce pain.

Chemical Burn

Contact poison center immediately and quickly do the following:

- Wet Chemicals: Rinse skin/eyes w cool tap water.

- Dry Chemicals: Brush off from skin/eyes.

- Bring substance to ED w you.

▶ Burn Assessment

Rule of Nines: A useful, quick method to estimate percentage of body surface areas that were burned.

Rules of Nines

Adult

   Palm of victim's hand, not including fingers = 1%

   Perineum = 1%

   Head/Neck = 9%

   Arm = 9%

   Leg= 18%

   Ant. trunk = 18%

   Post, trunk = 18%

▶ Burn Care

Immediate Care

- Pain: Tylenol.

- Pain/Swelling: Cold compress Q1D. (See Home Tx)

- Remove rings, bracelets, etc., only if you can do so easily. If not, you need to come in to have the items removed.
- Pain/Swelling: Raise the bum area above heart level.
- Don't use "Caines" or Benadryl sprays for bum—may cause a reaction.
- Check tetanus status. If you have a clean bum and your last tetanus shot was > 10 yr ago, you need a tetanus shot within 72 hr.

▶ Blister Care

- Don't break blisters. They are like "nature's Band-Aids" and will protect your skin from infection.
- If they break, leave them alone. Do not peel off skin from broken blisters.
- Cover w clean, dry dressing. Change as needed.
- Watch for signs and symptoms of infection. (See Bum Care; review with caller.)

TeleTriage Systems
Workflow Process

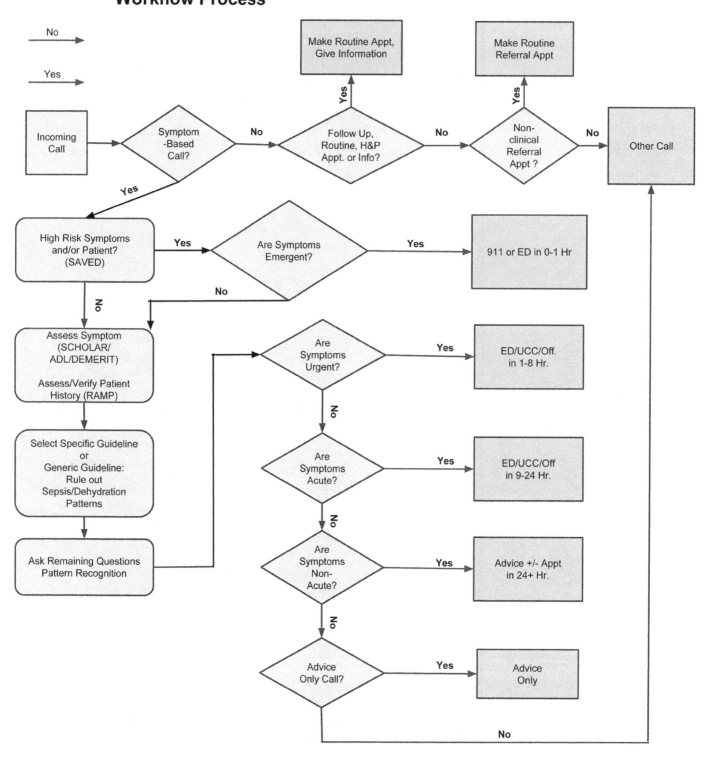

©2017 TeleTriage Systems

Disposition Options

FIVE-LEVEL TRIAGE APPROACH

The Five-level approach divides symptom patterns into five levels of Urgency, entitled as follows:

- Life Threatening
- Emergent
- Urgent
- Acute
- Non-Acute

Although the Adult Version of these guidelines has three general categories (Emergent, Urgent, Acute-Non-Acute), technically, it still delineates Five Tier Triage as described here.

Each level has a time frame and a range of sites to be further evaluated -- as appropriate and depending upon the time of day and day of the week. Each urgency level is intended as a flexible time frame within which the nurse must determine what is safe, timely and prudent. Nurses have a professional responsibility to use good judgment. A common rule of thumb to apply being "when in doubt, err on the side of caution, and bring patients in sooner rather than later".

EMERGENT

Life threatening symptoms always require paramedic transport to ED within minutes. They must be kept NPO. Remain on the line with the caller. Whenever possible, institute a three-way conference call with both parties (patient and EMS services, Suicide Prevention, Rape Crisis or Poison center, for example) as directed by your policies.

Emergent level symptoms always require ED services. Some must be kept NPO. Some patients will require paramedic transport; some may be brought by car by a person who can safely bring them in within the appropriate time frame (0-1 hour). Always notify Labor and Delivery or Emergency Department of pending arrivals of any patient coming via car.

URGENT

Urgent symptoms typically require evaluation within 1-8 hours (same-day appointment). Some may require evaluation within the hour and are instructed by guideline to "Come in now". Depending upon the time of day and day of the week, some patients may be directed, as appropriate, to Emergency Department, Urgent Care, or office settings for further evaluation.

Some patients in Urgent category may also require paramedic transport due to transportation problems. Some may require other reliable, timely transport as is practical, i.e. cabs, Uber, Lyft, etc. if there is no readily available car or if relatives are too anxious to drive them in. Always notify Labor and Delivery or Emergency Department of pending arrivals any patient arriving via car.

ACUTE-NON-ACUTE

Acute Symptoms typically require evaluation within an 8-24 hour time frame, or a next day appointment. Depending upon the time of day and day of the week, some patients may be directed, as appropriate, to Emergency Department, Urgent Care, or office settings for further evaluation. Always notify Labor and Delivery or Emergency Department of pending arrivals of any patient arriving via car.

Non-Acute Symptoms may require evaluation within a 24+ time frame or future appointment or advice only. Depending upon the time of day and day of the week (available access), these patients may be directed to Emergency Department, Urgent Care, or office settings for further evaluation, as appropriate.

Continuity of Care

To prevent patients with emergent to acute symptoms from "falling through the cracks", policies should require nurses to notify managers in Labor and Delivery or Emergency Department *via phone call*, about pending arrivals of any patient who is arriving via car.

After Hours Lack of Access requires that provisions for safe, timely access be in place. Depending upon the time of day (After hours) and day of the week (Holiday or weekend), nurses should direct some patients as appropriate, to Emergency Department, Urgent Care, or office settings for further evaluation.

Informed Consent

According to Dan Tennenhouse, MD, JD, (1993) nurses must apprise patients of the urgency of their symptoms" ("the duty to terrify"), in order to motivate patients to comply with disposition instructions in a timely way. Thus, explicit directives define the time frame (when) and place (where) and the level of urgency (why) patients need further evaluation in clear, concise and understandable terms – thereby lessening the chance of delay in care.

PATTERN RECOGNITION & MATCHING

Patients rarely present with the "classic picture" of any condition. People are unique individuals, symptoms vary, and the advice nurse must deal with a myriad of variables. In truth, MI may present in various ways: with one key symptom (like chest pain); a few ill-structured or vague symptoms (nausea, vomiting, sweating without chest pain); or the "classic picture" of key and associated symptoms (crushing chest pain accompanied by shortness of breath, nausea, vomiting, dizziness, sweating, anxiety). The RN must use his/her best professional judgment to determine what constitutes a "match."

DOCUMENTATION STRATEGIES

Always start the assessment process using the above questions and the Documentation Form (below), rather than the Protocol. The rationale is to get a mental image of the problem, using the form and key questions, then fill in details using the Protocol.

Patients often present symptoms in erratic and disorganized ways, and may focus on one symptom to the exclusion of other, more important ones. Start with the Master Guideline and Documentation Form for the "first pass" to reduce the risk of premature selection of a Protocol that can lead to mistriage. The RN must be investigative, starting with a "clean slate" and performing a preliminary assessment before choosing a Protocol.

FORMING AN "IMPRESSION" OR "WORKING DIAGNOSIS"

In regard to the diagnosis, the most an advice nurse can hope for is a "working diagnosis" or "impression." Forming a working diagnosis is no great mystery. Use the patient's chief complaint in their own words—"headache," "nosebleed," "vaginal bleeding," "earache," etc. Then add modifiers or qualifiers (See Appendix for Approved Abbreviations) that will designate the level of acuity. For example:

> Abdominal pain, 9 on scale of 10, sudden onset
> Ankle pain, 4 on scale of 10, trauma history

Documenting high-risk patients and symptoms using SAVED may help "defend" dispositions. For example:

> Headache, non-English-speaking, yelling
> Abd. Pain, Prev. Hx, ectopic

The final steps, treatment, and evaluation are addressed in the Protocol. The treatment plan, formed from the Protocol's disposition and advice, is always a provisional one. Evaluation is carried out when the nurse provides patient teaching for self-evaluation through follow-up instruction from the Protocol.

The Documentation Form is based on the concept of charting by inclusion. Charting by inclusion requires that the RN chart normal negatives (pertinent negatives) as well as abnormal findings. Pertinent negatives are "findings that are normal and significant" (e.g., "no black or bloody stools," etc.). If you are charting by inclusion, pertinent negative findings should always be written.

PERTINENT NEGATIVES

In telephone triage, the issue of charting by inclusion or exclusion is best addressed by in-house counsel and formal policies. This guide proposes no directives about charting except to encourage charting by inclusion, where feasible.

The most conservative approach is to documenT pertinent negatives, especially with head, chest, respiratory, abdomen, dizziness, and flu symptoms. However, with other, less serious-sounding problems, if it is obvious that no emergent symptoms are present and all answers regarding urgent (or acute, Nona cute) symptoms are answered "no," the pertinent negatives may be noted as follows: "Denies all urgent symptoms." If, for example, the patient answers "yes" to certain urgent questions, one might write: "Denies all urgent symptoms with exception of fever, shaking chills," or "Fever/chills"; denies all other urgent symptoms."

The Basic Assessment: Triage Form Key (See example next page)

1. All of the following demographic information is included here: Note vital statistics: Name, age, sex, and phone number, temperature, BP, weight, etc.
2. Immunization history: Elicit whether immunization is up to date and mark accordingly.
3. Chief complaint (CC).
4. "Key Questions": SCHOLAR, ADL are used to elicit detailed information about the chief complaint.
5. Note home care measures already tried.
6. Date of last normal menstrual period.
7. Note pregnancy status (circle one).
8. Note breastfeeding status (circle one).
9. Note allergies (circle one) and add if "Yes".
10. Note chronic illness (circle one) and describe.
11. Note emotional state.
12. Note medications (Rx, OTC, herbal, street, or recreational drugs).
13. Note recent injury or surgery and describe.
14. Note recent exposure to contagious illness.
15. Note recent possible ingestion of toxic substance.
Circle any/all emergent or urgent symptom patterns.
16. Note impression (working diagnosis), or circle one or more items in Emergent or urgent symptoms.
17. Note title of Protocol used, or note "Master Protocol."
18. Note any modifications to approved Protocol advice.
19. Mode of transport.
20. Note minutes or hour when patient to arrive at office, urgent care or ED.
21. Note date of appointment/time.
22. Note whether precaution was stated (circle one).
23. Note patient agreement to plan (circle one).
24. Signature/title.
25. Note time call ended.

NOTE: Boxes 5-15 relate to PAMPER.

TRIAGE/ADVICE FORM

1. Adult O Pediatric 0	Name
Age DOB M F	Date Time AM PM
Caller/Relation to Pt.	
T. Oral AX Rec. BP	2. Immz Up to Date? Y N (N = Needs Appt.)

3. Chief Complaint:

4

5. Home Tx Administered? Y N

6. *IMP?* 7. *Pregnant? YN*	8. *Breastfeeding?* Y *N*
9. *Allergies? YN*	10. *Chronic Illness? YN*
	11. *Emotional State?*
12. *Medications? YN*	13. *Recent Injury? Y N*
	14. *Recent Illness? YN*
	15. *Recent Ingestion? YN*

16. Impression: SAVED

EMERGENT SYMPTOMS	URGENT SYMPTOMS
1. Extreme, unusual, new, sudden, suspicious, emergent or urgent sounding symptoms? 2. Trauma with suspicious history? 3. Unusual pain or symptoms • postoperative • postpartum • postprocedure	1. Infection symptoms; temp > 104? 2. Infection symptoms after 48 hours on antibiotic? 3. Moderate symptoms in patient with • Extreme Age/Childbearing Age • Communication Barrier • Chronic Illness • Severe emotional Distress (Pt. or Caretaker)

17. Protocol Advice/18. Modifications:

19. Mode of Transport:	20. Advised to be here within Min. Hr.
21. Appt. Date Time	22. Disclaimer Stated? Y N
23. Client Agreement to Plan? Y N	24. RN Sig/Title 25. Time ended

Sidebar:

4
SCHOLAR
Sx
Char.
Course
Hx of Sx
Onset
Loc.
Ag. Fac.
Rcl. Fac.

4
ADL
Intake
Liquid
Solid
Output
Urine
BM
Emesis
Sleep
Activity
Color

How Should I Chart?

Charting must be complete but cryptic, and include accurate, timely observations in patient's own words. Nurses must use approved abbreviations and terminology as well.

Please review the charting sample for examples to make charting more complete, accurate, and detailed.

1. Quantify where possible—avoid vague expressions.
2. Time frames (8,16,24,48 hr) as related to symptoms or treatment
3. "Working diagnosis" or "impression"
4. Advice per Protocol name
5. Protocol deviations/override/modifications

Must I Ask Questions in a Specific Order or According to the Order on the Form?

Elicit information in any order that seems appropriate to the caller and the situation. It is not necessary to let the form dictate the order of data collection. In real-world situations, people volunteer information when initially describing their chief complaint. To interrupt and begin mechanically asking questions is counterproductive, may lead the caller in the wrong direction, and may actually lengthen the call. Take notes in the appropriate spot on the form as the caller volunteers information. Then fill in the gaps with follow-up questions.

What about Documenting the Caller's Consent?

Always end your call with the precaution statement and document it. The precaution helps to ensure that the patient has given informed consent—in other words, they understand the problem definition and proposed treatment *with the following understanding:*

a. This is an "impression," *not* a medical diagnosis.
b. The treatment is based on the impression.
c. The final decision to follow advice rests with the patient.
d. If patients disagree with the impression, they may have an appointment.
e. If symptoms become markedly worse or fail to respond to the home treatment, the patient agrees to call back or come in.

Elicit and document what the caller plans to do at the end of the call. This will demonstrate that there was agreement to a certain plan of action.

What Calls Must Be Documented?

Again, this is an area for in-house counsel to address through formal policies. It is best to document all calls involving advice and calls involving same-day or later appointments. Calls for information or referral probably do not need to be documented, provided the caller has no symptoms.

How Important Is It to Document Medications?

Always chart medications, whether current prescriptions, OTC, recreational drugs, or herbal remedies. All medications have the potential to cause side effects or to interact with other medications, food, or chronic conditions. With women of childbearing age, always elicit pregnancy and breastfeeding status before advising any OTC or herbal remedy.

Should I Leave Blanks or Fill in All Spaces?

Don't leave any blank spaces. Such omissions may be interpreted as failure to chart completely. Write N/A if the question is not applicable (as in pregnancy status, if the caller is male) or "unknown" if patient does not know the answer (as in whether they have allergies or whether they are pregnant).

The acronyms SCHOLAR, PAMPER, and ADL are incorporated into the Documentation Form to serve as "triggers" to remind nurses what Key Questions to ask.

Once the nurse has elicited this information, she/he is ready to choose a Protocol. In some cases, the nurse will use the General Protocol, a "core protocol" that serves as "infrastructure" for all other Protocols. Understanding this Protocol is one of the best ways to understand and appreciate the overall design.

The Triage Process

The concepts of picture-building and "drilling down" underlie the telephone triage process. The instructions below incorporate these concepts as well as the strategies introduced on the preceding pages.

First Steps

Start with a global approach (SAVED) and the Documentation Form. Unless it is clearly an emergency, follow this quick assessment with Key Questions (SCHOLAR, PAMPER, ADL) as appropriate. Use open-ended questions where possible. Do *not* start with a Protocol, lest you fall prey to the "wrong track" syndrome. Clawson and Democoeur (1998) states that "if you get on the wrong track at the station, no matter how fast you travel, you still end up in the wrong place." Without the symptom and patient history, you may not know which Protocol to use or you may waste valuable time in the wrong Protocol and either delay treatment and/or mistriage.

How Do I Know Which Protocol to Use?

Once you have a general sense of the problem(s), turn to the Table of Contents or divider tab. Use the Protocol that best matches the site and/or symptoms of the patient's presenting problem(s). If patients present with multiple symptoms, use the Protocol that has the highest likelihood of leading to an appointment, or ask the patient which symptom is the most bothersome. If there is no Protocol that relates to the presenting symptom, use the General Protocol.

What Is the Purpose of the General Protocol?

Because of the variation in symptom presentation in unique individuals, it is not feasible to develop a set of Protocols to cover every condition. Not having a Protocol to cover a condition leads to what is commonly known as the "out of Protocol" experience. This is where the General Protocol is useful.

The General Protocol is especially useful in two instances: (1) when the nurse does not know which Protocol to use and (2) when responding to calls about elderly, and poor historians whose presenting symptoms are vague or ill-structured. In such cases, you may use the General Protocol alone.

The General Protocol (See Key Assessment Tools tab) acts as a safety net to keep patients from falling through the cracks by organizing problems in a very broad way. Each box contains general categories of problems that are emergent to nonacute (severe pain, major trauma, fever, acute infection, minor self-limiting symptoms, (etc.). Also included are general categories of high-risk patients because of age, veracity, emotional distress, debilitation, and distance. While it does not address symptoms or patients in a detailed way, the General Protocol provides general guidelines for the "out of Protocol" experience. However, there is always a need for more detailed Protocols that cover symptoms in depth. This is where site-specific Protocols come into play (e.g., Ear Problems, Urinary Problems, etc.).

How Do I Use the Protocol?

Generally speaking, each Protocol is divided into two sections—a triage "chart" and Supplemental Information (SI). For patients describing symptoms, start with the triage chart, reading from left to right and top to bottom. Reviewing the Bum Protocols, start with Key Questions first. For instance, if the patient responds "yes" to "electrical bums," question, go right to the middle column in "emergent symptom patterns." Continue asking more specific questions related to electrical bums. If the answer to *one or more* of these questions is "yes," shift to the right again for appropriate disposition and first aid. Many Protocols start with the key question of "Trauma." Thus, if the caller denies trauma (or pain, discharge, etc.), skip all questions related to it (to the right with pluses in front of them).

Always rule out emergent symptoms first, either by asking specific questions or from the patient history. Symptom patterns are listed in the middle column in descending order of acuity from emergent to nonacute. Corresponding Dispositions are listed in the right-hand column, also in descending order of acuity. Work your way down the list, ruling out emergent to nonacute symptoms. If the patient answers "no" to all key questions (left-hand column), consult the cross-reference section for other possibilities.

Some problems require immediate first aid or home treatment. First aid instructions are usually located in the "disposition" column (far right) or under Supplemental Information. Specific home treatment instructions are in the Supplemental Information (SI) section, and common home remedies are located under Flome Treatment Supplemental Information in Appendix A. The SI section provides information regarding particular conditions or treatments or for answering questions unrelated to symptoms or about conditions that have been previously medically diagnosed only.

▶ General Reminders

Remember, the most important task of telephone triage is to reduce uncertainty and urgency by asking *enough* of the *right questions,* in the *right way* to elicit *enough* of the *right data,* and to choose the *right Protocol(s)* and *right disposition.* Pattern recognition requires eliciting sufficient contextual information. The more preliminary information gathered, the more obvious the pattern.

General guide: *When in doubt, always err on the side of caution.* RNs must rely on their best professional judgment and use every means at their disposal to ensure that patients are treated in a timely manner. Time frames designated on the template are intended as a *general* guide. When in doubt, have the patient come in *sooner rather than later.* With the exception of emergent level dispositions, *time frames are intended to be flexible,* allowing for professional judgment. For example, when presented with a problem corresponding with a disposition time frame of 1-8 hr (essentially a same-day appointment), the RN may direct a caller to come in within 2 hr, if in his/her professional judgment it is more prudent or reasonable to do so.

Upgrading/downgrading: RNs may upgrade dispositions as appropriate (i.e., from urgent to emergent; nonacute to acute). However, never downgrade (i.e., urgent to nonacute) without a physician consultation. If a patient is noncompliant, always seek advice from the physician on call.

Ask questions in any order, or simply let the caller tell their story first.

Beware of the developing disease: What starts out as vague abdominal pain with low-grade fever may quickly develop into the classic picture of appendicitis. Follow-up calls should be mandatory for possible developing diseases, and especially for Abdominal Pain, Respiratory Problem, Diarrhea, N/V, Fever, or Marked Change in Activities of Daily Living.

▶ OTC Medications

Just because a medicine is over the counter does not mean it is harmless. Herbal remedies can have side effects, as can megadoses of vitamins. Prolonged use of any drug, over the counter or prescription, can produce unwanted or even dangerous side effects. Sometimes people become "functionally dependent," meaning that a body function has ceased to work naturally because it has been altered by the drug and must have it in order to continue to function. Remind patients that drugs should be taken in the smallest dose for the shortest time possible.

Currently many drugs that previously required a prescription are being approved for over-the-counter status. In order to avoid the possibility of delayed diagnosis, flawed triage, and possible complications, nurses must remain alert to possible side effects and cautions regarding all medications. There are three ways in which problems can arise with any drug, either over the counter or prescription. A few common examples are:

- Drug/drug interactions: Aspirin can interact with anticoagulants to increase the effect of anticoagulation. When combined with alcohol, long-term use of Tylenol may have a toxic effect on the liver.

- Drug/food interactions: Certain antidepressants (MAO inhibitors) can interact with foods that contain tyramine (Chianti wine, homemade bread, sour cream, avocado, aged game, liver, canned meats, eggplant, and many others) to cause a life-threatening rise in blood pressure.

- Drug/disease interactions: Salicylates are contraindicated in persons with bleeding disorders, ulcer, gout, asthma.

General Instructions

- Advise all patients using folk remedies of risk of two medications acting together; might cause harm.
- Most OTC brands come in numerous preparations, e.g., Robitussin, DM, AC, etc.

Some Final Words

If telephone triage is to continue to evolve into a formally recognized subspecialty, then standards, Protocols, and training must keep pace with developments in managed care and technology. Telephone triage nurses are being challenged by economic forces to prove themselves to be a viable component of this service. Telephone triage nurses can continue to uphold their unique traditional role as patient advocate and upgrade their profession and practice through ongoing training and standards development.

References

Clawson, J.J., and Democoeur, K.B. (1998). *Principles of Emergency Medical Dispatch.* (2nd ed.). Salt Lake City, UT: Priority Press.

Daugird, A.J., and Spencer, D.C. (1989). Characteristics of patients who highly utilize telephone medical care in a private practice. *The Journal of Family Practice, 27,* 420-421.

Fillit, H., and Capello, C. (1994). Making geriatric assessment an asset to your primary care practice. *Geriatrics, 49{* 1), 27-30.

Finley, R. (1995). Telephone triage: Essentials for expert practice. *Polypharmacy and the Elderly.* Dublin, CA: Contemporary Forums.

► Pain Assessment Guidelines (ALL AGES)

"Pain is one of the most common reasons people seek medical attention" (JCAHO 2001).

Assessment Parameters/Descriptors

- Pain intensity
- Associated symptoms
- Characteristics (measure at present and at worst):
  —Quantity (8-10 on scale of 10; mild, moderate or extreme; worst or unbearable)
  —Quality (sharp, dull, throbbing, etc.)
- Onset/duration:
  —Sudden, gradual. How many hours, days, months?
- Location:
  —Local versus generalized (Have patient point to site and describe.)
- Aggravating factors:
  —What makes it worse? (Food, activity, position, etc.)
- Relieving factors:
  —What makes it better? (Meds, food, activity, position, etc.)
- Current Home Treatment
- Effects on daily life: Eating, sleeping, work, relationships, emotions, concentration

► Red Flags and Pain

"Red Flags" direct our attention to certain high-risk symptoms and populations (SAVED).

Severe

- Any severe, sudden or suspicious pain:
  —Awakens patient from sleep or keeps patient awake.
  —Described as "worst," "unexpected," "unusual," "sudden," "recurrent."
  —Any pain unrelieved by prescribed pain medication.
  —8-10 on scale of 10.
  —Sudden onset is considered to be more serious.
  —Localized pain is considered to be more serious.

Age Related

- Beware of pain symptoms in very young or very old.

Veracity

- Pain symptoms in non-English speaking children or poor historians

Emotional Distress

- Frequent calls about chronic, recurrent or unrelieved pain may signal emotional distress (Do not overlook physical problem, however.):
  —All ages with chronic pain have 40%-50% depression.
  —Untreated depression lowers ability to cope with pain.

Debilitation

- Pain in patients with history of chronic illness:
- Pain unrelieved by usual pain medication

- Pain in patients with recent surgical history
- Unusually bad postoperative pain

Rules of Thumb

- Localized pain *tends* to be more serious; diffuse pain tends to be less serious.
- Sudden onset of pain *tends* to be more serious; gradual onset, less serious.
- Recurrent episodes of pain may indicate high acuity.
- Take all patients' complaints of pain seriously.
- Severe pain is always treated as an emergency.
- Minority callers often fail to recognize acute symptoms, report fewer symptoms, or attribute them to other causes.
- Beware of any pain that awakens patient or keeps him or her awake at night.
- Ideally, preventive therapy starts the moment symptoms of pain appear.

Red Herrings

"Red Herrings" are common distractions (symptoms or situations) that lead the nurse astray, away from the main problem.

- Barriers to pain assessment:
  —Reluctance to discuss pain.
  —Denial of pain, when pain is likely to be present (postop, trauma, bums, cardiac emergencies).
- Remain vigilant to possible patient denial, minimization, and misinterpretation of symptoms.
- Regard with suspicion: all elderly callers and unusual sounding presentations, including pain that is new, sudden, or unexpectedly severe.
  —Patients who have been "seen recently" may still need to be seen today.
  —Don't be misled by concurrent complaints or patient self-explanation.
  —Symptom presentation may be early, late, silent, atypical, or novel.
  —Symptoms of two conditions may present concurrently, thereby causing confusion or misinterpretation.
  —Patients often misinterpret or stereotype their symptoms.

Pain Syndromes in the Elderly

In regard to pain management, the elderly are at risk for undertreatment and overtreatment. There is a common misperception that the elderly are less sensitive to pain. This is not true. While the elderly may be more accepting and resigned to pain, they have pain nonetheless. In regard to pain medications the elderly have a narrower range between therapeutic effect and drug toxicity, presenting the problems of polypharmacy.

The elderly have several conditions more likely to cause pain—cancer and shingles. The elderly comprise at least 80% of those with cancer and have significant pain with advanced cancer. Shingles affect about 40% of people over 70 yr of age; it is a major cause of suicide in the elderly. Cognitive impairment may create an obstacle to pain assessment. However, most elderly relate well to scales like "mild, moderate, or severe," or 1-10.

Pain Presentation in Comatose, Nonverbal Signs

- Comatose patients. The symptoms may be subtle: agitation, restlessness, irregular breathing, pupil dilation, and sweating (Todd 1998).
- Nonverbal signs of pain include grimacing, groaning, guarded posture, favoring a limb, isolation, irritability, or fatigue (Todd 1998).

► Chronic Pain

Chronic pain lasts longer than expected, may be continuous, repetitive, or intermittent. It may become a primary problem or lead to structural change in the nervous system. This can further lead to the "wind-up phenomenon" that can cause increased pain and lowered threshold for pain (Todd 1998).

► Pain as the Fifth Vital Sign

According to the American Pain Society, pain is the "Fifth Vital Sign." APS (1999-2001) and now JCAHO (2001) has set forth standards that promote routine evaluation of pain.

► JCAHO Standards*

Pain is assessed in all patients. (JCAHO 2001) Pain measurement standards mandate the consistent assessment of each patient complaint of pain through the use of pain measurement scales, number, picture, and/or verbal descriptions.

Patients are involved in making care decisions, including managing pain effectively. To this end, structures are developed, approved and maintained, such as a framework for addressing issues related to care at the end of life, providing for managing pain aggressively and effectively.

End of life pain issues. The health care organization addresses care at the end of life. Dying patients have unique needs for respectful, responsive care. All staff are sensitized to the needs of the patient at the end of life. Concern for the patient's comfort and dignity should guide all aspects of care during the final stages of life. The health care organization's frameworks for addressing issues related to care at the end of life provide for managing pain aggressively and effectively.

Patients have the right to appropriate assessment and management of pain. Pain that is unrelieved has adverse physical and psychological effects. The patient's right to pain management is respected and supported. The organization plans, supports, and coordinates activities and resources to ensure the pain of all individuals is recognized and addressed appropriately. This includes

- Initial assessment and regular reassessment of pain.

- Education of patients and families, when appropriate, regarding their roles in managing pain as well as the potential limitation and side effects of pain treatments. Taking into account personal, cultural, spiritual, and/or ethnic beliefs communicates to patients and families that pain management is an important part of their care.

Postprocedure: The patient is monitored continuously throughout the postprocedure period. The following specific items are monitored:

- Impairments and functional status.

- Pain intensity and quality (for example, pain character, frequency, location, education, and response to treatments).

- Unusual events or postoperative complications and their management. Results of monitoring trigger key decisions, such as change of care due to a precipitous change in vital signs.

Patients are educated about pain and managing pain as part of treatment, as appropriate. When appropriate, patient and families are instructed about understanding pain, the risk for pain, the importance of effective pain management, the pain assessment process and methods for pain management, when identified as part of treatments. Data that the organization considers for collection to monitor performance include the appropriateness and effectiveness of pain management.

- All patients are asked the following screening or general question about the presence of pain: "Do you have pain now?"

EMERGENCY MEDICINE ACUITY CATEGORIES

The *Master Guideline* is designed to serve as a "fall back" or "contingency "guideline in cases where no guideline seems to fit the problem. In the left-hand column are definitions of acuity from the Model of the Clinical Practice of Emergency Medicine. In the right-hand column are corresponding categories of acuity from the Wheeler design with examples of symptoms that fit each category.

Emergency Medicine Acuity Categories and Definitions	Wheeler Acuity Categories and Examples
CRITICAL	**EMERGENT (0-1 Hr)**
Signs or symptoms of a life-threatening illness/injury with a high risk of mortality if immediate intervention is not begun to prevent further airway, respiratory, hemodynamic, and/or neurologic instability	Loss of consciousness Major trauma Shock or impending shock OB crises, Impending birth Sudden confusion, disorientation Loss or threat of loss of vital functions: Respiratory, circulatory, or sensory organs Caretaker/patient presents danger to self or others *RN feels symptoms are emergent*
EMERGENT	**URGENT (1-8 Hr)**
Signs or symptoms of an illness/injury that may progress in severity or result in complications with a high probability for morbidity if treatment is not begun quickly	Trauma Severe pain Any severe symptom (See SAVED) Acute infection symptoms Any infection requiring antibiotics *RN feels symptoms are urgent*
LOWER ACUITY	**ACUTE/NONACUTE (8+ Hr)**
Signs or symptoms of illness/injury with low probability to worsen to a more serious disease or to develop complications	Moderate symptoms in high risk patient (See SAVED) Failure to improve on home treatment Minor trauma Self limiting Sx. not markedly worsening

"The Core Content Task Force It created and endorsed the 2001 Model of the Clinical Practice of Emergency Medicine (EM Model) as published in the June 2001 *Annals of Emergency Medicine* and *Academic Emergency Medicine.*

Emergency Medicine Model Review Task Force. (2007). Emergency model. *Annals of Emergency Medicine.*

http://wtvw.abem.orn/PUBLIC/Dortal/alias Rainbow/lanu en US/tablD 3590/DesktopDefault.aspx

MASTER GUIDELINE

Acuity Level		Disposition
Key Symptom	**Emergent Symptom Patterns**	**911 or ED in 0-1 H**
Major Trauma?	Blunt Trauma/MVA/Fall > 15 FT	
Loss of Consciousness?		
Shock or Impending Shock?		
Severe Respiratory Distress?		
Presents danger to self/others? (Patient or caregiver)		
Disorientation, Confusion, Marked Behavior Change?		
Decompensation, or Threat of Decompensation of Vital Functions:	Neurological, Respiratory, Circulation Excretion, Mobility or Sensory (Hearing, Sight) Organs?	
Suspected or Confirmed Infection and ANY:	• Sudden change in mental state, confusion ■ Abdominal Pain ■ Marked decrease in Urine Output ■ Decreased capillary refill or mottling? *(Suspect Sepsis)*	
Severe Vomiting, Diarrhea or Extremely Low Intake and ANY:	• Extremely quiet/inactive/weak ■ Very difficult to arouse, confused • Skin: cool/mottled/blue, < Turgor/Tenting ■ Mucous membranes: Extremely dry, parched lips/tongue, difficult to swallow • Eyes: Sunken ■ Respirations: Mouth breathing - very fast ■ Intake: No fluids for 4-8 hr. ■ Output: Urine - No urine, or scanty amount *(Suspect Severe Dehydration)*	
Are severe pain, or suspicious or emergent symptoms ruled out?		

MASTER GUIDELINE

Key Symptom	Urgent Symptom Patterns	ED/UCC/Office 1-8 H First Aid or Home Tx
Trauma and ANY:	■ Suspicious History? (Possible Abuse)	COME TO ED NOW
Adult: Suspected or Confirmed Infection and ANY:	■ Temp > 38.5C or < 36 C ■ HR > 90 BPM ■ RR > 20 RPM ■ History/Risk Factors: • *Immunodeficienl:* Age > 65 Yr. • *Immunosuppression:* Chronic Disease (All), Cancer, Transplant • *Immunosuppressive Med/Tx:* Chemo/Corticosteroid/Radiation • *Implant, Invasive* Post-Op/Post-Partum, Post-Procedure/Trauma/Large Bum • *International* Travel • Alcohol/Substance Abuse • Antibiotic therapy (ongoing) *(Suspect Sepsis)*	COME TO ED NOW
Pain or Unusual Symptoms and ANY:	■ Fever > 40°C or 104°F? ■ Post-Op, Post-Partum, or Post-Procedure? (Suspect Complications/Infection) ■ Recent Injury	COME TO ED NOW
Symptoms of Infection and ANY:	■ Failure To Improve On Antibiotics X 48 Hr.? *(Ineffective Rx)*	
Decreased intake +/- moderate vomiting/diarrhea and ANY:	• Drowsy, Weak, Dizzy? • Skin: Pale, Decreased Turgor? • Mucous Membranes: Very Diy Lips/ Tongue? • Respirations: Moderately Fast? • Unable to hold down sm. amt. fluids X 2-3 H • Urine - Dark yellow, Decreased *(Suspect Mod - Severe Dehydration)*	COME TO ED NOW
Possible Exposure: Inhalation, Ingestion, Eye/Skin Irritation or ANY:	Exposure to ANY Toxin, Adverse Dmg Reaction, New Medication, Drug-Drug, Drug-Disease, Dmg-Food Interactions, Intentional or Accidental Ingestion, Animal/Insect/Snake, Food or Mushroom Poisoning or Dmg reaction?	
ANY Condition	With the potential to result in admission to ED/ hospital within 24 hours (ACEP)	
Urgent symptoms ruled out?		

MASTER GUIDELINE

Key Symptom	Acute Symptom Patterns	ED/UCC/Office 9-24 H First Aid or Home Tx
Moderate Symptoms and ANY:	■ High Risk Patient: - Extremes of age - Communication barrier - Emotional distress - Chronic illness History	Possible Upgrade to Urgent?
Decreased Intake, Mild Diarrhea/Vomiting and ANY :	■ Fatigue, low energy, irritable ■ Skin: Color-Normal, Turgor-WNL ■ Mucous membranes: Moist - si. dry ■ Respirations: WNL ■ Intake: Able to take small frequent amounts of fluid ■ Output: Urine slight decrease ■ BM: Infrequent, small, watery stools (Suspect Mild Dehydration)	
Moderate Symptoms and ANY:	■ Persistent, worsening, or failure to improve on home treatment X 24-48 hr.	Possible upgrade to Urgent (> Risk)?
Acute symptoms ruled out?		
Key Symptom	Non Acute Symptom Patterns	Future Appt in 24 + H First Aid or Home Tx
Minor Symptoms and ANY:	■ Self-Limiting, Existing > 1 Week, Not Becoming Markedly Worse? ■ Improving on home treatment	

Rule of Thumb: Assess all Children and Elderly patients for symptoms of possible sepsis and dehydration.

Dehydration
- May be the result of *the combined effect* of several conditions including: Extreme Weather Conditions (Heat, Humidity), *Job Occupation or Exercise,* Fever orN/V, Diarrhea, Low or No Fluid Intake.
- Always consider risk factors such as Age, Chronic Disease, Degree and Duration of Fever, Past Medical Hx, Medication, etc.
- General descriptions of dehydration are based on alterations of Activities of Daily Living (ADL).

Acuity Definitions
- Emergent: S&S of life threatening illness/injury with *high risk of mortality* if immediate intervention is not begun to prevent further airway, respiratory, hemodynamic, and/or neurologic instability. ACEP
- Urgent: S&S of illness, injury that may progress in severity or result in complication with *high probability for morbidity* if treatment is not initiated quickly. *Any condition resulting in admission of the patient to a hospital within 24 hours* ACEP
- Acute: S&S of illness/injury with some *probability to worsen or develop complications.*
- Non-Acute: S&S of illness/injury with *low probability* to worsen or develop complications

ABDOMEN PROBLEM 1: UPPER AND GENERALIZED
Pain with or without Trauma

ASSESSMENT	ACUITY LEVEL	DISPOSITION/ADVICE
Key Questions	Emergent Symptom Patterns	ED 0 min-1 hr
Major Trauma	+ Weak, dizzy, cold/mottled, or pale skin, blue lips/nail beds, rapid/shallow breathing, unresponsive, loss of consciousness? (Trauma/Internal Hemorrhage) (See Shock)---------------------------------------.........	▪▶ All emergent abd. pain: Keep NPO
Pain w/o Trauma	+ Generalized, unbearable, sudden onset, radiating from chest or abdomen to back/legs. ± Hx of > BP? (Aortic Aneurysm)	
	+ Sudden onset, bloody/coffee ground emesis, or bloody diarrhea, melena (Black Stools), weakness, fainting, pale? (Upper GI Bleed)	
	+ Sudden onset. Hx of exposure to street drugs/Rx, poisonous plant, or inhalation/ingestion of toxic chemical or pesticide? (Toxic Exposure/Ingestion) —▶	Contact poison center; bring substance to ED w you
Pain w/o Trauma	+ (Severe) Sudden or gradual onset, guarding, ± fever/vomiting, confused, altered level of consciousness, weakness, dizziness? (Acute Abdomen w Systemic Symptoms)	

Key Questions	Urgent Symptom Patterns	ED/UCC/Office 1-8 hr
		All urgent abd. pain: keep NPO
Trauma	+ Lower abd. (Groin). Hx falls, > 65 yr, urinary retention? (Pelvic/Hip Fx)	
Pain	+ (Severe), Sudden, or gradual onset, ± trauma, guarding, + fever/vomiting? (Acute Abdomen)	
	+ Fever, localized or generalized tenderness, rigidity, involuntary guarding, ± vomiting, pain w movement? (Peritonitis)	
	+ Sudden, radiating from flank to groin/back, colicky then constant/severe, NV, ± hematuria ± urgency, ± painful urination? (Kidney Stone)	

(continued)

Key Questions	Urgent Symptom Patterns	ED/UCC/Office 1-8 hr
Pain (continued)	+ Abd./back/chest pain worsened w exertion? (Cardiac)	
	+ Burning, tightness, relieved by antacids? (Esophagitis)	
	+ Dull/sev., > w cold drink or alcohol? (Esophageal spasm)	
	+ Fever, ± jaundice, RUQ pain. ± Hx gallstones? (Acute Cholangitis, Cholecystitis)	
	+ (Sev.-Mod.), Radiating from abd./flank/back to groin, colicky then constant & severe, fever/chills, N/V, dysuria, ± hematuria, frequency/urgency? (Pyelonephritis)	
	+ Generalized, colicky, elderly, vomiting, abd., distention. Hx severe constipation, no appetite, not passing gas ± abd. surgery? (Bowel Obstruction)	
	+ RUQ, fever, N/V, ± Hx of ETOH abuse. Hx gallstones? (Pancreatitis)	
	+ Abd./chest/back pain + > w resp., fever/chills, + productive cough, difficult breathing, N/V, fatigue? (Pneumonia)	
	+ (Mod.), Crampy, watery stools, ± blood/mucus/pus, alternating w normal stools, ± N/V, fever, recent immigration, (x 1-2 yr). Hx of foreign travel, exposure to contaminated water, undercooked meat/seafood/poultry/improperly stored food, ± dehydration? (Infectious Diarrhea)	

Key Questions	Acute/Nonacute Symptom Patterns		FA 8+ hr ± Home Tx
Pain (Epigastric)	+ Burning/gnawing/aching on empty stomach. ± Hx ETOH abuse/stress? (Peptic Ulcer, GERD, Dyspepsia)---		➤ Sa: Pain relieved by food/milk/antacids? (Yes = +)
	+ Constant burning, ± N/V, diarrhea. Hx of ETOH/steroids/NSAIDs/ASA? (Acute Gastritis)		
Pain (RUQ)	+ Fever, N/V w/o dehydration. Sx: anorexia, yellow sclera, fatigue, swollen glands, clay-colored stools, dark urine, ± exp. to hepatitis? (Hepatitis)		
	+ Colicky, after rich meal, N/V, bloating, ± jaundice? (Cholelithiasis)		
Pain (Generalized)	+ (Crampy), N/V, diarrhea w/o dehydration. Sx: ± fever, joint pain, ± headache? (Gastroenteritis)		
	+ Prolonged, after milk products? (Lactose Intolerance)		

Cross-References
Abdomen Problem 2

Back Problem	Chest Pain	Hepatitis
Bowel Problem 1; 2	Fever	Urinary Problem

ABDOMEN PROBLEM 2: LOWER
Pain without Trauma

ASSESSMENT	ACUITY LEVEL	DISPOSITION/ADVICE
Key Questions	Emergent Symptom Patterns	Ed 0 min-1 hr
Pain (Severe)	+ Sharp, progressive, unilateral pelvic pain, ± radiates to shoulder, pale, lightheaded, fainting. Hx: STI, PID, any abdominal/tubal surgery, prior IUD use, missed period x 3-6 wk, spotting, painful intercourse? (Ectopic Pregnancy)	
Pain w/o Trauma	+ (Severe) Sudden or gradual onset, guarding, ± fever/vomiting, confused, altered level of consciousness, weakness, dizziness (Acute Abdomen with Systemic Symptoms)	
Key Questions	Urgent Symptom Patterns	ED/UCC/Office 1-8 hr
Pain	+ Constant, progressing from periumbilical to RLQ, mild fever, ± vomiting, ± anorexia, ± walks bent over? (Appendicitis)------------------------------------- --►> SA: Standing on tiptoes > Pain = +; Touching RLQ > Pain = +	
	+ Sudden, radiating from flank to groin/back, colicky then constant/severe, N/V, ± hematuria? (Kidney Stone)	
	+ (Sev.-mod.), radiating from abd./flank/back to groin, colicky then constant & severe, fever/chills, N/V, dysuria, ± hematuria, ffequency/urgency? (Pyelonephritis)	
Pain (Pelvic)	+ Vaginal discharge: foul smelling, bloody/any color; fever (> 38°C or 100.4°F)/chills, walks bent over. ± Hx of STD exp., ± IUD user? (PID)------------------- --►SA: Walks bent over = + "PID Shuffle"	
Pain (Groin) (severe)	+ W firm/tender bulge at groin/scrotum, N/V? (Incarcerated Hernia)	
Pain (LLQ/lower)	+ Varying or steady, =/- relieved by BM or gas, diarrhea alternating w constipation, bloating, fever, ± rectal bleeding? (Diverticulitis)	
Pain (LLQ or RLQ)	+ Female, low, unilateral. Hx of pain w intercourse/ BM/period? (Ovarian Cyst, Endometriosis)	

Key Questions	Acute/Nonacute Symptom Patterns		FA 8+hr ± HomeTx
Pain (Groin)	+ Bulge at groin, mild tenderness? (Inguinal Hernia)		
	+ Pre- or during menstrual period? (Menstrual Cramps)		

Cross-References Abdomen Problem 1	Back Problem Bowel Problem 1; 2	Fever Urinary Problem	Vaginal Problem: STI SI

ABDOMEN PROBLEM
Supplemental Information

Quick Reference ▶ General Advice ▶ Drug Side Effect (Abdominal Pain)

▶ Abdominal Pain ▶ Menstrual Cramps

▶ Appendicitis

▶ General Advice

® Pain in elderly (age > 70) is cause for concern.

- Abdominal pain localized in one area is more suggestive of severe problem.
- All abdominal pain—must not eat or drink before coming in = urgent/emergent level.

▶ Abdominal Pain

- Causes: Infection, trauma, anxiety, obstruction, hernia, ectopic pregnancy, menstrual cramps.
- Abdominal Pain Tax Goal: Relieve abdominal discomfort.
  —Heating pad, hot water bottle or bath, 20-30 min.
  —Lie down, rest.
  —Prevent gas: Avoid ASA, spicy foods, alcohol, caffeine, cigarettes.
  —Gas: Mylanta
  —Sips of fluid —» BRAT —> soft —» reg. diet (See Home Tx SI, Appendix A: "BRAT Diet", Clear Liquids, Soft Diet)

▶ Appendicitis

- Rules of Thumb:
  —Appendicitis is usually not present when fever occurs before pain.
  —Appendicitis is most common in ages 15-24.

® Signs and symptoms: See Protocol.

® Cause: Infection of part of bowel.

- Complications: Rupture, serious infection (Peritonitis).
- Tx: Surgery.

▶ Drug Side Effect: Abdominal Pain

- The most common drugs and classes of drugs:
  —Antibiotics (many), especially:
    ° Tetracycline (Doxycycline)
    ° Metronidazole (Flagyl)
  —Codeine
  —Erythromycin
  —Nonsteroidal anti-inflammatory drugs:
    o Advil
    o Aleve
    ° Ibuprofen

o Midol 200

o Motrin

o Nuprin

► **Menstrual Cramps**

(See Vaginal Bleeding)

- Signs and symptoms: Pain during period, low abdominal pain, dull/constant ache, may travel to back or legs
- Cause: Physical cause unknown; stress thought to make it worse
- Complication: None
- Tx

    —Motrin, Tylenol

    —Heating pad to abdomen 20-30 min pm

    —Exercise

ABUSE 1: SEXUAL
Reporting Tree

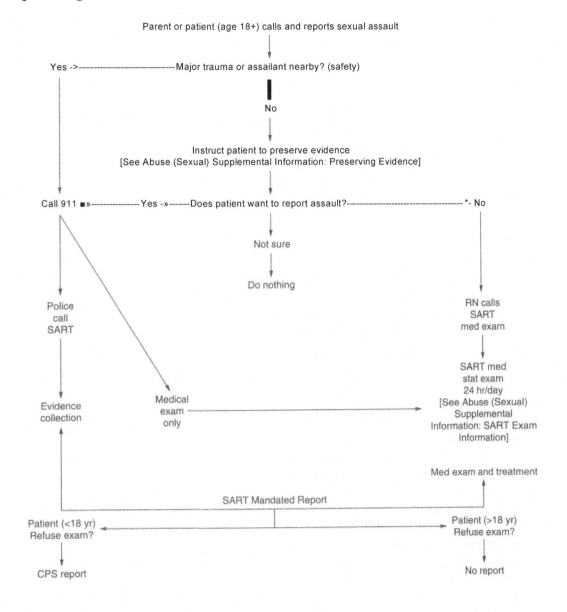

Parent or patient (age 18+) calls and reports sexual assault

Yes ->------------------------------Major trauma or assailant nearby? (safety)

No

Instruct patient to preserve evidence
[See Abuse (Sexual) Supplemental Information: Preserving Evidence]

Call 911 ■»---------------- Yes -»------Does patient want to report assault?-------------------------------- *- No

Not sure

Do nothing

Police
call
SART

RN calls
SART
med exam

Evidence
collection

Medical
exam
only

SART med
stat exam
24 hr/day
[See Abuse (Sexual)
Supplemental
Information: SART Exam
Information]

Med exam and treatment

SART Mandated Report

Patient (<18 yr)
Refuse exam?

Patient (>18 yr)
Refuse exam?

CPS report

No report

ABUSE 1: SEXUAL
Supplemental Information

Quick Reference ▶ Call Management for Sexual Abuse

Rules of Thumb

Instructions for Preserving Evidence

Information for the Survivor

Documentation and Reporting Guidelines

▶ Signs and Symptoms of Sexual Abuse

See also: Directory of Hotlines/Web Sites for Support Groups, Appendix E

▶ Call Management for Sexual Abuse

Rules of Thumb

- Most sexual abuse is inflicted on survivor by people known to survivor.
- High-risk groups include developmentally disabled, elderly, and teens.
- High-risk groups are less likely to disclose abuse.
- As with ED visits, a high percentage of calls may have a hidden agenda of abuse.
- Abuse crosses all sexual, economic, cultural, and racial lines.

Instructions for Preserving Evidence

- Comfort survivor.
- Do not shower, wash hands or face, or change clothes.
- Don't brush teeth.
- For women: Don't douche or remove tampon.
- Police may want to collect evidence in home or car (sheets, condom, etc.).
- Come with a friend.
- Bring change of clothes to ED. If you have changed, bring clothing worn at time of attack.

Information for the Survivor

Depending on the community, there may be a SART (Sexual Assault Response Team) or SANE (Sexual Assault Nurse Examiner).

- Examiner from SART, SANE, or Forensic Examiner may be available 24 hr for questions, intervention, advice, etc.
- Rape Crisis is called by SART, SANE, or Forensic Examiner for every case. They take care of most of the psycho/social intervention and follow-up care.
- SART or SANE nurse handles the medical exam.
- <72 hr: Preserve evidence: Don't do anything. Come as you are!
- >72 hr: Survivor may have medical exam.
- Pt. will be referred: Physical injury; counseling; pubic lice.
- Follow-up appt. w MD, SART coordinator, or CPS.
- STI risk/immunization: If possible, go to be evaluated within 24 hr.

—Tests may be done for gonorrhea, chlamydia, and syphilis. Follow-up tests for HIV and hepatitis may be done.

—Antibiotics: You will be given antibiotics for STIs.

—A pregnancy test will be done.

—You will be given a pill to prevent pregnancy called *morning-after pill.*

Documentation and Reporting Guidelines

- Consult with in-house counsel regarding developing written policies for reporting requirements to govern reporting of abuse suspected or verified through telephone triage.

- Nurses are legally required to report any incidents that they reasonably suspect or are told about. If a report is made by another staff member, the nurse is not required to make a report.

- Failure to report abuse may result in disciplinary action against one's license, a misdemeanor, and being held liable for damages suffered by survivors.

- Nurses who negligently or recklessly report abuse cannot be held liable.

- Assess suspected abuse cases carefully. Take care not to be too direct, while still encouraging them to come in.

- *Manage these calls carefully. Remember that patient safety is a priority.* Survivors of abuse may be placed at greater risk if law enforcement personnel intervene.

- Document in detail:

    —If survivor is in danger.

    —Name and relationship of person reporting suspected abuse.

    —Explicit details of injury (where, when, how).

    —Name of assailant if possible.

    —Previous history of abuse.

    —Elders: Review medication history, level of mental acuity, and physical mobility.

    —Use "survivor states" instead of "survivor alleges."

    —When referring to ED, you must inform ED of suspected abuse and have written documentation available.

▶ Signs and Symptoms of Sexual Abuse

Sexual assault on and sexual exploitation of adult. May be chronic or a single incident.

- STI symptoms in any adult.

- Genital injuries: Bruises, lacerations of rectum or vagina.

- Vaginal or urethral discharge or lesions.

- Rectal pain/bleeding.

- Mouth/tongue: Bruising or torn tissue under tongue or between upper lip and teeth ("classic injury").

- Bite marks.

- Bloody underclothing.

- Excessive anxiety/fear: Nightmares, depression, withdrawal, aggressive behavior.

- Change in toilet habits: Bed-wetting, encopresis.

- Survivor is known to be a survivor of other forms of abuse.

ABUSE 2: PHYSICAL
Supplemental Information

Quick Reference
▶ Community Alert
▶ Call Management for Physical Abuse (All Ages)
    Action Plan
    Documentation and Reporting Guidelines
    Prevention/Counseling
▶ Abuse: Spousal
    Rules of Thumb
    Signs of Physical Spousal Abuse
    Risk Factors
▶ Abuse: Elder
    Rules of Thumb
    Signs of Physical Elder Abuse
    Risk Factors
    Risk Factors for Financial Abuse

See also: Directory of Hotlines/Web Sites for Support Groups, Appendix E

▶ **Community Alert: Remain Aware of Precipitating Factors**
- Any community celebration: Sport events (e.g., Super Bowl), New Year's, etc., with or without alcohol or drug use.
- Natural disasters: Floods, earthquakes, hurricanes, etc.

▶ **Call Management for Physical Abuse**
(Note: Refer to this section first, whether you are dealing with Spousal or Elder Abuse.)

Action Plan
- When callers reveal that they have been abused: Patient's safety is primary focus.
  —Always tell the survivor that the police must and will be notified and will come to the site immediately.
  —Review escape plan. They should do the following:
    o Collect money and credit cards.
    ° Get children.
    o Collect important papers: Driver's license, passports, marriage certificate, birth certificates, leases, deeds,
    o Pack clothing.
    ° Call or go to a safe place or shelter for battered survivors.
- When referring to ED, you must inform them of suspected abuse situation and have written documentation available.

Documentation and Reporting Guidelines

- Consult with in-house counsel regarding developing written policies for reporting requirements to govern reporting of abuse suspected or verified through telephone triage.
- Nurses are legally required to report any incidents that they reasonably suspect or are told about. If a report is made by another staff member, the nurse is not required to make a report.
- Failure to report abuse may result in disciplinary action against one's license, a misdemeanor, and being held liable for damages suffered by survivors.
- Nurses who negligently or recklessly report abuse cannot be held liable.
- Assess suspected abuse cases carefully. Take care not to be too direct, while still encouraging them to come in.
- Manage these calls carefully. Remember that patient safety is a priority. Survivors of abuse may be placed at greater risk if law enforcement personnel intervene.
- Document (detailed documentation is essential):
  —If survivor is in danger.
  —Name and relationship of person reporting suspected abuse.
  —Explicit details of injury (where, when, how).
  —Name of assailant if possible.
  —Previous history of abuse.
  —Consult your organization's Policies and Procedures.
  —Elders: Review medication history, level of mental acuity, and physical mobility.
  —Use "survivor states" instead of "survivor alleges."

Prevention/Counseling

- Goals for prevention of domestic abuse:
  —Increase social support.
  —Decrease isolation.
  —Decrease burden of parenting and supporting family; encourage family to seek counseling.
- Goals for prevention of elder abuse:
  —Respite care
  —Adult day care
  —Board and care
  —Conservatorships
- Counseling:
  —Express caring concern, e.g., "I do not want you (your child, your parent) to be hurt," "I am concerned for your (their) health and safety."
  —Support survivor's decision to seek help.
  —Be aware of the potential barriers to leaving an abusive situation (e.g., threats from the assailant, fear of poverty, failure of police and others to effectively intervene, hope that the abuse will stop, hope that child abuse will stop, fear of losing custody of the child, relationship can work, etc.).
  —Explore ways to stay safe from future abuse. Provide a referral to self-help agencies.
  —Have legal aid information and telephone number available.
  —If possible, enhance parenting, caretaker, or spousal skills through classes or support groups.

► Abuse: Spousal—Domestic Violence

(See Abuse 2 SI, Call Management for Physical Abuse)

Rules of Thumb
- People who live with violence tend to normalize it. Abuse and denial go together. Be alert for minimization of injuries at all times (especially head injuries).
- All trauma involving women is suspect for possible abuse.
- Look for symptoms and history which are incongruent, "accidents" inconsistent with severity of injury.
- Like ED visits, a high percentage of calls may have a hidden agenda of abuse.
- Abuse crosses all sexual, economic, cultural, and racial lines.
- Pregnancy may either increase or decrease episodes of abuse, depending upon the attitude of the assailant.
- The moment of greatest danger to the survivor may be the moment she/he tries to leave for good.
- About 95% of survivors are female, about 5% are male.

Signs of Physical Spousal Abuse
- Abdomen: Punch injuries (more common in pregnant women).
- Arms: Defensive injuries (mid ulna of arms).
- Back: Whip/cord marks on back.
- Breast: Bite injuries to breast, nipples.
- Eardrum: Rupture from blow to ear/head.
- Face: Bruises, lacerations, abrasions, fractured nose, broken or missing teeth, jaw or orbital fractures.
- Hair: Pulled out.
- Neck: Bruising (from choking); stab/gunshot wound.
- Rape: (See Abuse 1, Call Management for Sexual Abuse)
- Hidden Injuries: Internal injuries w or w/o hemorrhage: Ruptured spleen, liver. Bruising of muscles and bones. Cigarette burns: Genitals, soles of feet, abdomen.

Risk Factors
- In assailant:
  —Learned behavior to use violence as a solution to frustration, fear, anger.
  —Drug/alcohol abuse.
  —History of family violence.
  —Guns in home.
  —Reaction to survivor defiance.
  —Unemployment/homelessness/poverty.
  —Gang activity: May have guns in home.
  —Military service people may be subject to multiple stressors: Frequent geographical moves, lack of control over work hours, separations, dangerous work, masculine culture, downsizing.
  —Abusive language.
  —Anger: Poor impulse control, acts out anger, frustration through violence.
  —Objectifies women as sex objects, "bitches."
  —Controlling behavior: Possessive, jealous; dictates dress, behavior, and with whom survivor may associate.
  —Recent accident, car or other.

- In survivor:
  —The survivor often takes on burden of guilt for assailant's behavior. Believes her/himself to be deserving of abusive behavior.

Red Flag
- Pregnancy is a high risk period for domestic abuse.

▶ Abuse: Elder—Physical, Financial, Emotional, Neglect
[See Abuse 2 SI, Call Management for Physical Abuse]

Rules of Thumb
- People who live with violence tend to normalize it. Abuse and denial go together. Be alert for minimization of injuries at all times (especially head injuries).
- All trauma involving women is suspect for possible abuse.
- Look for symptoms and history which are incongruent, "accidents" inconsistent with severity of injury.
- Like ED visits, a high percentage of calls may have a hidden agenda of abuse.
- Abuse crosses all sexual, economic, cultural, and racial lines.
- The moment of greatest danger to the survivor may be the moment she/he tries to leave for good.
- About 95% of survivors are female, about 5% are male.

Signs of Physical Elder Abuse
- Fractures, dislocations w questionable history.
- Bruises on thigh, trunk, hip.
- Burns.
- Bedsores.
- Vaginal bleeding. (See Abuse 1 SI, Signs and Symptoms of Sexual Abuse)
- "Chemical restraints": Caretaker may overmedicate w prescription drugs, OTC, or ETOH.
- Malnourishment symptoms.
- Failure to thrive.
- Extreme lethargy, barely responsive.
- Symptoms are not explained by previous documented mental status exam.

Risk Factors
- In assailant:
  —Learned behavior to use violence as a solution to frustration, fear, anger
- In survivor: Caregiver burden; isolated family.
  —Alzheimer's (late symptoms)
  —Dementia
  —Frail elderly
  —Incontinent
  —Physical burden

Risk Factors for Financial Abuse

- In assailant:
  - —Veteran
  - —Drug/alcohol abuse
- In survivor:
  - —Dependent is medical/Social Security recipient.
  - —Owns property, has money, pensions.

BACK PROBLEM: UPPER AND LOWER
Pain with or without Trauma

ASSESSMENT	ACUITY LEVEL	DISPOSITION/ADVICE
Key Questions	Emergent Symptom Patterns	ED 0 min-1 hr
Major Trauma	+ W or w/o pain. ± Hx diving/fall, loss of sensation/ ability to move/numbness & tingling, incontinence? (Spinal Trauma)--▶	> Don't move patient
Pain w/o Trauma	+ Sudden onset, generalized, unbearable, radiating from chest or abdomen to back/legs. ± Hx of > BP, + fainting episode? (Aortic Aneurysm)	

Key Questions	Urgent Symptom Patterns	ED/UCC/Office 1-8 hr
Pain w or w/o Trauma	+ Sudden onset, severe, "like toothache," cannot lie down/sleep, unable to stand upright? (Acute Low Back Strain)	
	+ Severe, radiates from buttocks & lower back to leg/unilateral? (Sciatica)	
	+ Pain, sudden/severe/or gradual, ± numbness in lower ext.? (Herniated Disk)	
	+ Persistent? (Vertebral Fracture)	
	+ Urinary retention, incontinence, impotence, < sensation in rectal/perineal area. ± Hx of tumor, stenosis, compression fracture? (Cauda Equina Syndrome)	
Pain w/o Trauma	+ Fever, ± limp? (Osteomyelitis, Discitis)	
	+ Back pain + fever w/o other bone/joint pain, history of IV drug abuse? (Osteomyelitis Epidura/Abscess)	
	+ Sudden, radiating from flank to groin/back, colicky then constant/severe, N/V, ± hematuria? (Kidney Stone)	
	+ Pain (sev.-mod.), radiating from abd./flank/back to groin, colicky then constant & severe, fever/chills, N/V, dysuria, ± hematuria, frequency/urgency? (Pyelonephritis, Prostatitis)	

(continued)

Key Questions	Urgent Symptom Patterns	ED/UCC/Office 1 -8 hr
Pain w/o Trauma (continued)	+ Male: chronic dysuria, urgency/ffequency? (Prostatitis)	
	+ Back/chest/abd./shoulder/arm/neck pain worsened w exertion? (Cardiac)	
	+ Worsening numbness, tingling, weakness in extremities? (Nerve or Spinal Compression)	
	+ Chest pain ± > w resp., fever, ± shaking chills, cough ± productive, difficult breathing, N/V, ± abd. pain, anorexia, fatigue? (Pneumonia: Bacterial, Viral, Aspiration)	
	+ Abd. pain, N/V. Hx ETOH abuse, Hx gallstones? (Pancreatitis)	

Key Questions	Acute/Nonacute Symptom Patterns	FA8 + hr± HomeTx
Pain w or w/o Trauma	+ High-risk patient: > 60 yr, any cancer, esp. breast, prostate; diabetes/immunosuppression/osteoporosis, prolonged steroid use Hx? (Upgrade to Urgent)	
	+ > 50 yr, gradual onset, weakness, fatigue, ± headache, ± fever, ± urinary retention, incontinence. ± Hx of cancer, Hx wt loss? (Neoplastic Disease)	
Pain	+ (Skin) Lesion, linear/painful, follows the path of nerve, unilateral, begins as cluster of bumps, becomes blisters, then dry crust, ± severe itching? (Herpes Zoster/Shingles)	
	+ Recent history of unusual activity—lifting, straining? (Low Back Strain)	
	+ Pregnancy? (See Pregnancy Problem)	
	+ Menstrual cycle? (See Vaginal Bleeding)	
	+ Gradual onset, not related to physical activity. Hx of degenerative arthritis? (Degenerative Arthritis)	
	+ Work-related back injury?	

Cross-References		
Abdomen Problem 1	Pregnancy Problem SI	Skin Problem
Abuse	Respiratory Problem	Urinary Problem

BACK PROBLEM
Supplemental Information

Quick Reference
- ▶ Acute Back Injury Treatment
- ▶ Activity Modification: Acute Phase
- ▶ Chronic Recurrent Back Pain Syndrome
- ▶ Back Pain Tutorial

▶ Acute Back Injury Treatment (See below for Chronic Phase)

- First aid: Use heat or cold on the injured area—*whichever seems to help the most.* Be careful not to burn yourself.
  - —First 48-72 hr: Usually cold feels best for acute injuries. Put ice pack on area x 20-40 min q 2 hr x 48-72 hr. (See Home Tx SI, Appendix A: Ice Pack)
  - —After 72 hr: Alternate ice pack and hot pack x 20 min q 2 hr x 48 hr. (See Home Tx SI, Appendix A: Hot Pack; Ice Pack) Do not leave heating pad on while sleeping. It can cause a serious burn.
- Back pain treatment goal: To relieve pain, restore function.
  - —Pain: Ibuprofen (Motrin, aspirin, etc.) q 4 hr (unless history of allergy, pregnant, ulcers, asthma, bleeding disorder, taking anticoagulants, or NSAIDs). Medication will only reduce pain, not cause healing.
  - —Take medications w small meal to prevent stomach upset or irritation.
  - —Stop medications and call MD if food with medications does not help.
  - —Avoid alcohol.
  - —Avoid strenuous activity. Return to your normal routines and activities as soon as you are able.
- Back pain treatment: This is a way to help reduce tension, muscle spasms, or pain.
  - —For this exercise, you will be lying on the floor on a thick towel or rug.
  - —You will lie on your back with your lower legs resting on the seat of a chair or sofa.
  - —Make the room temperature comfortable so you don't get cold during the exercise.
  - —Keep a blanket nearby to use in case you get cold.
  - —You will need a firm pillow and bath towel.
  - —Fanfold the towel about 3-4 in wide so it is 1/2 to 1 in thick, whatever feels best.
  - —Try out the towel by placing it in the small of your back.
  - —Some people feel better without the lumbar pad, so try again in a few weeks as needed.
  - —When it feels comfortable, put tapes around it and slip it into a pillowcase, so it is ready every time.
  - —Lie on carpeted floor with lower legs bent over the seat of a chair or couch.
  - —Put folded towel in small of back before lying down and put pillow behind head.
  - —Rest quietly for 5-10 min or read. You may do this exercise as often as you like, *with or without the towel.*

▶ Activity Modification: Acute Phase

- Rest as much as possible for the first three days. Do not stay in bed all day. It helps to walk around for a brief period every day.

- Adult Protocols

  - No unsupported sitting > 20 min.
  - Do not do any heavy lifting or bending and twisting while lifting.
  - Don't do anything that causes the pain. Do not drive, if possible.
  - Relax as much as possible. Tension makes the problem worse.
  - Take a warm shower or bath; drink warm tea. Do whatever helps you to relax.
  - Gentle but firm massage will relax the muscles and will help to get rid of the soreness.
  - Homemade Ice Pack:
    —In large Ziploc bag, put three cups water and one cup rubbing alcohol. Place in freezer until it has a mushy consistency. Wrap in thin cloth (dishtowel, pillowcase) before using. Put two or three in freezer, so you can rotate them.
  - Towel Compress:
    —In a large Ziploc bag, neatly fold a small wet, cold towel. Place it behind your back as you lie on back in relaxation position. (See earlier.)

▶ Chronic Recurrent Back Pain Syndrome (See above for Acute Phase)
  - Definition: A vicious cycle in which injury causes muscle spasm; spasm causes pain; and pain causes more spasm. Pain usually lasts 48-72 hr followed by days or weeks of less severe pain.
  - Cause: Injury; poor posture.
  - Complication. 50%-70% of patients will have a recurrence within 1 yr.
  - Prevention:
    —Don't do anything that causes pain.
    —Always bend knees when lifting.
  - Taking care of your back:
    —Driving: Put a rolled-up towel or pillow behind the small of your back. Stop hourly and walk for 5 min.
    —Exercise: Bed rest is helpful when you first hurt your back. However, avoid spending the day in bed. It is important not to get out of shape when your back flares up. Gentle exercise is now recommended when people have back injuries. Exercise helps you feel better physically and emotionally. It increases the chemicals in your brain that make you feel good.
    —The following exercises are usually safe to do when you have back problems. Start with 5-10 min periods and increase them slowly, 5 min at a time.
      ° Walk daily for 20-30 min
      ° Bicycling (stationary or gentle incline)
      ° Swimming
    —Shoes: Wear low-heeled, comfortable shoes.
    —Sleeping: Sleep on your back with two or three pillows under your knees, or sleep on your side with your knees bent and a pillow between them.
    —Work Station: Be sure that your desk is at the right height for you to work,
      o If you sit for long periods of time, rest one foot on a low stool.
      ° If you stand for long periods of time, rest one foot on a low stool.
      ° Take frequent short breaks. Get up and move around and stretch.
    —Alternative Therapies: It is important to see the doctor to be examined and get an explanation for your back pain. You might also discuss other kinds of therapy, like massage, chiropractic/physical therapy, and exercises to do at home, and possibly acupuncture.

➤ Back Pain Tutorial

Red Flags

- Be suspicious of any patient with back pain and a history of
    - —Cancer
    - —Infection
        - ° Chills, fever
        - ° Unexplained weight loss
        - o Risk factors
        - o Any recent bacterial infection: UTI
        - ° IV drug abuse
        - ° Immune suppression (Steroids, Transplant, HIV)
    - —Trauma
        - ° All major: MVA, fall > 6 ft
        - ° Minor: Age > 50 or < 20
    - —Pain, unusual
        - ° Worse when supine, at night
        - ° Unusually severe postoperative pain
        - ₒ Bilateral sciatica in any patient > 50 yr

Rules of Thumb

- Nontraumatic back pain associated with fainting (or near fainting) in patients > 50 yr is considered to be a dissecting aortic aneurysm until proven otherwise (Clawson and Dernocoeur 1998).
- Postoperative pain unrelieved by prescribed medications should be evaluated further.
- Failure to respond to treatment: Needs follow-up appointment.

Red Herrings

- Beware of other medical illness simulating acute back problem.
- Postoperative pain may be a symptom of postoperative complications.
- Patients who have been "seen recently" may still need to be seen today.

Assessment Tips

- Get a good history. Always determine if the symptoms preceded the trauma, or vice versa. It makes a difference in how the problem is triaged.
- Assessing Pain Severity: Always ask about the effect of the pain on sleep, appetite, energy, work/school/activity, mobility, relationships, mood.

BOWEL PROBLEM 1
Diarrhea; Incontinence; Bloody Stools

ASSESSMENT	ACUITY LEVEL	DISPOSITION/ADVICE
Key Questions	Emergent Symptom Patterns	ED 0 min-1 hr
Diarrhea (Severe)	+ Fever, N/V, sev. intractable diarrhea, rash, muscle aches, headache, confusion, dizziness, fainting? (Sepsis Syndrome)	
Black/Bloody Stools	+ ± Sx of shock? (Internal Bleeding/Meckel Diverticulum)	
	+ Black/bloody or tarry BMs (large amt.), weakness, fainting, pale, shock symptoms? (GI bleeding)	
Diarrhea	+ Severe abdomen pain, sudden or gradual onset of pain, guarding, ± fever/vomiting, confused, altered level of consciousness, weakness, dizziness (Acute Abdomen with Systemic Symptoms)	

Key Questions	Urgent Symptom Patterns	ED/UCC/Office 1-8 hr
Bloody Stool	+ ± Abdominal pain, w/o shock Sx, NOT elderly (Lower GI Bleed)	
Diarrhea (Severe-Mod.)	+ Listless, dizziness, no urine output x 8 hr, dry mouth, sunken eyes, frail elderly, bedridden? (Dehydration)	
Diarrhea	+ Abd. pain (severe), colicky, vomiting, abd. distention, Hx of major change in bowel habits? (Bowel Obstruction)	
	+ Watery stools ± blood/mucus/pus, alternating w normal stools, crampy abd. pain; N/V, fever, recent (x 1-2 yr) immigration. Hx of foreign travel, exposure to contaminated water, undercooked meat/seafood/poultry/improperly stored food? (Infectious Diarrhea, Food Poisoning)	
	+ Hx antibiotics? *(Clostridium Difficile)*	

Key Questions	Acute/Nonacute Symptom Patterns	FA 8 + hr ± Home Tx
Diarrhea	+ Weight loss, chronic blood/pus in stool. ± Hx Crohn/ulcerative colitis? (Inflammatory Bowel Disease)	
	+ W/o dehydration. Sx: crampy abd. pain, N/V, ± fever, ± joint pain, ± headache? (Gastroenteritis)	
	+ On antibiotics/antacids, laxatives? (Drug Side Effects) (See Bowel Problem SI)	
	+ Alternating w constipation, mucus, pain, bloating, all ages/esp. young adult? (Irritable Bowel Syndrome)	
	+ Chronic diarrhea + Hx of HIV? (> Risk)	
	+ Related to milk products? (Lactose Intolerance)	
Large, Oily, Foul BMs	+ Hx of bowel surgery/pancreatitis? (Malabsorption Syndrome)	

Cross-References		
Abdomen Problem 1; 2	Dehydration Assessment	Rectal Problem
Bowel Problem 2	Fever	Vomiting/Nausea

BOWEL PROBLEM 2
Constipation; Stool Color Change

ASSESSMENT	ACUITY LEVEL	DISPOSITION/ADVICE
Key Questions	Emergent Symptom Patterns	ED 0 min-1 hr
Color Change	+ Black/bloody/maroon, tarry stools (large amt.), w weakness, fainting, pale? (GI Bleeding)	
Key Questions	Urgent Symptom Patterns	ED/UCC/Office 1-8 hr
Constipation	+ Abd. pain, colicky, elderly, abd. distention. Hx severe constipation, ± abd. surgery, not passing gas? (Bowel Obstruction/Tumor)	
Key Questions	Acute/Nonacute Symptom Patterns	FA 8+ Hr ± Home Tx
Color Change	+ Fever, N/V, anorexia, yellow skin, yellow sclera, itching, fatigue, swollen glands, clay-colored stools, dark urine, ± exp. to hepatitis? (Hepatitis)	
	+ Food related? (See SI)	
	+ Med. related? (See SI)	
Constipation	+ Hx spinal cord injury? (Autonomic Hyperreflexia)	
	+ Dry, hard stools w varying frequency to "ribbon-like," w or w/o abd. pain. Hx < mobility, bed rest or < fluid intake, elderly or immobilized? (Impaction)	
	+ Post-BE or proctoscopy? (Complication)	
	+ Alternating w diarrhea, mucus, abd. pain, bloating, all ages/esp. young adult? (Irritable Bowel Syndrome)	
	+ Hx of hemorrhoid/fissure? (Hemorrhoid/Fissure) (See Rectal Problem)	
	+ Hx high carbohydrate, low fiber diet, < exercise? (Diet-Induced)	
	+ Overuse of laxatives? (Drug Effect)	

Cross-References
Abdomen Problem

Bowel Problem 1		Hepatitis	Rectal Problem

BOWEL PROBLEM
Supplemental Information

Quick Reference	▶ BM Color Change
	▶ Constipation
	▶ Dehydration
	▶ Diarrhea
	▶ Drug Side Effect (Constipation)
	▶ Drug Side Effect (Diarrhea)
	▶ HIV or AIDS Patients w Diarrhea
	▶ Infectious Diarrhea (Food Poisoning)
	▶ Lactose Intolerance

See also: Directory of Hotlines/Web Sites for Support Groups, Appendix E

▶ BM Color Change
- Food effect: Foods and juices that may cause BM color change: Red—Grape juice, beets, tomatoes. Black—Licorice, spinach. Red and Green—Jello: red and green.
- Disease effect
  —Hepatitis (clay-colored stools)
- Drug effect
  —ASA (black)
  —Antacids (yellow/white)
  —Iron Supplements (black stools)
  —Pepto Bismol (black stools)

▶ Constipation
- Definition: Hard, dry BMs that are hard to pass
- Causes: Lack of fiber in diet (raw fruit and vegetables). Not drinking enough water. Not doing enough exercise. Sometimes travel and stress cause constipation.
- Complication: Bowels get clogged and stretched.
- Prevention/Tx
  —More fiber in diet. Eat raw fruits, vegetables, cereals 3 x day. (Fruit: Prunes, dates, raisins, all fruits w skin. Veg.: Lettuce, all veg. raw. Cereals: Bran flakes, muffins, whole wheat bread, shredded wheat.)
  —Drink 8 glasses of water or juice daily.
  —Prune juice w 7-Up (half of each)
  —Don't intake milk, ice cream, cheese, yogurt—makes constipation worse.
  —Don't take too many laxatives. This can make constipation worse.
  —> Exercise. Walk 3 x wk.
  —Cardiac history patients should not bear down for BM. (Vasovagal reflex = > Risk fainting)
  —Fleet enema

► **Dehydration**
- Definition: Not enough water in body. May be very serious in frail elderly.
- Signs and symptoms: Scant, dark urine, dizziness, weak, dry lips/tongue, great thirst, nausea, exhaustion.
  —Loss of skin turgor: Pinch skin on forearm—should snap back in place quickly.
- Complications: Loss or imbalance of minerals in the circulatory system.
- Prevention/Tx: Drink 6-8 glasses/day of clear liquids or oral dehydration solution. (See Home Tx SI, Appendix A: Clear Liquids)

► **Diarrhea**
- Definitions: Bowel movements that are frequent, watery, hard to control, or that cause abdominal pain
- Causes: Infection, inflammation, or irritation of bowel. Usually caused by bacteria, virus, or parasite.
- Complication: Dehydration
- Prevention: Diarrhea can be made worse or will last longer if you eat the wrong foods. Cook and refrigerate foods well. Wash your hands to prevent spread of infection. Don't drink any water that is not clean. (See Home Tx SI, Appendix A: Clear Liquids, Soft Diet)
- Diarrhea Tx Goal: Rest the bowels. Stop diarrhea. Prevent dehydration.
  —Drink 8 or more glasses of water daily.
  —Clear liquids x 24 hr (See Home Tx SI, Appendix A: Clear Liquids)
  —"BRAT" diet (See Home Tx SI, Appendix A: "BRAT" Diet)
  —No coffee, sodas w caffeine (e.g., Coke), ETOH.
  —No milk, cheese, yogurt, or ice cream x 3 days.
  —OTC Kaopectate, Imodium.
  —Rest as much as possible.
  —Watch for signs and Sx of dehydration. (Review)
- Additional teaching
  —Mild diarrhea w vomiting can result from excess alcohol or food.
  —Restaurant workers should not return to work until diarrhea is gone.
  —Antibiotics can cause mild diarrhea. You don't need to stop taking them, unless diarrhea is more than every 3 hr. Eat yogurt w active cultures to help soothe bowels.

► **Drug Side Effect: Constipation**
- Drugs that may cause constipation:
  —Antacids w aluminum (also yellow/white stools)
  —Antihistamines
  —Diphenhydramine (Benadryl, Nytol, Sominex, Sleep-Eze)
  —Calcium
  —Carafate (Sucralfate)
  —Codeine
  —Cough mixtures
  —Morphine and other opiates
  —Verapamil (Isoptin)
  —Vitamins or supplements w iron (also black stools)

► Drug Side Effect: Diarrhea

- May still occur 1-10 days after antibiotic Rx. Most common drugs and classes of drugs that may cause diarrhea:

  —Antibiotics (all)

  —Ampicillin

  —Antacids, magnesium based

  —Erythromycin

  —Tetracyclines

► HIV or AIDS Patients w Diarrhea

- Rule of Thumb: Patients w HIV or AIDS often have chronic diarrhea (any amount). Always watch for dehydration.
- Causes: HIV virus, secondary infection (1 or more germs).
- Complications: Dehydration, weight loss
- Tx: Imodium. If no improvement in 1 day, see MD.

► Infectious Diarrhea (Food Poisoning)

- Signs and symptoms: See Protocol.
- Cause: Bacteria, toxins, parasites in food, water, stool.
- Complications: Dehydration; weight loss. (See Dehydration above)
- Prevention:

  —Wash hands before eating.

  —Avoid contaminated water, raw or uncooked seafood.

  —Eat only well-cooked foods.

- Tx: Medications prescribed by MD.

► Lactose intolerance

- Rule of Thumb: All milk products can cause diarrhea.
- Definition: Inability to digest milk, cheese, etc.
- Causes: Some People are not able to digest milk products.
- Complications: Diarrhea, weight loss, poor nutrition.
- Prevention: Avoid milk products—use products w added lactase (e.g., milk w acidophilus). You may take over the counter medications that help you digest milk products. Follow the directions on the bottle.

CHEST PAIN
Pressure/Pain; with or without Trauma

ASSESSMENT	ACUITY LEVEL	DISPOSITION/ADVICE
Key Questions	Emergent Symptom Patterns	ED 0 min-1 hr
Major Trauma	+ Weak, dizzy, cold/mottled/or pale skin, blue lips/nail beds, rapid/shallow breathing, unresponsive, loss of consciousness? (Cardiac Tamponade, Shock) (See Shock)	
	+ Sudden, sharp chest pain, dyspnea, dry hacking cough, cyanosis, Child: history of cystic fibrosis, asthma? (Pneumothorax)	
	+ Penetrating object*-- - - - ▶	Do not remove impaled object
Pain w/o Trauma	+ Pain/discomfort originating from substernal/ epigastric area, radiates to back/neck/jaw/arm/shoulder (left/right/both), and described as dull ache, pressure, heaviness, fullness, tightness, squeezing, crushing, burning, aching, arm heaviness or chest discomfort ± exertion. Associated Sx: SOB, sweating, pale, lightheaded, dizzy, unexplained indigestion, belching or heartburn, N/V, anxious, restless, sense of impending doom, nx or illicit cirug usct (MI/Angina;----------------▪▶	Chew ur pieK-c ullv.ll.ı ıuııguc adult 1 tablet (325 mg) or 4 baby ASA if no history of aneurysm, ulcer, abd. pain, black or bloody stools, or other bleeding disorder
	+ SOB/fast breathing/cough/wheezing, sob at rest/ exertion, pain with inspiration, anxious, restless, sweating, faintness, calf or thigh pain/swelling, wheezing. Hx of surgery/postpartum/BCP/phlebitis/ immobilization, or Hx > 4 hr air/car travel? (Pulmonary Embolus)	
	+ Generalized, unbearable between shoulder blades, sudden onset, radiates to back/legs, fainting, sweating, restlessness	
	+ Tearing/ripping pain in back/flank/abdomen. Older Male + > BP + smoking Hx. Young Adult with Marfanoid appearance, pregnancy w Hx Marfan syndrome, family Hx aortic aneurysm? (Aortic Aneurysm)	
	+ Hx of sickle cell disease, spider bite? (Sickle Cell Crisis, Black Widow Bite)	

Key Questions	Urgent Symptom Patterns	ED/UCC/Office 1 -8 hr
Trauma	+ Suspicious history? (Abuse) (Possible Abuse)	
	+ Any chest pain w trauma? (> Risk Complications)--*-Come to ED Now!	
Pain w/o Trauma	+ Any back/shoulder/neck/jaw/arm/shoulder pain w/o pain between shoulder blades, worsened w extension? (Cardiac)----------------------------------- - - -*-Chew or place under tongue	adult 1 tablet (325 mg) or 4 baby ASA if no history of aneurysm, ulcer, abd. pain, black or bloody stools, or other bleeding disorder
	+ Substernal, worse w eating or lying down, + vomiting, fullness after eating, regurgitation. Relieved by antacids? (Esophagitis, Hiatal Hernia, GE Reflux, Esophageal Spasm)	
	+ Burning, tightness relieved by antacids? (Esophagitis)	
	+ Dull/sev., > w cold drink or alcohol? (Esophageal Spasm)	
	+ (Sev.) Crushing, sharp, SOB, > resp. Hx of sickle cell disease? (Sickle Cell Crisis)	
	+ SOB, anxiety. ± Hx of cardiac disease? (> Risk Cardiac Complications)	
	+ Hx of chronic cough, FB aspiration? (Foreign Body)	
	+ Sudden or gradual SOB, chest tightness, wheezing, coughing, retractions, nasal flaring? (Asthma)	
	+ Cough, SOB, respiratory chest pain, fever/chills? (Pleuritis: Bacterial, Viral, Fungal)	
	+ Chest/abd. pain, ± > w resp., fever, ± shaking chills, cough ± productive, difficult breathing, N/V, ± abd. pain, anorexia, fatigue? (Pneumonia: Bacterial; Viral, Aspiration)	
	+ Feeling of unreality, fear of going crazy/dying/being out of control, distorted perceptions, irrational fear, SOB, gasping, palpitations, dizzy, > respiration (rapid, shallow), chest pressure, choking sensation, lump in throat, numbness, tingling: face/ fingertips/toes? (Hyperventilation Syndrome, Severe Anxiety) (See Emotional Problem 2)	

(continued)

Key Questions	Urgent Symptom Patterns	ED/UCC/Office 1-8 hr
Pain w/o Trauma (continued)	+ Sharp/dull, ± radiates to neck or shoulder, > w inspiration movement/cough, repeat viral infection? (Pericarditis)----------------------------------	→SA: Pain < by sitting up & leaning forward? (Yes = +)
	+ Dull, steady, worse w movement, age > 50 or diabetic? (> Risk due to prev. history)	
	+ Sharp, intermittent, worse w breathing/movement? ѴѴ^obiocnonåriubChest ѴѴdíf oyñiirumej -------	→ SA: Press on painful area (> Pain = +)

Cross-References		
	Emotional Problem 2	Respiratory Problem

CHEST PAIN
Supplemental Information

Quick Reference	► Acute Myocardial Infarction
	► Costochondritis
	► Marfan Syndrome
	► Tutorial: Telephone Triage of Cardiovascular Patients

See also: Directory of Hotlines/Web Sites for Support Groups, Appendix E

► **Acute Myocardial Infarction (AMI)**
- Coronary heart disease is the No. 1 cause of death in the United States.
- Acute myocardial infarction pain is chest pain that lasts more than a few minutes, or that goes away and comes back.
- Signs and symptoms: See Protocol.
  —Acute myocardial infarction pain duration varies > 15 min to hr(s).
- Cause: A heart attack occurs in people with heart disease when the heart muscle doesn't get enough blood and oxygen because there is a block in a blood vessel.
- Complications: Heart muscle may be seriously damaged, the heart can stop beating, leading to death. Severe damage to heart muscle can lead to heart failure.
- Prevention/Treatment:
  —Seek prompt medical attention if you have *any* symptoms of chest pain to find out the cause of it.

► **Costochondritis (Age: Teen 30 yr)**
  ® Signs and symptoms: See Protocol.
- Causes: A virus can cause irritation and pain in the muscles of the rib cage.
- Complications: None.
- Treatment goal: Prevent pain/complications.
  —Pain: ASA, Tylenol, Motrin.
  —Heat, rest. Don't do anything that hurts.
  —If symptoms persist or >, call for appt.

► **Marfan Syndrome**
  Tall with long, thin arms and legs and spider-like fingers. When they stretch out their arms, the length of their arms is significantly greater than their height.

► **Tutorial: Telephone Triage of Cardiovascular Patients**
  Red Flags
- Cardiac disease risk factors:
  —Smoking
  —Hypertension

—High cholesterol

—Previous heart disease

—Diabetes

—Family history of:

° Heart disease

° Stroke

° Diabetes

- Other risk factors:

—Age/sex

° Males > 45 yrs

° Females > 55 yrs

—Congestive heart failure history

—Obesity

—Physical inactivity

—Stress

- *Smokers* have 2-3 times the risk of dying from coronary heart disease and double their risk for stroke.
- *Hypertension* includes anyone with a BP > 140/90 or who is on BP meds.
- *Abnormal cholesterol* increases the risk for heart disease.
- *Diabetes:* Diabetes is a risk factor for coronary heart disease; people with diabetes have the same risk for a heart attack as someone who already has CHD.
- Heart disease death rates 2 to 4 times higher in diabetics than those without diabetes

® *Family history of premature CHD:* First-degree relative male: < 55 yr, Female, 65 yr.

Triggers: Four "F's" of Chest Pain

- Exercise/exertion
- Emotional stress
- Excessive eating
- Extremes of weather: Cold or heat

Rest, with exercise/exertion; increased stress, cold weather or combination, or after a heavy meal. History of previous MI/angina/recent procedure (stent, CABG), history of illicit drug use-—cocaine and methamphetamine.

Rules of Thumb

- Treatment delayed is treatment denied.
- Patients with suspected acute coronary syndrome with chest discomfort or other symptoms *at rest for greater than 20 min, or recent syncope or presyncope* should come to ED immediately.
- Women may present with typical symptoms, but are more likely than men to experience shortness of breath, nausea/vomiting, and back or jaw pain.
- Diabetic patients may have atypical presentations due to autonomic dysfunction.
- Elderly patients may have atypical symptoms such as generalized weakness, stroke, syncope, or a change in mental status.
- Time is muscle. Outcome is significantly improved if care can be accessed within the first hour.
- Trauma: All chest trauma is considered urgent until proven differently.
- A little chest pain may be as bad as a lot (Clawson and Dernocoeur 1998).

- All pain between nose and navel should be regarded as chest pain until proven differently (Bartlett, 1998).
- Any chest pain in high-risk caller (see Red Flags) should be treated as myocardial infarction until proven otherwise.
- Beware atypical or novel presentations (see Soft Symptoms)
- Acute MI symptoms in older people, women, and people with diabetes may be vague, silent, or atypical.
- Age > 70 yr. Patients over 70 may not have chest pain, or present atypically.
- Minority callers often fail to recognize acute MI symptoms, report fewer symptoms, or attribute them to other causes.
- Beware of any pain that awakens patients or keeps them awake at night.
- Smokers who have acute MI are more likely to die and die suddenly (within the hour).

Red Herrings

- Remain vigilant to possible patient denial, minimization, and misinterpretation.
- Regard with suspicion: all elderly callers and unusual sounding presentations, including symptoms that are described as "the flu," or are new, sudden, or unexpected.
- Patients who have been "seen recently" may still need to be seen today.
- Don't be misled by concurrent musculoskeletal, epigastric complaints or patient self-explanation.

Assessment Tips

- Regard with suspicion: all recent trauma, childbirth, surgery, amphetamine or cocaine use, and history of blood clotting problems.
- Prodromal angina or acute myocardial infarction (soft symptoms).
- Reminder: 20% of all people with acute myocardial infarction have *no chest pain*.
  —Weakness
  —Sweating
  —Nausea
  —Dizziness
  —Shortness of breath
  —Palpitations

Angina Pectoris

Angina pectoris (or *angina)* is chest pain or discomfort that usually happens upon exertion. Angina may happen during exercise, strong emotions, or extreme temperatures. Some people, such as those who experience coronary artery spasm, may have angina when they're resting. Angina is a sign that someone is at increased risk of heart attack, cardiac arrest, and sudden cardiac death.

Stable angina (or chronic stable angina) is chest pain that is usually predictable. It happens on exertion (such as running to catch a bus) or under mental or emotional stress. *Normally the chest discomfort is relieved with rest, nitroglycerin, or both. See NTG cautions.*

Unstable angina is the chest pain that is unexpected and usually occurs while at rest. The discomfort maybe worse or last longer than typical angina or be the first time a person has angina. Unstable angina should be treated as an emergency. People with new, worsening or persistent chest discomfort should go to the hospital emergency department immediately. They're at increased risk for heart attack, severe cardiac arrhythmias, or cardiac arrest leading to sudden death.

Nitroglycerin

PLEASE NOTE: *Pt. may take NTG if available, but do not delay going to ED or calling 911. Do not take NTG if you recently took medications for erectile dysfunction (Viagra, Cialis, or others.). Check with MD or come to ED.*

Nitroglycerin (NTG) is the most common drug for angina. It causes blood vessels to relax. This causes the blood flow to improve, and gets oxygen and nutrients to the heart muscle. By relaxing the veins, it eases the heart's workload.

Nitroglycerin instructions:

- If a patient has been prescribed NTG, they should:

    —Take 1 NTG dose sublingually promptly for chest discomfort/pain.

- If symptoms are unimproved or worsen 5 min after taking 1 NTG dose:

    —The patient should call 911 immediately to access EMS.

- While awaiting ambulance arrival, if the patient tolerates NTG the patient may:

    —Take additional NTG every 5 min up to 3 doses.

Red Herring Potential: Self-treatment with prescription medication, including nitrates, and with nonprescription medication (e.g., antacids) has been documented as frequent cause of delay among patients with ACS, including those with a history of MI or angina.

Although the traditional recommendation is for patients to take 1 NTG dose sublingually, 5 min apart, for up to 3 doses before calling for emergency evaluation, this recommendation has been modified to encourage earlier contacting of EMS by patients with symptoms suggestive of ACS.

Implantable Cardioverter Defibrillator (ICD)

An ICD is used to prevent sudden death in patients with known, sustained ventricular tachycardia or fibrillation. The defibrillator detects dangerous heart rhythms and shocks the heart to restore the normal rhythm.

If patients feel a shock from their defibrillator, they should call 911 only if they do not feel well, they are anxious, or they are having repeated shocks—even if they feel well, they should let their cardiologist know their defibrillator was activated.

Pacemakers

Pacemaker or "artificial pacemaker" is a small, battery-operated device that helps the heart beat in a regular rhythm. Some are permanent (internal) and some are temporary (external). A pacemaker uses batteries to send electrical impulses to the heart to help it pump properly. If you have a pacemaker or defibrillator, some devices may interfere with it. *If you are unsure always ask the doctor. See the following list for common sources of interference.*

Home appliances

- CB radios, electric drills, electric blankets, electric shavers, ham radios, heating pads, metal detectors, microwave ovens, TV transmitters, and remote control TV changers, do not damage defibrillators or pacemakers.
- Power-generating equipment, arc welding equipment, and powerful magnets (as in heavy equipment or motors) can harm or damage your defibrillator or pacemaker. Patients who work with or near such equipment should know that their pacemakers might not work properly in those conditions.

Cellphones

- *Currently* cell phones don't seem to affect pacemakers or defibrillators. This may change as technology changes and becomes more powerful.

Medical equipment

- Carry a wallet ID card with you. Always tell healthcare workers that you have a pacemaker or defibrillator, since many diagnostic tests (like an MRI) can damage the pacemaker or defibrillator.

COLD EXPOSURE
Hypothermia; Frostbite

ASSESSMENT	ACUITY LEVEL	DISPOSITION/ADVICE
Key Questions	Emergent Symptom Patterns	ED 0 min-1 hr
Cold Exposure	– ▶	See Hypothermia First Aid.
	+ Progressive picture—shivering, feeling numb, fatigue, sleepiness; Skin: cold, gray/blue/pale, slurred/difficult speech; Activity: slow uncoordinated movements/clumsiness; staggering/uncoordinated gait: generalized blue/gray coloring, slow breathing/pulse, rigid muscles/posture, no shivering, temp. < 35°C or 95°F, coma? (Profound Hypothermia)	+ Handle comatose patient very little or not at all! Hypothermia = > Risk Dysrhythmias.

Key Questions	Urgent Symptom Patterns	ED/UCC/Office 1-8 hr
ⅴ_/0ⅰʹJ .Cxpоsⅼlｉ̇c ̇т rvⅼSｉ̇ｙpuuｉ̇ciｉiｉｕd *rʹｉ̇ｉｏк̇ ⅼaci (Urban Hypothermia) – – – – ▶	(See SI, Frostbite First Aid)	
Factors?		
	+ *Severe Cold Stress: Any* cold and windy weather, esp. extremes, length of exposure; homelessness/social isolation/poverty; inadequate home heating/housing or clothing	
	+ *Age/Gender:* > 65 yr, esp. > 85-yr male	
	+ *Veracity:* Poor historians, nonverbal patients, confusion	
	+ *Emotional/Neurological Problems:* Mental illness, confusion, dementia/Alzheimer's, any memory disorders	
	+ *Debilitation/PMH:* Homelessness, malnutrition/underweight; medical vulnerability: HIV, pneumonia, septicemia, hypothyroidism, hypopituitarism, diabetes, Parkinson, stroke, cardiac problems, impairment of shivering or cold perception	
	+ *Medications:* Overmedication, drug overdose, antianxiety, phenothiazines, tricyclic antidepressants, alcohol, sedatives	

(continued)

Key Questions	Acute/Nonacute Symptom Patterns	FA 8 + hr ± HomeTx
Cold Exposure + Risk Factors? (continued)	+ *Recent Injury, Ingestion, Illness:* Trauma, head injury/CVA, fall in home, sepsis, dehydration, any illness confining mobility	
	+ *Activities Associated with Hypothermia:* Hiking, hunting, homelessness	
Cold Injury (Finger, Toes, Face, Nose, Ears)?	+ Blisters, numbness/tingling, cold, white, waxy appearance, firm/hard to "frozen feeling," swelling of entire extremity? (Deep or Late Cold Injury)--------■▶	See SI, Frostbite First Aid

Key Questions	Acute/Nonacute Symptom Patterns	FA 8 + hr ± Home Tx
Cold Injury (Fingers, Toes, Face, Nose, Ears)?	+ Blanching, < feeling/sensation, skin soft? (Superficial or Early Cold Injury)-----------------------◀▶	(See SI, Frostbite First Aid)

Cross-Reference
Shock

COLD EXPOSURE
Supplemental Information

Quick Reference:
- ► Hypothermia First Aid
- ► Hypothermia Rules of Thumb
- ► Hypothermia

- ► Frostbite First Aid
- ► Frostbite Rules of Thumb
- ► Frostbite

► **Hypothermia First Aid**
- Handle injury as little as possible; cover the victim's head
- Keep warm, dry and protected from wind, cold, rain
- *Carefully* remove wet or constrictive clothing/shoes
- Wrap in warm blankets, sleeping bag
- Cover with plastic sheet/garbage bag to keep heat in
- Give warm fluids only if person is conscious
- Do not massage skin or rub affected area
- Do not give alcohol or caffeine
- Do not break blisters

► **Hypothermia Rules of Thumb**
- Extremes of age add to the risk of hypothermia. Err on the side of caution with adults > 60 yr.
- Extreme cold temperatures may aggravate other medical problems. Don't overlook other possible medical conditions that may be present.
- The longer the cold exposure, the higher the risk for hypothermia; although any patient can develop hypothermia in a very short time.
- Hypothermia can be fatal within several hours.
- Hypothermia may be misinterpreted as drug/alcohol intoxication.
- Profound hypothermia (See Hypothermia below): The heart is extremely sensitive to ventricular fibrillation and standstill. Handle stuporous and comatose patients with extreme caution and care.
- "No one is dead until warm and dead." EMD axiom. Until patient is warmed, to 35°C or 95°F, they may be successfully resuscitated.
- Unlike frostbite, hypothermia can occur at temperatures well above freezing, because of wind and rain.

► **Hypothermia**
- Definitions:
  —Mild hypothermia: Core temperature is 90°-96.8°F (32°-36°C).
  —Profound hypothermia: Core temperature is below 90°F (32°C).
- Signs and Symptoms: (See Protocol)
- Causes: There are two ways hypothermia can happen:
  —In healthy people: Overexposure to cold temperatures due to lack of preparation.
  —When any condition or disease lowers the body temperature, like a near drowning, head or spinal cord injury, sepsis, drug ingestion, shock, or diseases such as hypothyroidism, heart disease, diabetes.
- Complications: Coma, death

► Frostbite First Aid

- Warm soak (temp, tolerable to rescuer's elbow)
- Do not rub or massage area; Do not apply direct heat.
- Raise area on pillows to cut down on swelling
- Pain: Tylenol prn; Check tetanus status

► Frostbite Rules of Thumb

- Initial appearance and sensation may not correlate well with extent of injury. Always consider contributing factors such as temperature, duration of exposure, dampness of environment and/or clothing.
- Do not attempt to rewarm deep frostbite, unless a lengthy transport is anticipated. It may be hazardous and should be performed under controlled conditions.

► Frostbite

- Signs and symptoms: See Protocol.
- Causes: Prolonged exposure to damp, cold temperatures. Other conditions or diseases may also lower the body temperature: drowning, head or spinal cord injury, sepsis, drug ingestion, shock or diseases such as hypothyroidism, heart disease, diabetes.
- Complications: Blister formation, nerve damage, infection, gangrene, amputation of extremities.
- Prevention/treatment:
  —Remove wet clothing.
  —Wear loose-fitting, layered wool or synthetic clothing. Wool retains heat when wet.
  —Wear waterproof outer clothing to protect from wind and rain.
  —Keep your head warm at all times. A lot of heat may be lost from your head. Wear a wool stocking cap.
  —For children, especially infants < 3 mo: In cool weather, they need knit caps because their body's ability to stay warm is not well developed.

CONFUSION
Sudden; Chronic

ASSESSMENT ACUITY LEVEL		DISPOSITION/ADVICE
Key Questions	Emergent Symptom Patterns	ED 0 min-1 hr

Confusion (Sudden + Progressively anxious, weak, dizzy, thirsty, N/V;
Onset) w or w/o Trauma Skin: pale, blotchy/discolored/cool or cold, sweaty;
                         Lips/Nailbed: blue; Pulse: weak/fast; Breathing: rapid/
                         shallow, unresponsive, loss of consciousness? (Shock)
                         (See Shock)

               + Headache, dizziness, N/V?
                  (Carbon Monoxide Poisoning)

               + Drug ingestion: Accidental/purposeful; street drugs/
                  Rx/barbiturates, poisonous plant, toxic chemical,
                  or pesticide? (Toxic Exposure/Ingestion)----------------▶ Contact poison center
Bring plant/poison/
pills/chemical to
ED w you.

               + Headache, sudden/severe, pupil changes, N/V,
                  respiratory changes, stupor, disorientation, slurred
                  speech, blurred/double vision, unsteady gait,
                  confusion, numbness/weakness/tingling in
                  extremities, loss of urine or bowel control, tongue
                  biting, history of BCP/atrial fib/> BP? (CVA,
                  Aneurysm, Lesion, Abscess)

               + Headache ± trauma (sudden/sharp or gradual/dull/
                  throbbing), neck pain/stiffness, resp. changes;
                  progressing: irritable/lethargic/± loss of
                  consciousness; visual changes, weakness, N/V,
                  staggering, slurred speech? (Intracranial Hemorrhage,
                  Lesion, Abscess)

               + Headache, neck pain, photophobia, fever/chills, N/V,
                  ± confusion, restlessness, somnolence, ± history
                  of HIV? (Meningitis, Encephalitis)

               + Fever > 40°C or 104°F? (Delirium)

               + History of head injury? (See Head Problem 1)

               + History of diabetes? (Insulin Reaction, DKA, Coma) -■▶ If conscious, give a glass of
fruit juice, or water with 3 tbsp.
table sugar.

Key Questions	Urgent Symptom Patterns	ED/UCC/Office 1 -8 hr
Confusion (Sudden) (continued)	+ Poor attention span, changing (fluctuating) level of consciousness, overactive, visual hallucinations, impaired judgment? (Delirium)	
	+ Deterioration of thought process, affective response and ability to be in touch w reality? History of psychiatric disorder, failure to take psych, meds.? (Relapse, Noncompliance, Psychosis)------------------- ▶	SA: Hearing voices = + Combative behavior = + Delusions = +
	+ Frail elderly? (Pneumonia, Sepsis, Overmedication, Drug Reaction, Idiosyncratic Reaction to OTC Med., Elder Abuse)--- •▶	Rule of Thumb: In elderly persons, confusion may be the only sign of underlying pneumonia, sepsis, or overmedication
	+ History of trauma (days, months), dizziness, ± N/V, sensitivity to noise/light? (Postconcussive Syndrome)	
	+ History: Recent seizure? (Postictal State)	
	+ History: Renal failure, or hepatic failure? (Encephalopathy)	

Key Questions	Acute/Nonacute Symptom Patterns	FA 8+ hr ± Home Tx
Confusion (Chronic)	+ Any major change from everyday behavior = poss. upgrade?-- -i▶	SA: Does patient know: own name? Caretaker's name? Can patient perform personal care activities?
	+ Slow onset, increases over time, impaired judgment, no underlying disease, sleep/wake cycle disruption, progressive memory loss, HIV history? (Chronic Dementia)	

Cross-References			
Dizziness	Emotional Problem 2 Fainting	Head Problem 2	Seizures

CONFUSION
Supplemental Information

Quick Reference
- ▶ Rules of Thumb
- ▶ Infections Related to Confusion
- ▶ Chronic Conditions
- ▶ Drug Side Effect: (Confusion)

See also: Directory of Hotlines/Web Sites for Support Groups, Appendix E

▶ **Rules of Thumb**
- Adolescent: Always rule out possible accidental or purposeful ingestion or inhalation.
- Severe confusion with agitation is most often caused by accidental or purposeful inhalation or ingestion.
- Elderly: All sudden confusion in frail elderly is urgent.

▶ **Infections Related to Confusion**
- Elderly: Confusion may be the *only* sign of underlying pneumonia, sepsis, other infection.
- Meningitis.
- Herpes encephalitis.
- Cat scratch fever.
- Lyme disease/Rocky Mountain spotted fever.
- Child: Reye syndrome.
- Child: Measles, encephalitis.
- Infant: Sepsis in newborn.

▶ **Chronic Conditions Presenting with Confusion**
- Congestive heart failure (congenital heart disease)
- Endocrine disorders (adrenal/thyroid disease)
- Hypernatremia (severe dehydration secondary to diarrhea/vomiting)
- Diabetes (hypoglycemia, insulin overdose)
- Liver/kidney disease (hepatic/hypertensive/uremic encephalopathy)

▶ **Drug Side Effect: Confusion**
This is not an exhaustive list of substances causing confusion. Most commonly known are:

Prescription/OTC Drugs	Toxins	Illicit Street Drugs
Adrenal steroids	Chemical poisons	Alcohol
Anticonvulsants	CO_2	Amphetamines
Antidepressants	Glue	Cocaine
Antipsychotics	Lead	LSD
Barbiturates	Paint thinner	Marijuana
Insulin overdose	Pesticides	Mescaline
Isoniazid (INH)	Poisonous plants	
Salicylate:	Mushrooms	
• Aspirin		
• Bismuth subsalicylate		
• (Pepto Bismol)		
Tranquilizers		
Tricyclic antidepressants		

DIZZINESS
With or without Trauma

ASSESSMENT ACUITY LEVEL		DISPOSITION/ADVICE
Key Questions	**Emergent Symptom Patterns**	**ED 0 min-1 hr**
Dizziness w or w/o Trauma	+ Trauma, head injury? (See Head Problem 1; SI)	
	+ Headache (sudden/sharp or gradual/dull/throbbing), neck pain/stiffness, resp. changes; Progressing: Irritable/lethargic ± loss of consciousness; visual changes, weakness, N/V, staggering, slurred speech? (Intracranial Hemorrhage)	
	+ Fever, N/V, sev. intractable diarrhea, rash, muscle aches, headache, confusion, dizziness, fainting? (Sepsis Syndrome)	
	+ Double vision; facial numbness, extremity weakness, hemibody lack of coordination? (Brainstem Cerebellar Lesions)	
	+ Hx heat exposure? (See Heat Exposure)	
	+ Hx of accidental exposure/purposeful ingestion: street drugs/Rx, poisonous plant, or inhalation/ingestion of toxic chemical or pesticide? (Toxic Exposure/Ingestion)------------------------------→	Contact poison center; bring substance w you to ED

Unsteady Gait, Staggering + Sudden onset? (Stroke, Mass/Lesion)

Key Questions	**Urgent Symptom Patterns**	**ED/UCC/Office 1-8 hr**
Dizziness w/o Trauma	+ New onset, age > 60, ± chest pain, ± nausea, ± sweating? (Cardiac)	
	+ Confusion, unilateral weakness, difficulty speaking? (TIA)	
	+ Hx of new Rx? (Drug Reaction)	
	+ Sudden onset, N/V, jerky eye movement, ± HxURI, ± hearing loss? (Labyrinthitis, Meniere syndrome, Vestibular Neuronitis)	
	+ Fever, ear pain, irritability, ± N/V, ± HxURI? (Otitis Media w Effusion)	
	+ Acute onset: ± vision change, unilateral weakness, w/o N/V, elderly? (Brainstem Dysfunction)	

(continued)

Key Questions	Acute Nonacute Symptom Patterns	FA 8 + hr ± Home Tx
Dizziness w/o Trauma (continued)	+ Sudden onset, N/V, jerky eye movement ± Hx URI, ± hearing loss? (Labyrinthitis, Vestibular Neuronitis)	
	+ Standing for long period ± w/o moving, ± heat exp.? ("Parade Square Faint," Venous Pooling)	
	+ ± Hx prolonged bed rest? (Venous Pooling)	
	+ (Gradual onset), persistent, ± headache, ± seizures? (Mass/Lesion)	
	+ Hx ototoxic drugs? (See Dizziness; Fainting SI)-------- •▶ Stop med	
	+ Gradual onset: hearing loss, unilateral? (Acoustic Neuroma)	
	+ > w Positional changes (esp. rotation of head), recurrent, short duration? (Benign Positional Vertigo)	
	+ Assoc, w car, plane, boat travel, ± N/V? (Motion Sickness)	

Cross-References		
Confusion	Ear Problem 1; 2 Fainting	Head Problem 2

FAINTING

ASSESSMENT	ACUITY LEVEL	DISPOSITION/ADVICE
Key Questions	Emergent Symptom Patterns	ED 0 min-1 hr
Fainting	Sudden brief loss of consciousness? -.............—............ ■▶	(See Dizziness; Fainting SI, First Aid)
Major Trauma (Listed below are possible causes of fainting)	+ Head injury? (See Head Problem 1; SI)	
Fainting	+ Hx heart disease, chest pain, irregular heartbeat? (Dysrhythmia, Acute Coronary Syndrome, Aortic Dissection)	
	+ Trauma? (Hemorrhage)	
	+ GI bleeding, ruptured ectopic pregnancy? (Hemorrhage)	
	+ Severe N/V, diarrhea Hx diuretics, vasodilators? (Drug Reaction: Dehydration)	
	+ Hx of accidental exposure/purposeful ingestion: street drugs/Rx, poisonous plant, or inhalation/ ingestion of toxic chemical or pesticide? (Toxic Exposure/Ingestion)----------------------------- ▶	Contact poison center; Bring substance w you
	+ Headache ± trauma (sudden/sharp or gradual/ dull/throbbing), neck pain/stiffness, resp. changes. Progressing: irritable/lethargic/± loss of consciousness; visual changes, weakness, N/V, staggering, slurred speech? (CVA/TIA, Intracranial Hemorrhage)	
	+ Chest pain/SOB/cough; anxious, restless, sweating, faintness. Hx BCP/phlebitis/immobilization/calf pain/surgery/postpartum? (Pulmonary Embolus)	
	+ Hunger, pallor, sweating, confusion? (Hypoglycemia) --▶	If conscious, give small amt. of sugar
	+ Thirst, vomiting, flushed skin, > resp., fruity breath, confusion, > urination? (Hyperglycemia)	
	+ Tremors, sweating, headache. Hx DM? (Insulin Reaction)--- ▶	If conscious, give small amt. of sugar

(continued)

Key Questions	Urgent Symptom Patterns	ED/UCC/0ffice/-8 hr
Fainting (continued)	+ Hx sudden pain/fright, preceded by nausea, yawning, weakness, blurred vision? (Vasovagal Syncope)	
	+ Assoc, w cough/urination or bearing down during BM? (Valsalva, < Venous Return)	
	+ Standing for long period w/o moving, ± heat exp.? ("Parade Square Faint," Venous Pooling)	
	+ ± Fix prolonged bed rest? (Venous Pooling)	
	+ Pleat Exposure? (Heat Syncope)	
	+ Palpitations, racing pulse, dizzy, lightheaded, > respiration (rapid, shallow), ± chest pressure, choking sensation, gasping, numbness/tingling in face, fingers, toes (Hyperventilation Syndrome)	
	+ Hx antihypertensive/antidepressant? (Medication Related) (See Dizziness; Fainting SI)	
	+ Pallor, fatigue, dizziness, lightheaded, palpitation? (Anemia)	

Cross-References

Confusion	Dizziness	Vaginal Bleeding
	Seizures	

DIZZINESS; FAINTING
Supplemental Information

Quick Reference ▶ First Aid: Dizziness/Fainting

▶ Drug Side Effect (Dizziness)

▶ Drug Side Effect (Fainting/Hypotension)

▶ Motion Sickness

▶   First Aid: Dizziness/Fainting

- Lay patient flat. Elevate legs higher than heart.
- Loosen tight clothing.
- Remove noxious stimuli.
- Apply cool cloth.
- Do not slap or shake.
- Don't let victim stand up.

▶   Drug Side Effect: Dizziness

Most common drugs and classes of drugs that may cause dizziness:

- Amitriptyline (Elavil)
- Desipramine
- Dilantin (Phenytoin)
- Doxepin
- Ethacrynic acid (Edecrin)
- Imipramine
- Furosemide (Lasix)
- Neomycin
- Nortriptyline
- Protriptyline
- Risperidone (Risperdal)
- Steroids
- Streptomycin

▶   Drug Side Effect: Fainting/Hypotension

Common drugs and classes of drugs related to fainting/hypotension:

- Diltiazem (Cardizem)
- Doxazosin
- Nifedipine
- Prazosin (Minipres)
- Terazosin (Hytrin)
- Vasodilators
- Verapamil (Isoptin)

- Adult Protocols

► Motion Sickness

Patient feels nauseated when traveling in car, plane, boat.

• Prevention/Tx:

—Have patient lie flat.

—Try to limit head movement.

—No reading.

—Open windows, fresh air helps.

—No alcohol or large, rich meals before travel.

—Small sips of water, ice chips, soda.

—Simple foods help settle stomach (e.g., crackers, pasta w/o sauce, rice, cereal).

EAR PROBLEM 1
Pain with Trauma; FB; Hearing Loss; Ringing; Earlobe Trauma

ASSESSMENT	ACUITY LEVEL	DISPOSITION/ADVICE
Key Questions	**Emergent Symptom Patterns**	**ED 0 min-1 hr**
Major Trauma	+ Clear or bloody drainage? (See Head Problem 1)	
Chemical in Ear	- ➤	Contact poison center; Bring substance w you
Hearing Loss (sudden)	+ Pain in back of head or neck, spinning feeling, unsteady gait, feeling off balance or uncoordinated, other neurologic symptoms? (CVA/TIA/Vascular Event)	
Key Questions	**Urgent Symptom Patterns**	**ED/UCC/Office 1 -8 hr**
Trauma	+ Penetrating (Q-tip, pencil), + bloody drainage? (Laceration/Perforation/Ruptured TM)	
	+ Sudden onset hearing loss, failure to respond to voice/noise, behavior change, N/V, dizziness? (Embolism, Hemorrhage, Blood behind Eardrum)	
Trauma/Laceration	+ Earlobe/pinna? - ➤	Apply cool compress; firm pressure
Pain	+ < Hearing, ± discharge, "digging at ear"? (Foreign Body)- ➤ (Poss. Complications/Infection) (Ineffective Rx)	• Do not try to remove object!
Key Questions	**Acute/Nonacute Symptom Patterns**	**FA 8 + hr ± Home Tx**
Pain	+ Following blow or blast of noise? (Ruptured eardrum)	
Hearing Loss (acute onset)	+ Hx Furosemide, Mycins, Quinine, Ethacrynic Acid? (Ototoxic Meds) (See SI).................---..................... ➤	Check w MD to see if pt. should stop meds
Ringing	+ Hx ASA, Quinidine use? (Drug OD) (See SI)............. ➤	Check w MD to see if pt. should stop meds
Hearing Loss (gradual onset)	+ Hx of long exposure to loud noise? (> Risk Hearing Loss)	
	+ Hx of excessive earwax? (Impacted Earwax)	
Cross-References Dizziness	Ear Problem 2	Face/Jaw Problem

EAR PROBLEM 2
Pain without Trauma; Discharge; Congestion; Earlobe Swelling

ASSESSMENT	ACUITY LEVEL	DISPOSITION/ADVICE
Key Questions	Urgent Symptom Patterns	ED/UCC/Office 1-8 hr
Pain	+ Persistent, throbbing, in or behind ear, fever, creamy/profuse discharge, Hx of OM, tenderness, swelling behind ear, < hearing? (Mastoiditis)--------- -•▶	Apply pressure behind ear. Describe results (Exquisite pain = +)
Swollen Earlobe	+ Red w or w/o streaking, tender, hot; ± discharge, often w fever, swollen nodes. Hx of trauma/bite/ local infection, recent ear piercing? (Auricular Cellulitis)	
Key Questions	Acute/Nonacute Symptom Patterns	FA 8 + hr ± Home Tx
Pain Congestion	+ Unilateral, deep, Hx URI, ear feels full? (Otitis Media)	
	+ W discharge, foul odor, Hx of seborrhea, swimmer? (Otitis Externa) (See SI)..»-	SA: Have patient pull on earlobe and describe result (> Pain = +)
	+ W hot/cold foods, chewing? (Dental Abscess)	
	+ Hx URI, deep sea diving, postflight, worse on descent? (Otitic Barotrauma)	
	+ Temporary, due to cold, wind, lack of cover?	
	+ Dizziness, tinnitus, popping, crackling sound while chewing, < hearing, itching, FB sensation, jaw click? (Temporomandibular Joint Syndrome) (See Face/Jaw)	
Cross-References Dizziness	Ear Problem 1	Face/Jaw Problem

EAR PROBLEM
Supplemental Information

Quick Reference:
- ▶ Rule of Thumb
- ▶ General Advice
- *- Drug Side Effect (Hearing Loss and Tinnitus)
- ▶ Ear Infection
- ▶ Ear Pain
- ▶ Earwax Instructions
- ▶ Ringing in Ear (Tinnitus)
- ▶ Sudden Hearing Loss
- ▶ Swimmer's Ear (External Ear Infection)

See also: Directory of Hotlines/Web Sites for Support Groups, Appendix E

▶ **Rule of Thumb**

Pain from other areas such as the jaw or teeth often gets referred to the ear.

▶ **General Advice**
- Never insert anything in ear (may perforate eardrum).
- Wear earplugs when around loud noise.
- Avoid blowing nose too hard.
- Mild earaches may develop in cold weather or wind.
- After swimming, dry ears; turn head to side, and pull earlobe for drainage.
- Have only qualified person pierce ears.

▶ **Drug Side Effect: Hearing Loss and Tinnitus**

Drugs and classes of drugs that may cause tinnitus and hearing loss:
- Antibiotics
  —Gentamicin
  —Neomycin
  —Streptomycin
  —Tobramycin
  —Vancomycin
  —Ethacrynic Acid
- Diuretics (all)
- Quinine
- Salicylates
  —Aspirin
  —Pepto Bismol (bismuth subsalicylate)

▶ **Ear Infection**
- Signs and symptoms: Pain, fever, poor appetite, ear feels full
- Cause: Bacterial or viral
- Complication: Hearing loss
- Prevention/Tx:
  —Follow-up appointment after infection is important.
  —Take all antibiotic pills.

▶ **Ear Pain**
- Ear pain Tx goal: Relieve pain. Relieve congestion.
- Pain.
  —Warm damp compress to ear p.r.n. (See Home Tx SI, Appendix A: Warm Compress)
  —Tylenol
  —Fluids (See Home Tx SI, Appendix A: Increase Fluids)

▶ **Earwax Instructions**
- Earwax instructions are not to be given before being seen and diagnosed (i.e., advice for follow-up visits only).
- For earwax: apply Debrox, or 1:1 mineral oil and H_2O_2—2 gtts in ear 2 x day.
- Do not use ear drops in the following conditions:
  —After ear surgery
  —Drainage
  —Pain
  —Irritation
  —Rash
  —Dizziness
- General instructions for earwax removal:
  —Tilt head to the side. Apply 2 to 3 drops Debrox (or other brand name) into the ear that has wax in it.
  —Keep head tilted to side for a few minutes, or place cotton in ear to keep drops in ear.
  —Put drops in 2 x day. Use them before you come to see MD as directed.
  —Ear drops are sold over the counter.

▶ **Ringing in Ear (Tinnitus)**
- Signs and symptoms: Sensation of "ringing" or buzzing in ear.
- Causes
  —Wax in ear
  —Diminished hearing Sx of elderly (presbycusis)
  —Damage to eardrum
  —Diseases of the inner ear (i.e., otosclerosis, Méni6re disease)
  —Abnormalities of the auditory nerve and its connection within the brain
  —Drug side effect (e.g., aspirin, quinine); one of the first Sx produced by an ototoxic drug

- Complication: Possible hearing loss. Persistent and severe tinnitus can interfere w the ability to perform daily activities. Can prevent pt. from getting sufficient sleep/rest. Can be incapacitating.
- Tx: No Rx. Try to determine underlying cause and treat the cause. If no cause found, some relief may be found by:
  —Background soft music
  —Other masking noise
  —Biofeedback
- Referral: American Tinnitus Association, P.O. Box 5, Portland, OR 97207

► Sudden Hearing Loss

- Rules of Thumb
  —May be caused by viruses of influenza, chickenpox, mononucleosis.
  —Hearing usually returns in 10-14 days.

► Swimmer's Ear (External Ear Infection)

- Signs and symptoms: Itching, pain, swelling, foul smell, drainage
- Cause: Bacteria or fungus, from getting water or other irritant into the canal.
  Irritation from cleaning or scratching canal can start the infection.
- Complication: Severe pain, < hearing. Can lead to further infection (spreading cellulitis).
- Prevention
  —Dry ears completely with hair dryer after swimming.
  —Q-Tip w $^1/_2$ + V_2 vinegar and water into outer ear canal to dry.
  —Keep ears dry/clean.
  —Wear earplugs when swimming.
  —Do not try to clean inside the ear. Ears are "self-cleaning."

EMOTIONAL PROBLEM 1

Behavioral Emergency: Suicide In Progress; Threat; Ideation

ASSESSMENT	ACUITY LEVEL	DISPOSITION/ADVICE
Key Questions	**Emergent Symptom Patterns**	**ED 0 min-1 hr**
Suicide in Progress	+ Any ingestion, regardless of substance; loaded gun; has rope, knife, razors, or other weapon in hand; rigged car for asphyxiation; is poised to jump? (Extreme Risk)..* ▶	(See Suicide SI, Management Instructions, Suicide in Progress)
	+ Characteristics of emergent suicide always include a plan, means, and access to means = Extreme risk	
	+ Remember, teens are more impulsive and may not have a plan	
Key Questions	**Urgent Symptom Patterns**	**ED/UCC/Office 1-8 hr**
Suicidal Threat: Plan Only	+ No means, no prior history; but has developed a plan: suicide note, setting time and place? (Urgent Risk)------------------------------------- »-	(See Suicide SI, Management Instructions, Suicidal Threat)
	+ Multiple risk factors? (Upgrade to Emergent)	
	+ High-risk teen behaviors? (Upgrade to Emergent)	
	+ Peer violence?	
	+ Dangerous driving?	
	+ Unsafe sex?	
Suicidal Ideation (chronic or new)	+ No plan, no means, no prior history, but is thinking about suicide? (Moderate Risk)	
Cross-Reference Abuse		

SUICIDE
Supplemental Information

Quick Reference:
> ► Management Instructions
>> Suicide in Progress
>> Suicidal Threat
>
> ► Lethality Scale
> ► Risk Factors
> ► Suicide Tutorial
> ► Assessment/Management Tips

See also: Directory of Hotlines/Web Sites for Support Groups, Appendix E

Please Note: The recommendations presented below are based on empirical findings in the literature and collective clinical experience. They are meant to be aids and suggestions for evaluating and managing suicidal patients who are at immediate risk. Like all of medicine, these guidelines are evolving as more knowledge is accrued to inform them. The instructions given herein are not intended as a substitute for formal training in suicide intervention. This specialized training is recommended and customarily available through your local Suicide Prevention Agency.

Duty of Care: The nurse's duty of care is to provide ordinary and reasonable care to the patient. In some cases, explicit contracts are not possible, as sometimes happens in outpatient settings, when unexpected emergency telephone calls occur during which the nurse learns that the patient is in need of immediate and urgent attention. The professional undertakes the treatment of the patient and provides "interim first aid."

Call Tracing: Establish a policy and procedure for call tracing. It currently takes an average of 45 min to trace a call, and cell phones may be more difficult to trace. As appropriate, attempt to elicit as much information prior to tracing. See what information the caller gives you.

► Management Instructions

Suicide in Progress

- Goal: Immediate face-to-face contact for 72 hr.
- Remain with caller! Don't hang up/transfer!
- Summon partner (attract attention of colleague without alerting the caller) to trace call as necessary.
- Elicit plan/accessibility
  —What weapon? Where is it now? Loaded?
- Buy time by putting distance between caller and weapon/method.
  —Management Instructions until transport arrives.
- Engage caller. (Elicit, validate, and reflect emotion to establish trust relationship.)
  —Elicit feelings of pain, recent loss, and meaning of loss.
- Negotiate. (Form an "information bank" to identify potential options.)
- Formulate a contract. (Reach a mutual agreement to begin cycle again in future as needed.)

Suicidal Threat

- Management instructions. (Goal: Appointment within 0-8 hr with therapist)
- Elicit plan: How, where, when will suicide take place?

- Elicit risk factors for possible upgrade to emergent.
- Engage caller. (Elicit, validate, and reflect emotion to establish trust relationship.)
- Negotiate. (Form an "information bank" to identify potential options.)
- Formulate a contract. (Reach a mutual agreement to begin cycle again in future as needed.)
- Assess for weapon and plan even if history of multiple threats only.
- Follow Management Instructions above.
- Elicit risk factors for possible upgrade to emergent.
- Appointment within 8 hr w therapist.

► Lethality Scale (Organized by highest to lowest lethality)

Extreme Risk

- The patient has a plan, means, and access to means. This group of callers is at extreme risk because they have "resolved plans and preparation." In other words, they not only have a plan, but also have a means or method in hand and are ready to act—a suicide in progress.

Urgent Risk

- Patient has a plan only, but no means or access to means. This group lacks the means (gun, rope, etc.) but has started to develop a plan. They may have a suicide note, set time, and place. *Remember* that teens are more impulsive and may not have a plan.

Moderate Risk

- No plan or means. This group lacks plan or means, but mentions ideation or alludes to ideation (See Red Flags). This group may include the elderly who have actually made complex plans, but are concealing them (i.e., suicide is a hidden agenda), in which case, once discovered, should be upgraded. It may also include teens, looking for someone to trust before revealing their intent.

► Risk Factors

Situations, objects, or relationships that influence (positively or negatively) the vulnerability of the caller to act in a suicidal manner. There are three types: proximal, distal, and mitigating.

Note: Risk factors listed below must be taken into consideration for possible upgrade of callers.

Proximal Risk

- Proximal risks are short-term or precipitating, recent events. They are usually weighted heavily. The caller is in *acute stress* owing to loss, mental illness, or substance abuse.
- Loss (A caller's loss may be different from the following list and may not be what you might consider a loss.)
  - —Relationship/divorce
  - —Health
  - —Job
  - —Housing/car
  - —Legal problems
  - —Death of pet
  - —Self-image or other
  - —Isolation (essentially loss of friends, family, community) plays a large role in the following:

- ° Transients/homeless/loners
- ° Teens: Gays/lesbians, especially from minority culture and/or younger age who have recently admitted to themselves that they are gay, but who have not "come out" and are therefore very isolated.
- Mental illness (Recent onset or exacerbation, possibly by discontinuing medication):
  —Mood disorders (intolerable pain, when not medically managed)
  - ° Depression
  - ° Bipolar disorders
  - ° Postpartum psychosis up to 3 yr
  —Thought disorders
  - ° Psychosis
  - ° Schizophrenia
  —Anxiety disorders
  - ° Panic disorder
  - ° Obsessive-compulsive disorder
- Substance abuse: Is an indicator of emotional pain, managed by self-medication to suppress depression and anxiety with street drugs, alcohol, and prescription medications.
- Proximal risk factors specific to teens: In general, teens are at higher risk owing to the fact that they:
  —Have less tolerance for emotional pain than adults do.
  —Are sensitive to any negative change in the environment that can trigger suicidal thoughts.
  —Are more difficult to manage by medication, because of their changeable physiological state, i.e., growth and hormonal fluctuations.
  —Have not lived very long, making proximal and distal risks the same. (See below)
- Proximal risk factors specific to both teens and adults
  —Feel isolation or rejection from school or peer group
  —Divorce
  —Sexual abuse
  —Serious illness in family
  —Legal involvement
  —Witnessing violence
  —Failing grades
  —College rejection
  —First sexual experience
  —Inability to refuse sex
  —Mother returning to work
  —Drug/alcohol dependency (self or parent)
- Predisposing or distal risk (adults and teens): These are long-standing or invariable conditions.
  —Prior history of attempt
  - ° Self-destructive modeling pattern created by caller or family member or school peer. They have broken their own taboo, making it easier to do it again.
  —History of chronic controlled or uncontrolled mood/thought/anxiety disorder. (See above)
  —Substance abuse/alcoholism.
  —Posttraumatic stress disorder (combat or violence related).
  —Abuse (physical, sexual, emotional, childhood, or domestic violence).

—Severe illness (life threatening).

—Season: Spring/fall/April/holidays.

—Day: Anniversaries remind them of the pain of loss.

- Mitigating or protective risk factors (adults and teens): If present, reduce risk of suicide. If they are weak or absent, it may increase risk.

—Responsible for, or parent/caretaker of child under age 18

—Religion or belief in God or spiritual system

—Social support system: family, friends, job

—*Any* emotional, financial, social strengths that give life meaning: interests, hobbies, pets

—Positive occasions: celebrations, birthdays, holidays

► Suicide Tutorial

- Identified Suicide Risk and Time Frames: Eve Meyer, Director of San Francisco Suicide Prevention, stresses the importance of focusing on the immediate risk and thinking in terms of "a clock running" the moment the suicidal intent is revealed. The nurse should be thinking, "How much time do I have?" The critical tasks are to establish trust while determining whether the caller is a "one-hour" or "one-day" type of management. The presence of a weapon or other means for carrying out suicide always represents an extreme risk.

- Triage vs. Trust Building: The suicidal call requires exquisite balances of triage and trust building. Triage involves eliciting essential information such as the caller's plan, means, access to that means, and risk factors. Establishing trust is a vital function and involves asking questions, acknowledging or validating emotional pain, but not judging it. This can be accomplished by asking what effect the pain has on a person's life. A balance of information gathering and the forging of a working alliance is key to achieving the goal of immediate observation.

Red Flags

- Suspicious verbalizations: There are two types of verbal alerts: direct and indirect declarations of suicidal intent and ideation. Always ask, "Are you considering suicide?" if you hear indirect Red Flag phrases such as

—"... When I'm gone ..."

—"... Going away.. ."

—"..Be over soon ..."

—"..Better off dead ..."

—"... End it all..."

- Second party caller (friend, relative calls about patient): Second party calls are a serious predictor of lethality. Assess these calls as if for first party, gathering as much information as you can regarding plan, means, and access to means.

- Lethality of means:

—*Always* ask about the presence of guns in the home.

—Gun lethality: 60% of all *suicide deaths* are gun related.

—Suicide via ingestion in age 5-14 is 5 times more common than all forms of meningitis.

—Drug ingestion is most common: 80% of all *suicide attempts* are pill ingestions.

Rules of Thumb

- Risk factors: The higher the number of risk factors (proximal and distal), the greater the need to upgrade.

- Teens: *Any* teenager who is depressed is at risk for suicide! Err on the side of caution—teens are highly impulsive and find emotional pain intolerable.

Red Herrings

- Myths about suicide: Beware of the many myths surrounding suicide. Asking about suicidal intent will not cause the caller to commit suicide or "give the caller ideas." Rather, it is very liberating for the caller to finally be able to speak honestly and openly with a sympathetic person. Conversely, the myth that "those who threaten never carry it out" is also a dangerous misperception.

- ® Elderly: Contrary to some stereotypes, old age can be a high-risk period for depression and suicide. Thus, age by itself carries an implied risk for suicide. No other age group must face so many multiple losses—health, spouse, home, friends, mobility, etc. The elderly often have undiagnosed depression, which masquerades in physical symptoms of no known origin—frequent physical complaints, for which no cause can be found. They often make appointments to see the physician before attempting suicide. In preparing for suicide, the elderly often form elaborate plans; however, they don't reveal them to others. With the elderly, always err on the side of caution and remain suspicious.

► Assessment/Management Tips

- The assessment process described below is not intended to be followed as a step-by-step process. Rather, it contains general directives. Nurses must be sensitive, sophisticated, intuitive, inventive, and resourceful with these calls, striking a balance of triage versus trust building.

Assessment/Management Tips (Action/Goal)	Question/Response (Sample Verbiage)
Remain with Caller Don't hang up or transfer call. Summon partner to trace call. Explore indirect or implied risk:	"I'm glad you called. This has been a terribly painful time. Are you considering suicide?"
Elicit Plan, Means, Accessibility *Find out HOW (plan) before WHY (reasons):* Elicit method and accessibility to find out how much time you have to save the caller and to gain maximum amount of time.	"Have you ever been suicidal? Are you suicidal now? Do you have a weapon? Where is it now? Is it loaded?"
Put distance between caller and weapon: Makes person safer when police arrive. "Suicide by cop" may be a method they are considering. Also reduces the "hypnotic effect" of the weapon. Have them put it where they cannot see it—in another room.	"Could you unload the gun and put it (knife, rope) in another room (close the window and move away from it) just while we are talking? It makes me nervous. It makes it harder to talk to you."
Engage Caller If crying:	"It's okay to cry. I'll wait until you are ready to talk."
Elicit Risk Factors Get as much information as possible: (Information can be a "hook" with which you can begin to forge a contract with the caller.) Focus on ambivalence:	"It sounds like you arc in terrible pain, what happened?" "You are having trouble deciding what to do. It sounds like part of you wants to live and part wants to die."

(continued)

Assessment/Management Tips (Action/Goal)	Question/Response (Sample Verbiage)
Explore emotional pain/recent loss:	"What did losing your job (divorce, losing your partner, health, etc.) mean to you?"
Validate feelings without adding your own: (Restate to check own understanding.) *Resist the impulse to give advice.*	"You were really angry (sad, upset) when ..."
Elicit Mitigating Factors: • Parent/caretaker of child under age 18. • Religion or belief in God or spiritual system. • Social support system: family, friends, job. • *Any* emotional, financial, social strengths that give life meaning: interests, hobbies, pets. • *Any* upcoming happy event: celebrations, birthdays, holidays (things to look forward to).	"Do you have children, family, friends?" "Do you practice a faith?" "Do you have interests, pets?"
Formulate a Contract (Weave mitigating factors into plan.) Reduce helplessness by bolstering control: Use food as protective factor: Elicit dream/faith/belief: (Reduce hopelessness by supporting dream.)	"What has helped in the past?" "When did you last eat?" "What would life be like if you weren't depressed?" "Where were you heading, What was going on before this happened?" "Do you ever pray (go to church, temple)?" "What about your friends/family?"
Elicit support system: (Reduce isolation by encouraging support.) Tips for Contracting: Always remain collaborative: "Personalize" the care. What you will do ...	"Listen, here's what we're going to do ..." "How would it be if you got some crackers and soda while we talk?"
What we/they will do ...	"I want you to come to the ED and see Dr. Jones. I know him. He's a really good doctor. I think you can be helped. That book you mentioned—I have a copy, and I'll send it down to you when you come."
"No Suicide" Pact	"Would you promise me not to harm yourself without calling here first?"
Always end the call with contract that must be verbalized by caller. (It is best if it is in his/her own words.)	

EMOTIONAL PROBLEM 2
Panic; Depression; Anxiety; Agitation; Aggression; Withdrawal; Hallucination

ASSESSMENT	ACUITY LEVEL	DISPOSITION/ADVICE
Key Questions	**Emergent Symptom Patterns**	ED 0 min-1 hr
Suicidal Thoughts, Threats in Progress?	(See Emotional Problem 1)	
Agitation/Aggression	+ Behavior threatening to others, self-destructive, severely disruptive behavior, hostility? (Psychosis)	
Withdrawal	+ Extremely unresponsive? (Catatonic State)	
Hallucinations	+ Confused, speech rambling or incoherent, disoriented? (Psychosis)	
	+ History of drug/alcohol/Rx abuse (recent/past)? (Drug Reaction)	
Key Questions	**Urgent Symptom Patterns**	ED/UCC/Office 1-8 hr
Emotional Problem (all)	+ Carrying weapons, hurting animals, plans to commit violence, marked increase in: violent behavior, risk taking, property damage, loss of temper? (Extreme Violence Risk)----------------------- ▪▶ Come to ED now!	
Anxiety (sudden onset) (4 or more)	+ Feeling of unreality, fear of going crazy/dying/ being out of control, distorted perceptions, irrational fear, SOB, gasping, palpitations, dizzy, > respiration (rapid, shallow), chest pressure, choking sensation, lump in throat, numbness, tingling (face/fingertips/toes)? (Panic Attack)---------- ▶ Come to ED now!	
Depression	+ Nearly all symptoms of depression, almost always keep pt. from doing daily activities? (See Emotional Problem 2 SI)	

Key Questions	Acute/Nonacute Symptom Patterns	FA 8 + hr ± Home Tx
Depression (moderate)	+ Many symptoms of depression, often keeps pt. from doing daily activities? (See SI)	
Anxiety (low-grade)	+ Feeling uncomfortable w/o knowing why; feeling fear, forgetful, confused, irritable, restless; history of recent hospitalization, Chronic illness, loss? (See SI)	
	+ Trouble sleeping, stomach upset, hot/cold, sweating? (Anxiety Disorder)	
Depression (mild)	+ Some symptoms of depression, takes extra effort to do daily activities? (See SI)	

Cross-References

Confusion	Emotional Problem 1	Postpartum Emotional Problem

EMOTIONAL PROBLEM
Supplemental Information

Quick Reference:
- ▶ Bipolar Disorder/Depression
- ▶ Drug Side Effect (Depression)
- ▶ Loss/Grief
- ▶ Obsessive Compulsive Disorder
- ▶ Panic Disorder
- ▶ Schizophrenia
- ▶ Violence Warning Signs

See also: Directory of Hotlines/Web Sites for Support Groups, Appendix E

▶ Bipolar Disorder/Depression

° Definition: Serious mood disorder. Also known as *manic depression.* The person's mood swings from overly "high" to extremely sad and back again. There are normal moods in between. It begins in adolescence or early adulthood. It is often not recognized or treated for many years. It tends to run in families.

Manic Phase

s Signs and symptoms:
- —High energy, restlessness, racing thoughts, rapid talking
- —Extreme feelings of well-being, happiness
- —Extreme irritability and distractibility
- —Needs little sleep
- —Feels extremely powerful
- —Poor judgment
- —Increased sex drive
- —Substance abuse
- —Aggressive behavior
- —Periods of behavior that are different from usual behavior
- —Denial that there is anything wrong

Depression

o Definition: Serious mood disorder. Depression is not just "feeling blue" or "down in the dumps." It is more than being sad or feeling grief after a loss. Depression is a medical disorder (like diabetes, high blood pressure, or heart disease) that day after day affects your thoughts, feelings, physical health, and behaviors.

• Signs and symptoms: Five or more of these symptoms, including at least one of first two, nearly all day every day x 2 wk:
- —Loss of interest in things you used to enjoy, including sex.
- —Feeling sad, blue, or down in the dumps.
- —Feeling slowed down or restless and unable to sit still.

—Feeling worthless or guilty.

—Changes in appetite or weight loss or gain.

—Thoughts of death or suicide; suicide attempts.

—Problems concentrating, thinking, remembering, or making decisions.

—Trouble sleeping or sleeping too much.

—Loss of energy or feeling tired all of the time.

- Severe depression is present when a person has nearly all of the symptoms of depression, and the depression almost always keeps them from doing their regular day-to-day activities (Urgent Level).

- Moderate depression is present when a person has many symptoms of depression that often keep them from doing things that they need to do (Acute Level).

- Mild depression is present when a person has some of the symptoms of depression and it takes extra effort to do the things they need to do. (Nonacute Level).

- Causes:

—Extreme stress or grief may bring out a natural psychological or biological tendency.

—May be inherited tendency.

—Drugs and alcohol abuse can cause depression (e.g., alcohol, codeine, cocaine, and marijuana). (See also Drug Side Effect below)

—Certain medications.

—Other emotional illness.

- Complications: Marital breakup, job loss, substance abuse, and suicide.

- Prevention/Tx: Medication, counseling, support groups. Avoid alcohol and drugs!

Depression Symptoms in Children/Adolescents

(See also Violence Warning Signs)
- Signs and symptoms:

—Absenteeism, truancy

—Anger, hostility, irritability

—Boredom

—Fall in grades

—Isolation, poor communication, difficult relationships

—Lack of interest in playing with friends

—Physical complaints: headaches, stomachaches, fatigue, muscle aches

—Reckless behavior, reckless driving, increases in risk-taking behavior

—Running away from home

—Substance abuse

—Unsafe sex

► Drug Side Effect: Depression

- ACTH
- Amphetamines (withdrawal)
- Anabolic steroids
- Benzodiazepines
- Cimetidine
- Clonidine

- Cocaine (withdrawal)
- Cycloserine
- Digitalis
- Glucocorticoids
- L-dopa
- NS AIDs
- Oral contraceptives
- Propranolol
- Reserpine
- Sulfonamides
- Thiazide diuretics

► Loss/Grief (Esp. death of loved one)

- Definition: Individual's physical and emotional response to loss of a highly valued person, object, or concept.
- Signs and symptoms:
  —Waves of sadness lasting 20-60 min.
  —Deep sighing.
  —Lack of strength.
  —Loss of appetite and sense of taste.
  —Tightness in throat.
  —Choking sensations accompanied by SOB.
  —Mentally preoccupied w death or loss of person/object/concept, or w thoughts of death/loss.
  —Daydreaming; feels like going insane. Feels guilt, anger, shock, and numbness.
- Cause: Emotions trigger physical reactions within the body.
- Complications: Distorted grief reactions.
  —Clinical depression.
  —Extreme hostility.
  —Excessive activity w/o sense of loss.
  —Physical symptoms of deceased person.
- Prevention of complications:
  —Understand grief is normal.
  —Know that denial, anger, bargaining, depression, and acceptance is normal pattern of grief. It can last one to two years.
  —Get counseling: Contact Center for Living & Dying for grief support group.

► Obsessive Compulsive Disorder

- Definition: Obsessive Compulsive Disorder (OCD) is a type of anxiety disorder. It can last throughout a person's life. People who have OCD may have repeated unpleasant or upsetting thoughts, called obsessions. They sometimes perform repetitious actions—like handwashing or checking things. This type of behavior is known as compulsion. These thoughts may be extreme enough to interfere with daily life.
- Signs and symptoms:
  —Repeatedly arranging objects
  —Handwashing

—Mentally repeating phrases

—Thoughts of harming someone

—Recurrent thoughts that the gas was left on, etc.

- Cause: The experts believe that OCD is caused by a chemical imbalance in the brain.

- Complications: Sometimes people with OCD also have depression, substance abuse, or other anxiety disorders.

- Prevention of complications: People with this disorder need medications, therapy, and behavior therapy to help them overcome these actions.

▶ Panic Disorder

- Definition: A *panic attack* is a brief period of intense terror. It may last a few seconds to a few minutes, and usually fades over an hour. Some people with panic attacks have physical symptoms too. Panic attacks can happen often and without warning. If someone has three or more panic attacks within 3 wk without having also extreme physical exertion, life-threatening situations, or phobias, this means they have a panic disorder.

- Signs and symptoms: Initial attack may occur in the following situations:

—Accident history

—Childbirth history

—Illness, serious

—Stress, overworking

—Surgery history

—Linked to excessive use of:

  « Caffeine

  ° Cocaine

  ° Any stimulant

- Ongoing signs and symptoms: Four or more of the following:

—Distorted perceptions, agitation, terror, irrational fear, sense of impending doom

—Feeling of unreality

—Fear of going crazy, dying, or being out of control

—Chest pains

—Palpitations

—Dyspnea

—Choking or smothering feeling

—Vertigo, dizziness, or unsteadiness

—Feelings of faintness

—Tingling in the hands and feet

—Shaking or trembling

—Hot and cold flashes

—Diaphoresis

- Cause: There are several theories about the cause of panic disorder. Panic disorder runs in families. Some experts believe it is caused by brain and biochemical problems.

- Complications: People with panic disorder may be unable to do life's activities and have physical signs of illness.

- Prevention/Tx:

—Psychotherapy

—Cognitive-behavioral therapy

—Medication

—Combination therapies (two of the above)

—Self-help and support groups

► Schizophrenia

- Definition: Schizophrenia is a complex mental disorder. It may involve *psychosis*—having hallucinations.
- Signs and symptoms:

  —Hallucinations: Seeing things that are not there.

  —Delusions: Belief in things that are not rational. For example, someone might believe that people from outer space are controlling their thoughts.

  —Disordered thinking: Inability to think straight or organize thoughts in a normal way.

  —Emotional expression: Inappropriate or severe lack of emotion, an expressionless face.

- Cause: The experts believe that schizophrenia is inherited and caused by genetic factors. There might also be a chemical imbalance in the brain.
- Complications: Schizophrenics are at risk for suicide.
- Prevention of complications: Schizophrenics must take medications to help them live a normal life. They also need psychotherapy and family therapy. Support and self-help groups are helpful as well.

► Violence Warning Signs

(See also Emotional Problem 1, Behavioral Emergency)

Indicators for Extreme Violence Risk

- Carrying weapons
- Hurting animals
- Increased:

  —Physical fighting

  —Substance abuse

  —Risk-taking behavior

  —Loss of temper (daily)

- Plans to commit violence
- Vandalism, property damage

Indicators for Potential Risk for Violence

- Access to, and fascination with weapons, esp. guns
- Bullying or victim of bullying
- Gang membership
- Isolation, feeling rejected/alone
- History of violent/aggressive behavior
- Poor school performance
- Problems with authority figures
- Serious substance abuse

EXTREMITIES PROBLEM 1: UPPER
Pain with or without Trauma; Fractures; Lacerations; Swelling

ASSESSMENT	ACUITY LEVEL	DISPOSITION/ADVICE
Key Questions	Emergent Symptom Patterns	ED 0 min-1 hr
Major Trauma	+ All amputations? (See Shock)----------------------------	Control bleeding: Save body part; wrap in clean cloth (place in plastic bag & place on ice) (See Extremities Problem 4 SI, First Aid)
	+ Weak, dizzy, cold/mottled/pale skin, blue lips/nail beds, rapid/shallow breathing, unresponsive, loss of consciousness? (Shock) (See Shock.)	
	+ Open wound w bone visible? (Open Fracture, > Risk Infection)---	Cover w clean cloth. Keep very still; do not move.
	+ 2 or more Fx? (> Risk Hemorrhage)	
Pain (Arm/Shoulder) w/o Trauma	+ Chest pain: ± exertion (dull ache, pressure, squeezing, crushing, radiates to neck/jaw/arms), SOB, sweating, dizziness, lightheaded, N/V, pale, anxiety, sense of impending doom? (MI/Angina) (See Chest Pain)	
	+ Hx fracture, difficulty breathing, SOB, petechial rash (upper trunk/extremities), high fever, jaundice, confusion? (Fat Embolism)	
Weakness	+ Unilateral, ± leg involvement, ± slurred speech, ± headache, ± unsteady gait, confusion, ± Hx HTN/ DM/smoker/previous CVA? (CVA, Cerebral Hemorrhage)	

Key Questions	Urgent Symptom Patterns	ED/UCC/Office 1-8 hr
Trauma	+ Suspicious history? (Possible Abuse)	
	+ All severe, increasing, uncontrolled pain? (> Risk)	
Swelling/Pain w Trauma	+ Lacerations (all) w severe uncontrolled bleeding, Hx of bleeding disorder, kidney/liver disease, anticoagulants cancer, chemo, radiation? (> Risk Hemorrhage)...	*-Control bleeding (See Extremities Problem 4 SI, First Aid)

(continued)

Key Questions	Urgent Symptom Patterns	ED/UCC/Office 1-8 hr
Swelling/Pain w Trauma (continued)	+ Open fracture/laceration/IV abuser Hx, high fever, swelling, redness, disproportionate pain, area is red, shiny, swollen, exquisitely tender w subcutaneous crepitation? (Necrotizing Fasciitis)	
	+ Swelling, deformity, discoloration, < ROM or refusal to use? (Fracture)--------------------------------- ►	SA: W fingers, gently press along bone to find injury
	+ Pain (sev.), numb, pale skin, Hx of recent trauma/ surgery, cast application, pain unrelieved by ice, evaluation, pain meds? (Cast Problem/Compartment Syndrome)--- ►	SA: Pain > w passive stretching of muscles? (Yes = +).
Swelling/Pain w/o Trauma	+ (Skin) Red ± streaking, swollen, tender, hot; ± discharge, often w fever, swollen nodes, hx of trauma/bite/local infection? (Cellulitis/ Lymphangitis)	
	+ Fever, point tenderness, unilateral, nonuse, hx of recent infection? (Osteomyelitis)	

Key Questions	Acute/Nonacute Symptom Patterns	FA 8 + hr ± Home Tx
Shoulder Pain	+ Hx trauma 6-12 hr prior, sudden onset, deltoid area, arm hanging limp? (Rotator Cuff Tear)	
Wrist Pain	+ Chronic radiates to hand, forearm, > w repetitive motion? (Carpal Tunnel Syndrome)	
Finger Pain	+ Hx trauma, blood under nail, discoloration? (Subungual Hematoma)	
	+ Dull, red, swelling of cuticle, nail fold? (Paronychia)	
Arm Pain	+ Chronic or acute, aggravated by any movement? (Tendonitis)	

Cross-References Extremities Problem 2	Joint Problem	Skin Problem: Laceration/ Wound	Skin Problem: Lesion/Lump/ Swelling

EXTREMITIES PROBLEM 2: LOWER

Pain with and without Trauma; Fractures; Lacerations; Swelling, Weakness, Limp

ASSESSMENT	ACUITY LEVEL	DISPOSITION/ADVICE
Key Questions	Emergent Symptom Patterns	ED 0 min-1 hr
Major Trauma	+ All amputations? (Shock) (See Shock.)----------------- -▶	Control bleeding; save body part; wrap in clean cloth, (place in plastic bag on top of ice); (See Extremities Problem 4 SI, First Aid)
	+ Weak, dizzy, cold/mottled/pale skin, blue lips/ nailbeds, rapid/shallow breathing, unresponsive, loss of consciousness? (Shock) (See Shock)	
	+ Open wound w bone visible? (Compound Fracture, > Risk Infection)----------------- -▶	(See SI, First Aid) Cover w clean cloth. Keep very still; do not move.
	+ 2 or more Fx or all femur Fx? (> Risk Hemorrhage) - - SA:	W fingers, gently press along bone to find injury. (> pain = +) Unable to bear weight? (Yes = +) (See Extremities Problem 4 SI, First Aid)
	+ Hx fracture, difficulty breathing, SOB, petechial rash (upper trunk/extremities), high fever, jaundice, confusion? (Fat Embolism)	
	+ Hip pain, inability to move/bear weight on extremity, distorted/shortened extremities, external rotation of leg? (Hip Fracture)	
Weakness	+ Unilateral, ± leg involvement, ± slurred speech, ± headache, ± unsteady gait, confusion, ± Hx HTN/DM/smoker/previous CVA? (CVA, Cerebral Hemorrhage)	

Key Questions	Urgent Symptom Patterns	ED/UCC/Office 1-8 hr
Pain/Swelling w Trauma	+ All severe, increasing, uncontrolled pain? (> Risk) + (Sev.) pain, numb, pale skin, Hx of recent trauma/ surgery, cast application, pain unrelieved by ice, elevation, pain meds? (Cast Problem/Compartment õyiiuiiuiiicj° -------------------------------▶	SA: > Pain with passive stretching of muscle? (Yes = +)
		(continued)

Key Questions	Urgent Symptom Patterns	ED/UCC/Office 1 -8 hr
Pain/Swelling w Trauma (continued)	+ Lacerations (all) w severe uncontrolled bleeding, Hx bleeding disorder, kidney/liver disease, Hx anticoagulants Hx cancer, chemo, radiation? (> Risk Hemorrhage)------------------------------------	Control bleeding (See Extremities Problem 4 SI, First Aid.)
	+ Pain above heel, sudden onset, assoc, w activity? (Achilles Tendon Rupture)	
	+ (Sudden onset) calf, swelling, unilateral, ± Hx of trauma/sport related? (Ruptured Gastrocnemius)	
	+ Swelling, < ROM, deformity, limp, unable to bear weight, point tenderness, discoloration? (Fracture)	
	+ Hx open ffacture/laceration/IV abuser Hx: high fever, swelling, redness, disproportionate pain, area is red, shiny, swollen, exquisitely tender w subcutaneous crepitation? (Necrotizing Fasciitis)	
Pain w/o Trauma	+ (Gradual onset) numbness, swelling, unilateral calf tenderness/warmth, past Hx deep vein thrombosis, BCP/HRT Hx, postop, postpartum, fracture, prolonged air travel/immobilization? (Ruptured Baker cyst, Deep Vein Thrombosis/ Thrombophlebitis) ---	Do not massage leg! SA: Pain in calf when flexes foot? (Yes = +)
	+ Hx of recent fall/trauma/surgery + large, tender, firm but swollen area over buttocks or muscle Hx cancer, chemo, radiation? (Possible Hematoma)	
Pain w/o Trauma (sudden onset)	+ (Severe) Unilateral, radiating from lower back? (Sciatica)--	SA: Straight leg raise > 60° (> Pain = +)
	+ All postop w fever, pain in calf or incision, foul smelling or puslike wound drainage, swelling, redness, warmth? (Postop Infection)	

Key Questions	Acute/Nonacute Symptom Patterns	FA 8+ hr ± Home Tx
Any Leg Problem	+ Hx diabetes, immunocompromised? (> Risk)	
Dull Ache	+ (Shin area), ± tenderness, hx of exercise? (Shin Splint/Stress Fx)	

Cross-References

Extremities Problem 1	Joint Problem	Postpartum Problem; SI	Skin Problem: Laceration/ Wound

EXTREMITIES PROBLEM 3: LOWER
Pain without Trauma; Swelling; Weakness; Limp

1 ASSESSMENT	ACUITY LEVEL	DISPOSITION/ADVICE
Key Questions	Emergent Symptom Patterns	ED 0 min-1 hr
Pain (± severe)	+ (Sudden onset) sev. pain, coldness, numbness, pale, blue skin? (Arterial Ischemia)	
Weakness	+ Unilateral, ± leg involvement, ± slurred speech, ± headache, ± unsteady gait, confusion, ± Hx HTN/DM/smoker/previous CVA? (CVA, Cerebral Hemorrhage)	
Key Questions	Urgent Symptom Patterns	ED/UCC/Office 1-8 hr
Pain (± severe)	+ All severe, increasing uncontrolled pain? (> Risk)	
	+ Numb, pale skin, Hx of recent trauma/surgery, cast application, pain unrelieved by ice, elevation, pain meds? (Cast Problem/Compartment Syndrome)	
	+ (Sudden onset) unilateral radiating from lower back, numbness, tingling toes/feet? (Sciatica)---------- ■▶	SA: Straight leg raise > 60°? (> Pain = +)
	+ (Sudden onset) sev. pain, coldness, numbness, pale, blue skin? (Arterial Ischemia)	
Limp/Nonuse	+ ± Fever, point tenderness, unilateral, nonuse, Hx of recent infection? (Osteomyelitis)	
Weakness/Staggering/ Difficulty Walking	+ (Legs) progressive, bilateral, < sensation, Hx recent infection, surgery, immz? (Guillain-Barre syndrome)	
	+ Toe walking, fatigues easily, ± muscle thinning? (Neuromuscular Disease)	
	+ ± Pain, ± bowel/bladder changes, numbness, tingling? (Spinal Cord Tumor)	
Swelling (leg)	+ (Skin) Red ± streaking, tender, hot; ± discharge, often w fever, swollen nodes, Hx of trauma/bite/ local infection? (Cellulitis/Lymphangitis)	
	+ (Gradual onset) numbness, swelling, unilateral calf tenderness/warmth, Hx of BCP, recent surgery/Fx/ recent prolonged immobilization? (Ruptured Baker Cyst, Deep Vein Thrombosis/Thrombophlebitis) - - s	▶ Don't massage leg!
Foot Problem (all)	+ Pain, discoloration, laceration, swelling, Hx of immunocompromised, diabetes? (> Risk Infection)	

Key Questions	Acute/Nonacute Symptom Patterns	FA 8+ hr ± Home Tx
Swelling (Ankle)	+ < w elevation, Hx heart failure, cardiac problem? (CHF)...	▶ SA: Press firmly on the bony area of the ankle for 1-2 sec.; describe results. (Severe Pitting = +)
Pain (Big Toe)	+ Sudden, warm, red, tender, male age > 40, female > 50, ± recent trauma? (Gout) (See Joint Problem)	
Numbness (Lower Legs)	+ < Sensation, Hx of DM/HIV/alcoholism? (Peripheral Neuropathy)	
Leg/Calf Pain	+ (Unilateral/bilateral) episodic, aching > w standing, local swelling of surface veins/discoloration? (Varicose Veins)---	▶ SA: Pain relieved by elevation or support hose? (Yes = +) SA: Pain > by standing? (Yes = +)
Leg Pain	+ Cramps, fatigue? (Claudication)--------------------------•■▶	SA: Pain/fatigue > by exercise? (Yes = +) SA: Pain relieved by rest? (Yes = +)
Shin Pain	+ Dull ache, Hx: exercise? (Shin Splints)	
Foot Problem (all)	+ Pain, discoloration, laceration, swelling, Hx of diabetes/immunocompromised? (> Risk Infection)	

Cross-References

Dizziness Extremities Problem 1; 2; 4	Joint Problem	Pregnancy Problem 2; SI	Skin Problem: Laceration/ Wound

EXTREMITIES PROBLEM 4: UPPER AND LOWER
Supplemental Information

Quick Reference:
- ▶ First Aid
  - Pressure Points
  - Fracture
- ▶ Cast Care
- ▶ Compartment Syndrome
- ▶ Fat Embolism
- ▶ Fracture
- ▶ Hematoma (Bruise)
- ▶ Ice and Heat Therapy for Injuries
- ▶ Leg Cramps/Pain
- ▶ Splints and Slings
- ▶ Sprain
- ▶ Strain

- ▶ Tx Goal for Fracture, Sprain, Bruise
- ▶ FAQs about Common Diagnostic Procedures:
  - Arthrogram
  - Bone Scan
  - CAT Scan
  - Discogram
  - Magnetic Resonance imaging
  - Myelogram
  - Nerve Conduction Velocity
  - X-Ray
- ▶ Tutorial

See also: Directory of Hotlines/Web Sites for Support Groups, Appendix E

▶ First Aid

Pressure Points
- Lay pt. down.
- Raise injured part above heart to decrease bleeding.
- Apply firm pressure with clean folded cloth.
- Arm wound: Apply pressure (firm and continuous) to pulse point inside the upper arm. Use four fingers. Apply pressure firmly against bone until you can no longer feel pulse.
- Leg wound: Place victim on back and feel for pulse in groin area—at top of leg where leg bends. Use the heel/palm of hand, keep arm straight, press artery against bone. If you need to, use both hands.

Fracture
- Take off all jewelry on injured part (possible swelling).
- Ice pack to injured part. (See Home Tx SI, Appendix A: Ice Pack)
- Do not move injured part.
- Do not eat or drink (preop).

▶ Cast Care

- If you have a cast, never let it get wet.
- Wait 48 hr for the cast to get strong. Don't walk or use the casted arm or leg until it is strong. If the cast is badly broken, indented, or wet, it must be changed.
- Raise cast up on pillows to stop swelling.

- Wiggle toes or fingers, if it does not cause pain. It will help prevent swelling.
- If the hand or foot swells or gets cold, blue, numb, or very painful, come in to be seen right away. If you have numbness, tingling, or burning that is not helped by raising the arm/leg on pillows and resting it for a few hours, come in to be seen right away.
- Bathing/showering: Put large, clean plastic bag over the cast while bathing or showering. Use a rubber band at the top to make it snug. Do not get the cast wet. If you do, make sure to dry it carefully.
- Painting the cast: Do not paint, tamper with, or get cast wet.
- Itching: Never put anything inside the cast (coat hanger, back scratcher) including your fingernails. Under the cast, the skin becomes very tender. Scratches can injure the skin under the cast and cause infection.
- Complications: If you notice pain or fever or a bad-smelling drainage coming from the skin under the cast, call the doctor. You may have an infection.

▶ **Compartment Syndrome**

Compartment syndrome symptoms include swelling and pressure in extremities or fingers. The swelling is so severe that it cuts off the blood supply to nerves and muscles. Compartment syndrome is a complication of surgery, postprocedure, or injury. This condition is very serious and may cause permanent damage. The most common places it occurs are in the lower leg, forearm, foot, and hand.

▶ **Fat Embolism**

Fat embolism is a serious condition. It can happen when fat enters the bloodstream after a fracture. It develops over a period of 24-72 hr. The most common cause of fat embolism is a fracture in the long bones. Fat embolism may occur in healthy patients. 1-2% of all fractures and 2-4% of all multiple fractures develop fat embolism.

▶ **Fracture**

- Signs and symptoms: (See Protocol)
- Causes: Trauma by twisting caused by muscle spasm, or disease
- Complications: Blood clot in lung, or elsewhere, gangrene, tetanus, nerve damage, and limb-threatening swelling
- Prevention/Tx: (See Cast Care above; Tx Goal for Fracture, Sprain, Bruise below).

▶ **Hematoma (Bruise)**

- Definition: A pocket of blood in the tissue
- Signs and symptoms: Discoloration of skin
- Causes: Trauma, surgery, or bleeding problem
- Complications: Infection/abscess (only if large amount)
- Tx Goal: Relieve pain, prevent complication. (See Also Tx Goal for Fracture, Sprain, Bruise)
- First aid for hematoma is "RICE": rest, ice, compression, and elevation. Large hematomas may go away in 1-2 days with this treatment. Compression with an Ace bandage and padding should be continued for 1 or 2 weeks. Normally, the blood is absorbed into the body tissues, and the clot disappears. In severe cases, the doctor may have to remove the blood using a needle and syringe.

  —Hot compress or ice pack—not directly on skin (See Home Tx SI, Appendix A: Hot Pack, Ice Pack)

  —NSAIDs.

  —Raise injured part above level of heart.

► Ice and Heat Therapy For Injuries

- Ice therapy is best for new, acute injuries or for overuse or sports injuries. The ice reduces swelling and inflammation, which helps ease the pain. Use ice in the first 48-72 hr or until swelling is gone (the swelling must be treated until it is gone). (See Home Tx SI, Appendix A: Ice Pack, Ice Massage). You may use ice packs for up to 1/2 hr over a period of up to 4 hr. You may do ice massage for 5-10 min.
  - —Complications: You may get frostbite if you leave the ice on too long. Be careful when using ice therapy on the elbow, knee, and foot.
  - —Elderly/Children: Use special care with ice packs for all elderly and children's injuries since they get frostbite more easily.
- Heat therapy is best for muscle, joint, and soft tissue injuries. It helps make joints and muscles more limber. However, don't use heat in the first few days after an injury. Use cold therapy at first, then use warm compress. (See Home Tx, Appendix A: Warm Compress).
  - —Complications: Heat can cause burns if left on too long. Be careful when using heat therapy on the elbow, knee, and foot.
  - —Elderly/Children: Use special care with heat therapy for all elderly and children's injuries since they get burns more easily.

► Leg Cramps/Pain

- Causes:
  - —Lack of calcium to muscle
  - —Excessive exercise
- Leg cramps are frequent in growing children. They are caused by fast growing and exercise (normal growing pains).
- Prevention/Tx:
  - —You need calcium. Drink milk; eat carrots, broccoli; take Turns.
  - —Take warm baths at bedtime.
  - —Avoid pointing your toes.
  - —Try to pull toes toward you.
  - —Put a pillow under the covers at the foot of bed to keep weight of blankets off feet.

► Splints and Slings

- Make a splint by using a rolled-up newspaper or magazine, an umbrella, stick, cane, or rolled-up blankets.
- Place the item next to or around the injured extremity.
- Hold it in place with several neckties, strips of cloth, tape, or belts in two or three places.
- Make sure the splint covers the joints above and below the fracture. This way it prevents movement and protects the fracture.
- Check the pulse before and after putting on a splint. If you cannot feel the pulse after the splint is on, it is too tight and must be loosened right away.
- Put a splint on only if you can do it without causing a lot of pain.
- *Injured leg:* Place padding between the legs to protect the skin. Loosely tape or tie the injured leg to the uninjured one.
- *Injured arm:* Place padding between the arm and body to protect the skin. Tape the injured arm to the chest if the elbow is bent, or to the side of the body if the elbow is straight. If the arm is bent, use a triangular piece of cloth or scarf. Place the arm in it. Tie the ends around the neck. Place the arm at the level of the heart.

- *Injured finger:* Wrap a paper clip with tape. Place the covered paper clip under the joint nearest to the finger injury. Tape lightly in two places.
- *Injured toe:* Place padding between the injured toe and the nearest unaffected one to protect the skin. Gently tape the injured toe to the next toe. Keep the padding dry.

► Sprain

- Signs and symptoms: Pain, swelling, difficult to use joint
- Causes: Trauma, wrenching or twisting of a joint, w or w/o partial tear of ligaments
- Complications: Damage to nearby blood vessels, muscles, tendons, and nerves
- Prevention/Tx: (See Tx Goal for Fracture, Sprain, Bruise below)

► Strain

- Signs and symptoms: Pain w/o swelling following overexertion of a muscle
- Causes: Overstretching of a muscle
- Complications: Rare
- Prevention/Tx: (See Tx Goal for Fracture, Sprain, Bruise below)

► Tx Goal for Fracture, Sprain, Bruise

Prevent swelling, pain. Prevent complications.

- Raise the injured part above heart to reduce swelling. Use pillows or blankets for comfort.
- Ice packs help cut down on swelling in the first 48 hr. (See Home Tx SI, Appendix A: Ice Pack.)
- If swollen, use Ace bandage.
- If you use an Ace (elastic) bandage, don't wrap it too tight. Always take it off when you sleep.
- Keep off injured area. Keep part still.
- Pain medication: Tylenol, Motrin, Advil, Anacin.

► FAQs About Common Diagnostic Procedures

Arthrogram

What is an arthrogram? An arthrogram is an invasive test that involves a series of x-rays of a joint (usually ankle, elbow, knee, hip, or shoulder). The doctor uses a special dye to see the inside of the joint.

Why is it done? An arthrogram is done to find out why there is joint pain or to discover what damage has been done to cartilage, ligaments, and bone.

Who should not have this test? Anyone with multiple allergies and/or allergies to iodine, shellfish, or other dyes used for x-rays should not have this test.

How is it done? A doctor or technician does it in the hospital, clinic, or diagnostic center. The doctor will inject Xylocaine into the skin with a needle, followed by the dye. The technician takes several x-rays of the joint. It takes about 30-45 min.

What do I have to do? After the procedure, you may need to take some OTC pain medication. You may want to do the "RICE" routine as well. You should rest the joint for the rest of the day. It may feel tight and/or click or crack for a few days.

Are there any complications or side effects? If you have rapid swelling and pain in the joint within the first few hours, call the doctor or go to the ED right away.

Bone Scan

What is a bone scan? A bone scan is used to diagnose disease of the bones and joints.

Why is it done? It is done to detect osteomyelitis, stress fractures, or cancer tumors. It is used to decide about future biopsy or surgery and to determine in what stage a cancer tumor is.

Who should not have this test? Anyone who has had any other tests using radiopaque dye for 1 -2 days before this exam should not have this test.

How is it done? A doctor or technician does it in the hospital, clinic, or diagnostic center, using a radiopaque dye. The dye is injected into your vein. Then, 3 hr later (after the dye is absorbed), several x-rays are taken while the dye is moving through the limb.

What do I have to do? Before the scan, the technician will take some blood. You may eat or drink as you wish before the scan. You might need some medication to help you stay very still while the scan is happening. You will need to drink 6 large glasses of water while you wait. You will be able to empty your bladder just before the scan begins. The procedure takes about 3-5 hr. After the scan, you cannot have any radionuclide tests for 48 hr.

Are there any complications or side effects? No.

CAT Scan

What is a CAT scan? A CAT scan is a test using an x-ray scan of extremities to show the details of bone and soft tissue.

Why is it done? This test is commonly used to evaluate tumors in the bone and soft tissue. It can also be used to evaluate bone/muscle damage after injury, to diagnose spinal cord and nerve abnormalities, fractures, infection, abscesses, and tumors.

Who should not have this test? People who should not have this test are those in traction or who have a cast, those who weigh more than 300 lb, and those who are very anxious or uncooperative.

How is it done? A doctor or technician does it in the hospital/diagnostic center. He or she may use a special dye. The dye is injected into your vein while the scan is being done.

What do I have to do? Drink fluids only for 4 hr before the test. Take all your usual medications. Take OTC or prescription medication for pain so you will not be uncomfortable during the test. You must lie very still during the test. The test takes about 1 hr. You may leave when it is done.

Are there any complications or side effects? No.

Discogram

What is a discogram? In a discogram, a radiopaque dye is injected into the spine to identify disc problems, injuries, or abnormalities.

Why is it done? This test is done to diagnose herniated discs. The doctor will stimulate your back to create a similar pain briefly to determine exactly where it is. The doctor also may do x-rays or CAT scan.

Who should not have this test? Anyone with multiple allergies and/or allergies to iodine, shellfish, or other dyes used for x-rays should not have this test.

How is it done? A radiologist or surgeon will start by injecting Xylocaine into the back. Then he or she will inject the dye into the disc.

What do I have to do? Before the test, you should discuss with your doctor how much or whether you should take pain medication before the test. You can help the doctor by telling him or her when the pain happens during the test. This will help the doctor tell where the pain is coming from. *Posttest:* You may want pain medication. It may be necessary to have someone drive you home.

Are there any complications or side effects? You may notice that your back or extremity pain is slightly worse after the exam. It will go away soon. In the meantime, take your usual pain medication.

Magnetic Resonance Imaging (MRI)

What is an MRI? An MRI is a noninvasive test that shows sections of a particular area in detail. It uses magnetic waves and a computer. It is better than an x-ray since it is so detailed.

Why is it done? MRIs are used to diagnose all types of orthopedic problems. It is especially good for diagnosing tumors and abnormalities of and injuries to muscles, bones, ligaments, or the spinal cord.

Who should not have this test? People with claustrophobia should talk to the doctor ahead of time about possible medication. The medication will help you relax and stay still during the procedure. Anyone with ANY metal fragments (clips/shunts/shrapnel), pacemaker, plates/screws from previous surgery may not be able to take this test. Please let the doctor know.

How is it done? You will lie on a cushioned bed. For the test, the part that needs to be examined must slide into a large circular-shaped magnet that surrounds the bed. There will be unfamiliar and perhaps loud noises during the exam—whirring and rhythmic clinking sounds. You may have either earplugs or a headset to muffle the noise. There might be an injection of a special dye in some patients. The procedure takes about an hour.

What do I have to do? Before the procedure, tell the doctor if you have fear of small places/elevators. Be sure to tell him or her about any metal fragments, pacemaker, plates/screws in your body. There is no special preparation. Wear loose, comfortable clothes without zippers. Remove all rings and jewelry. You will need to lie very flat and still for up to 1 hr. You may need to take some pain medicine or a sedative to help you remain still. Go to the bathroom just before the exam—it takes about 1-2 hr. After the procedure, you may drive home, but only if you have not had any medication that would impair driving, like a tranquilizer. Otherwise, someone will need to drive you home.

Are there any complications or side effects? No.

Myelogram

What is a myelogram? A myelogram is a test that uses a special dye to examine the spinal cord.

Why is it done? It is done to find spinal problems such as tumors or disc problems.

Who should not have this test? Anyone with multiple allergies and/or allergies to iodine, shellfish, or other dyes used for x-rays should not have this test.

How is it done? This procedure is done in a hospital or diagnostic center. You will lie flat on your back. The radiologist will perform a spinal tap and inject the dye into the spinal cord. He or she will then take the x-rays. It takes about 30-90 min.

What do I have to do? Before the test, drink more water/fluids than usual for 1 day. Drink clear liquids only on day of exam. If you are taking antidepressants or phenothiazines, talk to your doctor about stopping the medications for 2 days before and 2 days after the test. Medication can cause a reaction to the dye. Do not eat or drink anything after midnight the night before the test. After the test, take it easy for 1 day. Check with the doctor regarding the following instruction: For the first 6-8 hr, lie still with your head on several pillows raised to a 45° angle. Then you can lie flat after that. Also, drink at least 6-8 glasses of water for several days.

Are there any complications or side effects? Some people have some nausea and vomiting. If you have a backache, spasm, or discomfort in your arms/legs, it should not last longer than 1-2 days. If you have mild to severe headaches, there may be a small leak of spinal fluid. This is rarely serious. If symptoms do not go away, the leak can be sealed. This is done by the anesthesiologist.

Nerve Conduction Velocity (NCV)

What is an NCV? In an NCV, a small electrical impulse is used to stimulate certain nerves. It measures the time between the stimulation of the nerve and the response of the muscle.

Why is it done? It is used to diagnose muscle disorders or nerve damage, muscle weakness, Guillain-Barre, or nerve entrapment syndromes.

Who should not have this test? Patients who are agitated, uncooperative, or have a pacemaker or defibrillator should not take this test.

How is it done? The doctor places electrodes (needles or patches) in different muscles. The needles are very small and do not hurt. The electrical impulse shocks a certain muscle and the reaction is measured. The test takes about 1 hr.

What do I have to do? Before the procedure, you may take any medications or pain medicine that you normally take. You do not need to fast. Afterward, you may resume normal activity.

Are there any complications or side effects? No.

X-Ray

What is an x-ray? An x-ray is a noninvasive test that shows an image that is formed by the density of the tissue visualized. So, on x-rays, bone shows up more than air in the lungs or fat, for instance.

Why is it done? X-rays are done to evaluate injury to bones or joints.

Who should not have this test? Anyone who thinks or knows she is pregnant should not have this test. X-rays of very obese people may not be as clear due to the large amount of body fat.

How is it done? The x-ray is usually performed by a technician in a hospital, diagnostic center, or office. The technician places the part of the body to be evaluated on the x-ray plate. Since the x-ray shows only one angle, he or she must take a series of pictures from several angles in order to get a full picture of what is wrong.

What do I have to do? You must be able to hold still to have an x-ray taken of the position that the doctor needs. You may need to take pain medication, so you can hold still in that position.

Are there any complications or side effects? No.

► Tutorial

Assessment Tips

- Teens/Adolescents: Because of the accelerated rate of growth, injuries to extremities will more often result in fractures than in sprains or strains.

Red Flags

High-risk populations and symptoms for increased high risk in orthopedic problems (SAVED: severe symptoms, age, veracity, emotional distress, debilitation):

- Symptoms: Severe, sudden, or suspicious pain

  —Beware of pain that is more severe than expected or unrelenting.

  —Beware of any pain that awakens child or keeps him or her awake at night.

- Age:

  —Very old patients have increased risk of infection and fracture.

  —Childbearing age: Pregnant or postpartum women have a higher risk of deep vein thrombosis (DVT).

- Debilitation: Orthopedic problems occur more frequently for patients with diabetes, cardiac problems, or previous orthopedic problems.

- Recent injury: Local joint trauma predisposes for infection.

- Illness/infection: History of implants, chronic disease, IV drug abuse, local joint trauma, ALL immune deficiencies: AIDS/HIV, chemotherapy, diabetes, cystic fibrosis, asthma, splenectomy, steroid therapy, transplants, cancer; frail elderly or children are high-risk populations for infection.

Rules of Thumb

- The "5 P's" of compartment syndrome: pain, pallor, paresthesia, pulselessness, and paralysis.
- Tourniquet: The decision to apply a tourniquet is irreversible. (Use one only as last resort in life-threatening circumstances.)
- All severe pain must be seen within 8 hr or less.
- An open fracture has the greatest risk of infection.
- All orthopedic injuries: Chronic diseases lengthen the healing process.
- Minority callers may fail to recognize acute symptoms, report fewer symptoms, or attribute them to other causes.

Red Herrings

"Red herrings" are common distractions (symptoms or situations) that lead the nurse astray, away from the main problem.

- Remain vigilant to possible patient, parent, or caretaker denial, minimization, and misinterpretation of symptoms.
- Regard with suspicion: All unusual sounding presentations, including symptoms described as "the flu," or ones that are new, sudden, or unexpected.

- Patients who have been "seen recently" may still need to be seen today.
- Don't be misled by concurrent complaints or patient self-explanation.
- Patients "on medication" may be on the wrong medication (antibiotics).
- Symptom presentation may be early, late, silent, atypical, or novel.
- Symptoms of two conditions may present concurrently, causing confusion or misinterpretation.

EYE PROBLEM 1
Pain with Trauma; Burn; FB; Vision Changes; Blood in

ASSESSMENT	ACUITY LEVEL	DISPOSITION/ADVICE
Key Questions	Emergent Symptom Patterns	ED 0 min-1 hr
Major Trauma	- →	Consider head/neck injury with face/eye trauma
Trauma (All)	+ Penetration injury/flying object/FB, ± leaking fluid/ pain? (Globe Trauma, Hyphema)- - - - - - - - - - - - - - - →	Do not remove impaled object.
	+ (Face/head/eye) + vision change? (All)- - - - - - - - - - →	Do not lie down or bend over; have pt. sit up
	+ Sudden painless partial or complete loss of vision (veil, shadow, tiny dots)? (Detached Retina, Hemorrhage, Subluxated Lens)	
Burn	+ Welding? (Corneal Burn)- →	Pain may develop hours after injury.
	+ Chemical, toxic gas? (Corneal Burn) . . . . -▶	Contact poison center; bring substance w you (See Home Tx, Appendix A: Eyewash)

Key Questions	Urgent Symptom Patterns	ED/UCC/Office 1-8 hr
Eyelid Laceration?	- →	**Bring Child to E.D. Now** (w clean folded cloth— not cotton ball)
Pain w Trauma	+ Red eye, blurred vision, Hx of scratch, contact lens, FB? (Corneal Ulceration/Abrasion)	
FB/Contact Lens	+ Unable to remove at home? (> Risk of Abrasion) - -▶	Do not rub or touch eye

3

Key Questions	Acute/Nonacute Symptom Patterns	FA 8 + hr ± Home Tx
Trauma	+ Bruising eye area w/o vision change? (Lid Contusion, "Black Eye")	
Foreign Body (sand, dust, dirt, hair)	---■•▶	(See Eye Problem SI First Aid: Foreign Body).
Photophobia (See Eye Problem 2)		
Blood in Conjunctiva w/o Trauma	+ W/o pain, ± Hx of cough, sneeze, straining? (Subconjunctival Hemorrhage)	

Cross-References		
Eye Problem 2	Face/Jaw Problem	Head Problem

EYE PROBLEM 2
Pain without Trauma; Photophobia; Blood in; Discharge; Swelling; Vision Changes

ASSESSMENT	ACUITY LEVEL	DISPOSITION/ADVICE
Key Questions	Emergent Symptom Patterns	ED 0 min-1 hr
Blindness or Decreased Vision (sudden)	+ Headache, throbbing pain, N/V, blurred vision/halos, redness? (Acute Angle Closure Glaucoma)	
	+ Painless, unilateral? (Retinal Artery Occlusion)	
	+ Loss of vision, unilateral, brief episodes, double vision? (Intracranial pressure, Tumor, Stroke, TIA)	
Key Questions	Urgent Symptom Patterns	ED/UCC/Office 1-8 hr
Swelling Eyelids (extreme)	+ Conjunctiva? (Allergic Reaction)------------- ----------■►Benadryl	
	+ Poison oak exposure? (Allergic Reaction)-------------- ►Benadryl	
	+ Facial swelling, fever, fatigue, or pain w pressure on globe or eye movement? (Periorbital Cellulitis)	
Pain/Photophobia	+ Foreign body sensation, constant tearing, blinking, redness? (Corneal Ulcer/Herpes Keratitis)	
	+ Headache (sev.-mod.), throbbing, ± unilateral, N/V, abd. pain, > sensitivity to light & noise, Hx of similar headache in past, female, ± triggers, ± preceded by aura? (Migraine) (See Head Problem 2)	
Vision Change	+ Hazy vision, black floaters, redness? (Uveitis/Iritis)	
	+ painless, flashing lights, floaters, visual loss? (Retinal Detachment)	
Eyelid Droop	± Double vision progressive muscle weakness fatigability? (Myasthenia Gravis)	

Key Questions	Acute/Nonacute Symptom Patterns	FA 8 + hr ± Home Tx
Discharge	+ Red or pink eye, yellow discharge, eyelids stick together/esp. after sleeping; dried eye discharge on face, ± URI? (Conjunctivitis: Bacterial, Viral, Allergic, Chemical)	
	+ Purulent, red, itching, crusted, burning, ± Hx of recent swimming? (Conjunctivitis: Bacterial, Viral, Allergic, Chemical)	
	+ Watery, itching, swollen lid, Hx of allergy? (Allergic Response) (See Eye Problem SI)	
Vision Loss	+ Gradual? (Presbyopia)	
	+ Painless, gradual loss of vision, opaque Lens? (Cataract)	
Bleeding in Conjunctiva	+ w/o pain, ± Hx cough, sneeze, straining, no visual change, no fever? (Subconjunctival Hemorrhage)	
Pustule on Eyelid	+ Swelling, redness, tenderness, ± discharge on eyelid? (Sty/chalazion)	
Pain	+ Jabs of pain, "triggers" cause pain, severe spasms, brief, shooting pain, unilateral, shocklike pain, age > 50 yr? (Neuralgia) (See Face/Jaw Problem) —	S▸A : Does touching certain areas of face cause painful spasm? (Yes = +)
Vision Change (acute onset)	+ Halos around lights? (Open Angle Glaucoma)	
	+ Blurred vision, Hx diabetes, > BP, neuro problems, HIV? (Retinopathy)	
	+ Hx of retinotoxic Rx? (See Eye Problem SI, Drug Side Effect, Retinotoxicicty)	
	+ Recent ingestion drugs/alcohol? (OD/Side Effect)	
	+ Yellow/green halos around visual image? (Digitalis Toxicity)	

Cross-References
Eye Problem 1   Head Problem

EYE PROBLEM
Supplemental Information

Quick Reference:
- ► First Aid: Foreign Body
- ► General Advice
- ► Allergic Response
- ► Black Eye
- ► Blocked Tear Ducts
- ► Conjunctivitis
- ► Contact Lens Overwearing Syndrome
- ► Corneal Abrasion
- ► Drug Side Effect (Retinotoxicity)
- ► Spontaneous Conjunctival Hemorrhage
- Sty

See also: Directory of Hotlines/Websites for Support Groups, Appendix E

► **First Aid: Foreign Body**
- Comfort. Prevent further injury.
  —Tx: Clean gently around eye.
  —Eyewash. (See Home Tx SI, Appendix A: Eyewash)
- Pain
  —Tylenol
  —Cool compress. (See Home Tx SI, Appendix A: Cold/Cool Compress)

► **General Advice**
- Eye medication: Don't let tip of dropper touch the eye. It may spread infection to other eye.
- Eye patch: Driving with one eye covered is dangerous.

► **Allergic Response**
- Signs and symptoms: Discharge; tearing, itching, reddened, crusted, swollen eyelids; URI symptoms
- Causes: Pollens, irritants (chronic), mechanical or chemical
- Complications: Worsening of symptoms; chronic irritation; possible vision loss
- Home Tx:
  —antihistamines
  —compresses, warm or cold (See Home Tx SI, Appendix A: Cold/Cool Compress; Warm Compress)
  —natural tears
- Prevention: Elimination of irritating factors

► **Black Eye**
- Signs and symptoms: Bruising, swelling, pain, tenderness
- Cause: Injury
- Complications: Orbital Fx, infection
- Home Tx: Cold Compresses (See Home Tx SI, Appendix A: Cold/Cold Compress), Tylenol

► **Blocked Tear Ducts**
- HomeTx:
  —Massage inner eyelid gently q 2 hr.
  —Moist, warm compresses to area for 10 min, 3-4 x/day.

► **Conjunctivitis**
  - Signs and symptoms: See Protocol.
  - Conjunctivitis Tx Goal: Comfort. Treat infection. Prevent further infection. Wash hands with soap.
  - Causes: Bacterial, viral, allergic, chemical, or physical.
  - Complication: None.
  - Home Tx: Natural tears, Cold Compresses (See Home Tx, SI, Appendix A: Cold/Cool Compress).
  - Prevention:
    —Don't share eye makeup/towel/washcloth with others.
    —Wash hands frequently with soap.
    —Don't touch face or rub eyes.
    —Throw out old eye makeup.
    —Wash eye with warm washcloth. Don't use on the other eye.

► **Contact Lens Overwearing Syndrome**
  - Signs and symptoms: Severe pain after long flight, or wearing lens > 12 hr
  - Cause: Lack of tears carrying oxygen to cornea
  - Prevention: Remove contacts on flights > 4 hr. Drink more water, juice on flight.
  - Home Tx:
    —Rest. Warm or cool, damp washcloth to eyes q 2 hr.
    —Pain: Tylenol
    —Don't wear contacts x 4-5 days. Usually heals in 1 day.

► **Corneal Abrasion**
  - Signs and symptoms: Tearing, severe pain
  - Causes: Scratch or trauma
  - Complication: Possible vision loss
  - Home Tx: Needs to be seen by MD
  - Prevention: Use of safety glasses (when appropriate). Don't wear hard contact lenses > 12 hr.

► **Drug Side Effect: Retinotoxicity**
  Drugs and classes of drugs that may cause retinotoxicity:
  - Aralen (Chloroquine)—Blurred vision, difficulty focusing
  - Coco-Quinine (Quinine)—Blurred vision, difficulty focusing
  - Myambutol (Ethambutol)—Vision loss, loss of color (red/green) discrimination

► **Spontaneous Conjunctival Hemorrhage**
  - Definition: Leaking of blood into the white of the eye.
  - Causes: Cough, sneeze, vomit, standing on head, or straining (constipation).
  - Home Tx: No Tx. Will disappear in 2 wk. Reassurance.

► Sty

- Signs and symptoms: Pain, pimple-like lesion on the eyelid. May be at base of lid or deep within lid.
- Cause: Inflammation of one or more of the sebaceous glands of the eyelid.
- Complication: Infection spreads.
- Home Tx: Warm compresses for 15 min q 2 hr to promote drainage and help localize infection (See Home Tx SI, Appendix A: Warm Compress).

FACE/JAW PROBLEM
Pain with or without Trauma; Drooping; Swelling; Weakness

ASSESSMENT ACUITY LEVEL		DISPOSITION/ADVICE
Key Questions	Emergent Symptom Patterns	ED 0 min-1 hr
All Penetrating Trauma	---...-...............-*	• Do not remove penetrating object
Major Trauma	--- -▶	Always consider head/neck injury w face/jaw trauma
	+ Assoc, cervical spine trauma? (See Neck Problem) .. ..-▶	Do not move patient
Pain (Jaw) w/o Trauma	+ Chest pain: ± exertion (dull ache, pressure, squeezing, crushing, radiates to neck/jaw/arms), SOB, sweating, dizziness, lightheaded, N/V, pale, anxiety, sense of impending doom? (MI/Angina)	
Facial Drooping, Weakness w/o Trauma	+ Abrupt onset, sudden slurred speech, ± headache, double vision unsteady gait ± weakness in body, arms, legs, confusion, ± incontinence, Hx of BCP/atrial fib/> BP? (CVA, Cerebral Hemorrhage, Embolus)	
Facial Swelling w/o Trauma	+ SOB, wheezing, stridor, difficulty swallowing, agitation, anxiety, rash (itchy, raised, "hivelike"), swelling of face/tongue, Hx of allergies or exp. to allergen (meds, drug, food, chemical, substance, bite)? (Anaphylaxis)---	*- Benadryl

Key Questions	Urgent Symptom Patterns	ED/UCC/Office 1-8 hr
Facial Trauma	- -*-	Always consider head/neck injury w face/jaw trauma
	+ Asymmetry, severe/sharp pain, swelling, improper bite? (Fx Mandible/Maxilla/Zygoma)	
Facial Movements (unusual)	+ Involuntary (sudden onset) grimacing, chewing, wormlike tongue, drooling, Hx phenothiazines? (Tardive Dyskinesia)	
Face/jaw Pain w/o Trauma	+ Acute facial sinus pain, ± high fever, redness, swelling, esp. near eye, abnormal vision, severe headache, weak immune system, recent chemotherapy, Hx steroid medication, diabetic, recently hospitalized, mental status change? (Acute Bacterial Sinusitis/Preseptal/ Periorbital Cellulitis)	

(continued)

Key Questions	Urgent Symptom Patterns	ED/UCC/Office 1-8 hr
Face/Jaw Pain w/o Trauma (continued)	+ Swelling, tenderness, Hx toothache, redness, fever (> 38.5°C/101.3°F), warm to touch, drainage? (Dental Abscess)	
	+ (Skin) Red ± streaking, swollen, tender, hot; ± discharge, often w fever, swollen nodes, Hx of trauma/bite/local infection? (Cellulitis) (See also Eye Problem 2)	
Facial Weakness/ Numbness w/o Trauma	+ Sudden onset, unilateral drooping (face & mouth), drooling, feeling of fullness, swelling, pain, "crooked smile," irritated/dry/tearing eye, Hx of viral infection, unable to close eye (Bell Palsy)	

Key Questions	Acute/Nonacute Symptom Patterns	FA 8+ hr ± Home Tx
Facial Pain w/o Trauma	+ Jabs of pain "triggers" cause pain, severe spasms, brief, shooting pain, unilateral, shocklike pain, female, age > 50 yr? (Neuralgia)............................	*-SA: Does touching certain areas of face cause painful spasm (Yes = +)
	+ (Skin) lesion, linear/painful, follows the path of nerve, unilateral, begins as cluster of bumps, becomes blisters, then dry crust, ± sev. itching? (Herpes Zoster/Shingles)	
Facial/Jaw Pain	+ Facial/sinus pain, URI symptoms > 7-10 days, yellow/green nasal discharge, postnasal discharge, cough, pressure in teeth, bad breath, ± fever, swollen glands? (Rhinosinusitis)	
Jaw Pain	+ Popping crackling sound with pain in muscles wimc uicwuig, jdw CIICK: ^ nvij oyiiuiuiiicy	▶SA: L7iicKing sound wnen opening mouth = + chewing > pain = +

(continued)

Key Questions	Acute/Nonacute Symptom Patterns	FA 8+ hr ⋆ Home Tx
Facial Swelling (continued)	+ (Area below ear on cheek) chills, mod. fever, anorexia, malaise, pain on chewing/swallowing acidic fluids, exp. to mumps? (Mumps, Anterior Cervical Adenitis) + Hx of steroids, "moon face"? (Cushing Syndrome) + Any trimester of pregnancy? (See Pregnancy Problem)	

Cross-References		
Ear Problem 2 Eye Problem 2	Neck Problem Pregnancy Problem SI	Skin Problem: Lesion/Lump/ Swelling; SI Skin Problem: Laceration/ Wound

FACE/JAW PROBLEM
Supplemental Information

Quick Reference:
- ▶ Bell Palsy
- ▶ Cellulitis
- ▶ TMD (Temporomandibular Jaw)
- ▶ Trigeminal Neuralgia
- (Tic Douloureux)

▶ **Bell Palsy**

- Definition: Facial paralysis as a result of damage to the facial nerve. There may also be pain, tearing, drooling, or hypersensitivity to sound in the affected ear and impaired taste ability.
- Bell palsy is more common in pregnant women and people with diabetes, influenza, a cold, or upper respiratory infection.
- Signs and symptoms: Facial weakness/numbness, feeling of fullness, swelling, pain, "crooked smile," irritated/dry/tearing eye, sudden onset, unilateral drooping (face and mouth), drooling, Hx of viral infection, unable to close eye
- Causes:
  —Temporary nerve damage caused by virus.
  —The common cold sore virus, herpes simplex, and other herpes viruses are common causes of Bell palsy.
- Tx goals:
  —Steroid and pain medications.
  —Treatment is given to protect the eye from drying when sleeping.
  —Even without treatment, patients begin to get better within a few weeks.
  —Eighty percent recover completely within 3 months.
- Complications: In a rare case, the symptoms may never completely disappear.

▶ **Cellulitis**

See Skin Problem: Lesion/Lump/Swelling

▶ **TMD (TMJ Syndrome)**

- Definition: A disorder of the jaw muscles and joint. Symptoms include painful clicking, popping, or grating sounds when opening or closing the mouth, the jaw "locks," or there is limited jaw movement or a change in the "bite."
- Causes:
  —Severe injury to the jaw.
  —A fracture of the jaw.
  —Arthritis in the jaw joint.
  —Bad bite.
  —Stress may cause or worsen TMD.
  —People with TMD often clench or grind their teeth at night, which can tire the jaw muscles and lead to pain.
  —Women develop TMD twice as often as men.
- Signs and symptoms: Pain, popping or crackling sounds in ear when chewing; pain on side of face, tinnitus, < hearing, itching, or sensation of FB in ear.

- Complications: > Pain and symptoms.
- Prevention/Tx:
  —Limit yawning and movement of jaw.
  —Heat or ice to area.
  —Pain: Tylenol or NSAIDs.
  —"Nightguard" to prevent grinding.
  —Biofeedback.
  —Correction of "bite."
  —Surgery and injections are usually a last resort.

▶ Trigeminal Neuralgia (Tic Douloureux)

- Signs and symptoms: Severe pain in jaw lasting seconds to minutes, one-sided painful spasms.
- Definition: Damage to the facial nerve causing a sudden, severe, electric shocklike or stabbing pain on one side of the jaw or check.
  —Talking, brushing teeth, touching the face, chewing, or swallowing may trigger pain.
  —Trigeminal neuralgia is more common in women and people over age 50.
- Cause: Uncertain, possible compression of nerve by veins.
- Prevention/Tx: Needs appt. w MD.
  —Chew on unaffected side.
  —Gently brush teeth on affected side or not at all.
  —Use drinking straw.
  —Avoid cold drafts, chewing, drinking cold liquids, brushing hair, washing face.
- Tx: Anticonvulsant medication.
  —If medication fails to relieve pain, surgical treatment may be recommended.
- Complications:
  —Trigeminal neuralgia may come and go throughout the day.
  —The pain may last for days, weeks, or months.
  —Symptoms may disappear for months or years.
  —It may become worse.

FEVER
Fever with Associated Symptoms

ASSESSMENT ACUITY LEVEL		DISPOSITION/ADVICE
Key Questions	Emergent Symptom Patterns	ED 0 min-1 hr
Fever (±High)	+ Stiff neck, headache, N/V, extreme fatigue, ± pinpoint red purplish spots progressing to purple patches, extremely irritable or unresponsive, seizure? (Meningococcal Meningitis)......................................	*-SA: Touch chin to chest. (inability to perform = neck stiffness)
	+ Rapid onset high fever > 39.5°C or 103°F, toxic appearing, muffled voice, throat pain, drooling, insp. stridor, difficulty breathing/swallowing, sits very still w jaw extended? (Epiglottitis)----------------	Discourage opening mouth widely; nothing by mouth; do not use thermometer or give food/drink + First aid: Keep sitting upright and calm until you reach ED
	+ Confusion, dizziness, fainting? (Sepsis Syndrome)	
	+ Sore throat, difficulty breathing, nasal/pharyngeal infection, throat/neck swelling/pain, difficulty swallowing, drooling, neck pain w movement? (Retropharyngeal Abscess)	
	+ Heat/sun exposure or heat wave, ± extreme exercise (especially football) + low or no fluid intake, hot, dry skin, dizziness, weakness, headache, confusion, combativeness, ± loss of consciousness? (Heat Stroke) (See Heat Exposure)	
	+ Hx. psychiatric/antiemetic medication, altered mental status, muscle rigidity, sweating, fast pulse, rapid breathing? (Neuroleptic Malignant Syndrome)	

Key Questions	Urgent Symptom Patterns	ED/UCC/Office 1-8 hr
Fever (± Mod.)	+ Fatigue, ± weight loss, swollen lymph node, Hx viral infection? (Occult Neoplasm/Lymphoma/HIV/TB)	
	+ Chills, night sweats, fatigue, Hx of IV drug use/abuse, Hx or IV diagnostic procedures/central line, ± Hx heart murmur, heart valve surgery, ± recent dental work? (SBE)	

(continued)

Key Questions	Urgent Symptom Patterns	ED/UCC/Office 1 -8 hr
Fever (± Mod.) (continued)	+ High-risk groups: all immunocompromised, AIDS/HIV, chemo, diabetes, cystic fibrosis, asthma, sickle cell, splenectomy, steroid therapy, transplants, cancer, frail elderly (> Risk of Sepsis)	
	+ High-risk groups with diarrhea, < intake, ± < UA output/8 hr, weak, dizzy, dry mouth, sunken eyes, confusion, extreme thirst, frail elderly, bedridden, diabetes/HIV Hx, > 60 yr, > 101°F? (High-Risk Age Groups, > Risk Dehydration)	
	+ Abd./chest/back pain, ± respirations, difficulty breathing, chills, cough: ± productive, N/V, fatigue? (Pneumonia)	
	+ Abd. pain, constant, progresses from periumbilical to RLQ, ± vomiting, ± anorexia, ± holds abdomen, walks bent over? (Appendicitis)	
	+ Abdomen pain + vaginal discharge: foul smelling, bloody/any color; chills, walks bent over, ± Hx of STD exp., ± IUD user? (PID) (See also Abdomen Problem)	
	+ Severe facial/sinus pain, ± high fever, redness/ swelling, esp. around eye, abnormal vision, severe headache, mental status change, immunocom- promised: recent Hx: chemotherapy, steroids, diabetic, recently hospitalized? (Acute Bacterial Sinusitis/Preseptal/Periorbital Cellulitis)	
	+ N/V, dysuria, hematuria, ffequency/urgency, ± back pain, ± elderly (increased risk)? (Pyelonephritis, Urosepsis)	
	+ Male, chills, malaise, muscle aches, painful urination, pelvic/perineal pain, cloudy urine, dribbling, hesitancy, decreased urine output, ± vague/flulike symptoms? (Acute Prostatitis)	
	+ Localized musculoskeletal complaints (joints, bone, back), ± Hx IV drug abuse? (Septic Arthritis, Osteomyelitis, Epidural Abscess, Abscess, Rheumatologic, Neoplastic Diseases)	
	+ Breastfeeding ± "flulike" symptoms? (Possible Mastitis)	
	+ Seizure Hx = possible upgrade? (> Risk Seizure)	

(continued)

Key Questions	Urgent Symptom Patterns	ED/UCC/Office 1-8 hr
Fever (± Mod.) (continued)	+ Chemotherapy Hx ± diarrhea, stomatitis or respiratory symptoms? (Possible Chemotherapy Side Effect/Complications) + Yellow skin/eyes sclera? (Cholangitis, Liver Abscess) + N/V, anorexia, yellow sclera/skin, fatigue, swollen glands, clay colored stools, dark urine ± hepatitis exposure? (Hepatitis) + Fever 104°F-105°F in PM, normal in AM, sweating, fatigue, headache, enlarged lymph nodes, muscular pain, low back pain; wildlife or livestock contact: veterinarians, farmers, ranchers, slaughterhouse workers, meat inspectors, lab personnel? (Undulant Fever/Brucellosis) (See Bioterrorism Information, Appendix C) + Sudden onset of fever, headache, muscle pain, ± red rash? (Rocky Mountain Spotted Fever) + Any rash? (Infection)	
Fever (± Mild)	+ Recent foreign travel? (Acute/Chronic Tropical Infection) + Temp > 72 hr or recurrent after 24 hr? (Fever Unknown Origin) + New Rx or OTC med? (Drug-Induced Fever) (See revci oi)------------------------------	---➤ Rule of thumb: Drug fever often occurs 7-10 days after first dose

Key Questions	Acute/Nonacute Symptom Patterns	FA 8+ hr ± Home Tx
Fever	+ > Or several occasions, lasting 73 wk	

Cross-References			
Abdomen Problem Bowel Problem Breastfeeding Problem Chest Pain	Ear Problem Extremities Problem	Relevant Protocols Respiratory Problem Skin Problem	Urinary Problem Vaginal Problem: OB/GYN Procedures Vomiting/Nausea

TEMPERATURE-TAKING INSTRUCTIONS

The following instructions are written to be read to the caller, as appropriate:

GOAL: The most important thing is to be sure that the temperature you are getting is correct. Digital thermometers are the best kind. Always be sure the digital has a fresh battery; otherwise, it may not be correct.

Learning to take a temperature takes a little practice. If you have never taken a temperature before, it is a good idea to take it two or three times in a row. If the number is always the same, you are probably doing it right.

Types of Thermometers

DO NOT USE MERCURY THERMOMETERS, if at all possible. They can break and the fumes from the mercury inside can be poisonous. If you break a thermometer, call Poison Control for information about how to clean up the mercury and what to do. Never throw out a broken thermometer. You must take it to a waste facility. If you don't have one, wait until your community has waste management and take it there.

Mercury poisoning can affect the brain, nervous system, kidneys, and liver. It might cause tingling of fingers and toes, numbness sensation around the mouth and tunnel vision. Use nonmercury thermometers. They can be used for oral, rectal, or under the arm temperature-taking. Other kinds of thermometers include

- Digital electronic thermometers
- Glass alcohol thermometers
- Glass galinstan thermometers
- Digital thermometers
- Ear canal thermometers
- Pacifier thermometers
- Forehead thermometers

How To Take a Temperature

- Oral (digital or glass). This is the most accurate type.
- Armpit (digital or glass). Place the tip of the thermometer in the armpit. Hold arm down for the appropriate amount of time. This route is not very accurate.
- Rectal (digital or glass). Use some lubricant on the tip of the thermometer. Insert gently into the rectum (for adults insert 1 in). Hold the thermometer in for the appropriate amount of time.
- Ear (ear canal). If used correctly this is very accurate. It gives a reading within seconds. Follow instructions on package.
- Forehead (Fever strip only). These are only accurate for high fevers. Not recommended at this time.
- Mouth
  —Wait 10 min before taking the temperature, if the person has eaten or drunk anything hot or cold
  —Put the thermometer way under the tongue on one side.
  —Close mouth and keep it closed. Hold the thermometer with fingers.
  —Leave the thermometer inside for 1-2 min. You will hear a beep when it is ready.

Temperature Conversion Table

Centigrade	Fahrenheit
35°	95°
36°	96.8°
37°	98.6°
38°	100.4°
39°	102.2°
40°	104°
41°	105.8°

FEVER
Supplemental Information

Quick Reference:
- ▶ Dehydration
- ▶ Drug Side Effect (Fever)
- ▶ Fever
- ▶ Occult Infections
- ▶ Tutorial
- ▶ Surgical (Postoperative Fevers)
- ▶ Oncology

▶ Dehydration (See Home Tx SI, Appendix A: Rehydration Guidelines)
- Complication: Shock.
- Prevention/Tx: Drink fluids until urine is almost clear (See Home Tx SI, Appendix A: Clear Liquids).

▶ Drug Side Effect: Fever (Caused or Made Worse)
- Antitubercular drugs
- Barbiturates
- Cephalosporins
- Phenytoin (Dilantin)
- Erythromycin
- Ibuprofen
- Methyldopa (Aldomet)
- Penicillin
- Quinidine
- Quinine
- Septra, Bactrim, co-trimoxazole
- Streptomycin
- Sulfa drugs
- Sulindac (Clinoril)
- Chlorpromazine (Thorazine)
- Acetaminophen (Tylenol) (Paradoxical fever)

▶ Fever
- Signs and symptoms: Body temperature > 37.5°C or 99.0°F. It is not dangerous unless it is > 40°C or 104°F.
- Causes: Infection by a virus or bacteria. The fever is your body's way to help fight the infection. Viral infections are more common.
- Complication: Dehydration
- Home Tx:
  - —Goal: Reduce fever. Increase comfort.
  - —Fever: Tylenol q 4 hr.
  - —Fever record: Keep a record of the fever route. Take temperature every 4 hr (how you took it, when, how high). Check temperature 1 hr after medication. It should be lower or gone.
  - —Warm bath (See Home Tx SI, Appendix A: Warm [Tepid] Bath).

- **Adult Protocols**

  —Never use alcohol rub or bath to stop a fever. Fumes can be toxic (CNS depression).

  —Drink 8 or more glasses of cool or iced water, juice, soda, herb tea, etc. (except patients with change in level of consciousness, abdomen pain, CV disease, renal disease, diabetes insipidus).

  —Dress in single layer of clothing. Use sheet only.

  —Remove heavy blankets.

  —Rest.

► **Occult Infections**
  - Inflammatory bowel disease
  - Osteomyelitis
  - Prostatitis
  - Subacute bacterial endocarditis (SBE)
  - Sinusitis, dental abscess

► **Tutorial**

Red Flags

Populations and Symptoms which increase risk (SAVED: severe symptoms; high-risk populations: age, veracity, emotional distress, debilitation)

Indicators of acuity when considering fever:

- Any high fever; or fevers of long duration
- Immunocompromised status
- Poor response to antipyretics or home treatment
- Severe associated symptoms
- Similar symptoms or illness in contacts
- Sudden onset; quickly rising fever
- Dead tissue or blood leaked internally, i.e., heart attack, stroke, alcoholic hepatitis or pancreatitis, or blood in the belly

Rules of Thumb

- Elderly patients have decreased or absent febrile response to infection.
- "Temperature extremes often trigger medical problems" (Clawson and Dernocoeur, 1998).
- Minority callers may fail to recognize acute symptoms, report fewer symptoms, or attribute them to other causes.
- Fevers normally peak in late afternoon and evening.

Red Herrings

- Remain vigilant to possible patient denial, minimization and misinterpretation of symptoms.
- Regard with suspicion: All elderly callers and unusual sounding presentations, including symptoms that are described as "the flu," or new, sudden, or unexpected, or wakened caller from sleep.
- Patients who have been "seen recently" may still need to be seen today.
- Don't be misled by concurrent complaints or patient self-explanation.
- Don't be misled by the prospect of "normal postop fever" or patient self-explanation.
- Symptom presentation may be early, late, silent, atypical, or novel.
- Symptoms of two conditions may present concurrently, thereby causing confusion or misinterpretation.

- Illness rarely presents as a single symptom.
- Patients often misinterpret or stereotype their symptoms.

▶ Surgical: Postoperative Fevers

Common sources of postop fevers:

- Abscess
- Deep vein thrombosis due to restricted activity
- Phlebitis (because of IV)
- Respiratory infections: Most common source of fever in first 48 hours
- Urinary tract infections
- Wound infection

▶ Oncology

All chemotherapy patients with fevers must be evaluated within 8 hr or less, as appropriate, for possible neutropenia, stomatitis, and pulmonary or cardiac toxicity.

HEAD PROBLEM 1
Pain; Laceration; Level of Consciousness Change with Trauma

ASSESSMENT	ACUITY LEVEL	DISPOSITION/ADVICE
Key Questions	Emergent Symptom Patterns	ED 0 min-1 hr
Major Trauma	---	Always suspect spinalcord injury W head trauma (See Head Problem SI, First Aid)
	+ Penetrating object? (Intracerebral Bleed)--------- -------	Do not remove missile/fb
	+ Headache ± trauma (sudden/sharp or gradual/dull/ throbbing), neck pain/stiffness, resp. changes, progressing: irritable/lethargic/± loss of consciousness; visual changes, weakness, N/V, staggering, slurred speech? (Intracranial Hemorrhage/Cerebral Contusion/Subdural Hematoma)	
	+ Pain, tenderness, swelling over injured area, "racoon eyes" (bruising around eyes) ± blood, CSF coming from ear/nose, N/V, ± loss of consciousness, seizure, sev. weakness? (Skull Fx, Basilar Skull Fx)------------------------------------- ----▶	Rule of thumb: Usually assoc, w other severe injuries

Key Questions	Urgent Symptom Patterns	ED/UCC/Office 1-8 hr
Trauma	+ Repeated vomiting? (Intracranial Hemorrhage)	
Laceration	+ Persistent bleeding, ± Hx of bleeding disorder, kidney/liver disease, Hx of anticoagulants? (Laceration > Risk Hemorrhage)---------------------- - -	(See Head Problem SI, First Aid)
Pain w Trauma	+ N/V, dizziness, staggering, confusion, loss of memory and/or brief loss of consciousness? (Concussion) + Visual changes? (See Eye Problem)	

Key Questions	Acute/Nonacute Symptom Patterns	FA 8+ hr.* Home Tx
Pain w Trauma	+ Hx trauma (days to months), dizziness, confusion, ± N/V, sensitivity to noise/light? (Postconcussive Syndrome)	
Trauma (minor)	+ Headache (mild), nausea, sleepiness? (Minor Head Injury)	
	+ Swelling w/o other symptoms? ("Goose Egg" Hematoma)--■*- (See Head Problem SI, First Aid)	

Cross-References

Confusion	Eye Problem 1; 2	Head Problem 2
Dizziness	Fainting	Vomiting/Nausea

HEAD PROBLEM 2
Pain; Level of Consciousness Change without Trauma

ASSESSMENT	ACUITY LEVEL	DISPOSITION/ADVICE
Key Questions	Emergent Symptom Patterns	ED 0 min-1 hr
Headache (sudden/severe/ persistent) w/o Trauma	+ Sudden/sharp or gradual/dull/throbbing, "worst" or "first," neck pain/stiffness, resp. changes, progressing: irritable/lethargic/± loss of consciousness; visual changes, weakness, N/V, staggering, slurred speech ± worse with exertion? (Intracranial Hemorrhage)	
	+ Fever, stiff neck, N/V, extreme fatigue, ± pinpoint red purplish spots progressing to purple patches, extremely irritable or unresponsive, ± seizure? (Meningococcal Meningitis)	
	+ Vision change (sudden), throbbing pain, N/V, blurred vision/halos, redness? (Acute Angle Closure Glaucoma)	
	+ Dizziness, fatigue, ± nosebleed, ± Hx > BP, ± N/V, confusion? (Hypertensive Crisis)	
	+ 2nd/3rd trimester: blurred vision, Hx of rapid wt. gain, swelling (hands/feet/face), N/V, epigastric pain, fatigue, Hx of hypertension? (Preeclampsia)	
Headache	+ Neck pain, photophobia, fever/chills, N/V, ± confusion, restlessness, somnolence, ± Hx of TB/HIV/AIDS? (Meningitis, Encephalitis, Abscess)	
	+ Hx of exp. to street drugs/Rx, poisonous plant, or inhalation/ingestion of toxic chemical, pesticide? (Toxic Exposure)--	→ Contact poison center; bring substance w you
	+ Weakness, dizziness, SOB, drowsiness, faintness, N/V? (Carbon Monoxide Poisoning)	

Key Questions	Urgent Symptom Patterns	ED/UCC/Office 1 -8 hr
Headache (sev. to mod.)	+ New or sudden onset. Progressive worsening, ± Hx cancer persistent/severe drowsiness, vomiting, double vision, onset > 50 yr of age? (Mass, Lesion)	
	+ Throbbing, ± unilateral, N/V, abd. pain, > sensitivity to light & noise, Hx similar headaches in past, female, ± triggers, ± dizziness/staggering, ± preceded by aura? (Migraine) (See Head Problem SI)	
	+ (Unilateral), paroxysmal (repeated episodes, 1-hr attacks), periorbital, puffy eye, runny nose, > tearing, male? (Cluster Headache)	
	+ (Unilateral), chronic, muscle aches, weakness, elderly woman, < vision, fever (mild)? (Temporal Arteritis)	
	+ Acute facial sinus pain, ± high fever, redness, swelling, esp. near eye, abnormal vision, severe headache, weak immune system, recent chemotherapy, Hx. steroid medication, diabetic, recently hospitalized, mental status change? (Acute Bacterial Sinusitis/ Preseptal/Periorbital Cellulitis)	

Key Questions	Acute/Nonacute Symptom Patterns	FA 8+ Hr. ± Home Tx
Headache (mod. to mild)	+ Premenstrual, Hx of ERT, BCP? (Hormonal Headache)	
	+ Dull, nonthrobbing, persistent low intensity, "like tight band around head," tense facial/scalp/ neck muscles? (Tension Headache)	
	+ Recent lumbar puncture, > when sitting up? (Spinal Headache)	
	+ Hx of recent alcohol use, N/V, depression, thirst, irritability, fatigue? ("Hangover")	
	+ Hx of recent withdrawal from caffeine, chocolate, cigarettes? (Caffeine/Tyramine Withdrawal) (See Head Problem SI)	

(continued)

Key Questions	Acute/Nonacute Symptom Patterns		FA 8+ Hr. ± Home Tx
Headache (mild)	+ Facial/sinus pain, URI symptoms >7-10 days, yellow/green nasal discharge, postnasal discharge, cough, pressure in teeth, bad breath, ± fever, swollen glands? (Rhinosinusitis) + Hx fever, joint pain, N/V, diarrhea? (Viral Syndrome)		

Cross-References Head Problem 1 Lip/Mouth; Teeth/Gums; Tongue Problem	Nose/Sinus Problem	Pregnancy Problems	Vomiting/Nausea

HEAD PROBLEM
Supplemental Information

Quick Reference:
- ▶ First Aid
  - Neck Injury
  - Laceration
  - Cold Pack
- ▶ Rule of Thumb
- ▶ Caffeine Withdrawal

- ▶ Concussion
- ▶ Headache
- ▶ Drug Side Effect (Headache)
- ▶ Head Injury Instructions
- ▶ Migraine Headache
- ▶ Spinal Headache

See also: Directory of Hotlines/Web Sites for Support Groups, Appendix E

▶ **First Aid**

Neck Injury
- Do not move, unless absolutely necessary. Wait for help.
- Keep neck still.
- Place both hands on side of head to stabilize neck

Laceration
- Lay pt. down.
- Apply firm pressure w clean folded cloth.
- Keep pressure on until help arrives.

Cold Pack
- Apply ice pack. (See Home Tx SI, Appendix A: Ice Pack)
- Keep head elevated.
- Keep in sitting, semireclining position.

▶ **Rule of Thumb**
- Always elicit any Hx of recent (30 days) head trauma. (Any Hx: See Head Problem 1)

▶ **Caffeine Withdrawal**
- Signs and symptoms: Headache, irritability, restlessness.
- Causes: Sudden stop of caffeine intake.
- Complications: Severe headaches, N/V.
- Prevention/Tx: *Gradually* cut down on coffee, cola. Then do not use products that have caffeine, e.g., coffee, cola, chocolate, Excedrin, and other OTC med(s) that contain caffeine.

▶ **Concussion**
- Definition: Shaking of the brain caused by a blow to the head. This causes unconsciousness. Least serious form of head injury
- Complications: Nausea/vomiting, photophobia, hallucination
- Tx: Keep pt. lying down quietly. Cool compresses to head or neck. If pt. recovers quickly, may have headache for 12-72 hr (See Head Injury).

► **Drug Side Effect: Headache**
- Antihypertensive
- Vasodilators, e.g., nitroglycerin

► **Headache**
- Headache Tx goal: Relieve pain. Prevent recurrence.
  —Pain: Tylenol as appropriate.
  —Comfort: Rest in quiet, dark room w cool damp cloth on forehead. (See Home Tx, Cold, Appendix A: Cool Compress)
  —Relaxation techniques.

► **Head Injury Instructions**
- Tx:
  —Pain: Tylenol
  —Do not leave person alone for the next 24 hr.
  —It is normal for a person to vomit right after injury, and 1-2 times in the first 8 hr. If the person doesn't vomit right away, but then starts vomiting several hours after the injury, call right away.
  —Person should be easy to waken when sleeping.
  —Do not use any drug that could cause drowsiness X 48 hr (e.g., cough med, antihistamines).
  —Quiet activity x 72 hr.
  —Give person light meals: Soup, plain pasta, cereal.
- Complications: Wake pt. every 2 hr and check for and call right away if any of the following symptoms occur (even within several months):
  —Vomiting: Frequent (3 or more times), persistent, sudden
  —Stiff neck
  —Fever
  —Seizures or unconsciousness
  —Blurred vision or seeing double
  —Confusion, very sleepy, or very difficult to wake up
  —Stumbling or other problems w arms or legs
  —Ear or nose drainage in first 48 hr
  —Headache that is becoming worse or more frequent
- Do not use sedatives, narcotics, alcohol, or any other drug that could cause drowsiness x 48 hr. Ask patient specific questions: What is your address? Name of family dog, names of family members? Patient should be able to answer correctly.

► **Migraine Headache**

More common in women.
- Definition/signs and symptoms: AM headache awakens pt. Usually severe, progressive, unilateral, throbbing, N/V, photophobia, irritability, weakness, vertigo. Often preceded by a period of depression, chronic irritability, pain in eyes (aura).
- Causes: Vascular, involving constriction of the blood vessels. Can be hereditary. Some common triggers: too much sleep, physical exertion, dieting, heat, lights, estrogen levels, foods, alcohol, caffeine, MSG, yeast, ripened cheese, chocolate, meat w nitrate additive.

- Prevention: The earlier the drug is taken, the better the relief. Prescription med may be needed.
- Tx: See Home Tx in Protocol.

► Spinal Headache
- Tx:
  —Bedrest, increase fluids (See Home Tx, Appendix A: Increase Fluids)

HEAT EXPOSURE
Heat Stroke; Heat Exhaustion; Heat Cramps

ASSESSMENT	ACUITY LEVEL	DISPOSITION/ADVICE
Key Questions	Emergent Symptom Patterns	ED 0 min-1 hr
Heat Exposure ± Hx of increased exercise/ humidity + decreased fluid intake	+ Rapid onset: hot, dry skin, fever, > 105°F, marked change in behavior, hallucinations, confusion, combativeness, ± loss of consciousness, seizures?	(See Heat Exposure SI, First Aid)
Key Questions	Urgent Symptom Patterns	ED/UCC/Office 1 -8 hr
Heat Exposure ± Hx of > exercise/humidity + < fluid intake	+ ± Fever, thirst, skin: sweating (may be profuse), cool/clammy/pale/ashen, N/V, headache, muscle cramps, dizzy, weak, staggering? (Heat Exhaustion)------------------------------------ ■+- (See Heat Exposure SI, First Aid)	
	+ Previous medical Hx: cardiac disease, hypertension, thyroid disease, DM, cystic fibrosis, some dermatologic disorders, obesity? (> Risk Heat Exhaustion)	
	+ Medications: alcohol/street drugs/or Rx: antihypertensive, phenothiazines, thyroid, amphetamines? (> Risk Heat Exhaustion)	
Heat Exposure + high-risk age group stays	+ Elderly > 65 yr; frail elderly: listless, dizzy, no urine output x 8 hr, dry mouth, sunken eyes, bedridden? (> Risk Dehydration)	►+ SA: Pinch skin briefly and release. Describe: if skin pinched-looking = tenting or + for dehydration
Key Questions	Acute/Nonacute Symptom Patterns	FA 8 + hr ± Home Tx
Heat Exposure	+ Dehydration (mild)? (> Risk Dehydration)	
	+ Excessive water intake, muscle cramps (legs/abd.), lightheadedness, weakness, heavy perspiration? (Heat Cramps, Hyponatremia)	

Cross-References
Dizziness/Fainting   Seizures   Skin: Burn

HEAT EXPOSURE
Supplemental Information

Quick Reference:
- ▶ First Aid
- ▶ Community Alert
- ▶ High-Risk Populations
- ▶ High-Risk Occupations/Activities

- ▶ Drug Side Effect
  (Heat Exposure Worsened)
- ▶ Prevention

▶ First Aid
- Move to shade/cool area.
- Remove clothing.
- Spray, splash, or sponge and fan victim.
- Place covered ice packs or cold cloths: head/neck, groin, armpits.
- If victim is conscious and awake, give frequent sips of cool fluids, Gatorade, or commercial sports drink.
- Elevate legs.
- Do not give ASA or Tylenol.

▶ Community Alert
- Heat waves may increase incidence of heat stroke, *even in the absence of strenuous exercise.*
- The longer (in days) and more extreme the heat wave, the higher the incidence of heat stroke.
- Predisposition to heat stroke lasts for 24+ hours. Thus, heat stroke may depend on temperature of *the previous day.*

▶ High-Risk Populations
- Extremes of age add to the risk of hyperthermia. Err on the side of caution with adults > age 60.
- Heat extremes may aggravate other medical problems. Don't overlook other possible medical conditions that may be present.

▶ High-Risk Occupations

The following occupations are high risk due to intake exertion:
- Miners
- Heavy industry workers
- Military personnel

▶ High-Risk Occupations/Activities

The following occupations/activities are high risk due to impermeable garments.
- Wrestlers
- Dieters
- Firefighters
- Hazardous waste handlers

▶ Drug Side Effect: Heat Exposure Worsened

• Drugs and classes of drugs that may worsen heat exposure:

—Alcohol

—Amphetamines

—Anticholinergic agents

—Antihypertensives (e.g., diuretics)

—Beta-blockers

—Phenothiazines (decrease diaphoresis)

° Chlorpromazine (Thorazine)

° Prochlorperazine (Compazine)

° Thioridazine (Mellaril)

° Trifluoperazine (Stelazine)

—Thyroid (affects heat/cold tolerance)

° Synthroid

° Cytomel

▶ Prevention

- Avoid sun exposure between 10 AM-3 PM.
- Drink several glasses of water before and after exercising.
- Cover head with hat, wet cloth, or scarf. Cover neck with wet scarf.
- Eat salty foods, to replace salt lost through sweating.
- Stay in shade when possible.
- Avoid overdoing exercise. Rest when possible.
- Wear loose-fitting, light-colored, lightweight cotton clothes.
- Soak your T-shirt in cool water, wring out, and wear.
- If taking any medication, consult with your pharmacist regarding possible side effects related to heat. Remember, certain medical conditions, activities, or jobs may put you at higher risk for heat illness (review).

JOINT PROBLEM
Pain with or without Trauma; Swelling (Shoulder, Elbow, Wrist, Hip, Knee, Ankle); Limp

ASSESSMENT	ACUITY LEVEL	OISPOSITION/ADVICE
Key Questions	**Emergent Symptom Patterns**	**ED 0 min-1 hr**
Pain (Arm/Shoulder) w/o Trauma	+ Chest pain: ± exertion (dull ache, pressure, squeezing, crushing, radiates to neck/jaw/arms), SOB, sweating, dizziness, lightheaded, N/V, pale, anxiety, sense of impending doom? (MI/Angina) (See Chest Pain)	
Major Trauma	+ Hx fracture, difficulty breathing, SOB, petechial rash (upper trunk/extremities), high fever, jaundice, confusion? (Fat Embolism)	

Key Questions	**Urgent Symptom Patterns**	**ED/UCC/Office 1 -8 hr**
Joint Pain w Trauma	+ (All joints) swelling, deformity, skin discoloration, < range of motion, refusal to move, unable to bear weight? (Fx, Dislocation, Separation, Acute Sprain)	
	+ (Ankle/foot) swelling, discoloration, able to tolerate some weight bearing? (Sprain, Strain)----------------- ➤	First aid: Rest on pillow, elevate feet above heart, if possible; + Ace wrap, if available
	+ (Knee, hip) gradual onset, walks leaning over. Affected hip, limp, ± trauma? (Slipped Capital Femoral Epiphysis)	
	+ (Shoulder) Fix trauma 6-12 hr prior, sudden onset, deltoid area, arm hanging limp? (Rotator Cuff Tear)	
	+ Open fracture/laceration/IV abuse Fix, high fever, swelling, redness, disproportionate pain. Area is red, shiny, swollen, exquisitely tender w subcutaneous crepitation? (Necrotizing Fasciitis)	
	+ (Sev.) Pain, numb, pale skin, Hx of recent trauma/ surgery, cast application, pain unrelieved by ice, elevation, pain meds? (Cast Problem/Compartment Syndrome)	

(continued)

Key Questions	Urgent Symptom Patterns	ED/UCC/Office 1 -8 hr
Joint Pain w/o Trauma	+ ± Fever, Hx of sickle cell disease? (Sickle Cell Crisis)	
	+ Swelling/tenderness, Hx of hemophilia? (Hemarthrosis)	
	+ Fever/chills, fatigue, intense joint pain/tenderness, refusal to move limb, extreme pain on movement; high risk: HIV, elderly, etc.? (Septic Arthritis)	
Limp/Nonuse	+ + Fever, point tenderness, unilateral, nonuse, Hx of recent infection? (Osteomyelitis)	
	+ Sudden onset, fever, chills, tenderness, joint swelling, skin warm to touch? (Septic Arthritis, Septic joint)	

Key Questions	Acute/Nonacute Symptom Patterns	FA 8 + hr ± Home Tx
Joint Pain w/Trauma	+ (Base of thumb), > w movement? (De Quervain Disease)	
	+ (Palm/base) 3rd & 4th fingers? (Dupuytren Contracture)	
Joint Pain w or w/o Trauma	+ (Great toe) sudden onset, warm, red, tender, male age > 40, female > age 50? (Gout) (See Joint Problem SI)	
	+ (Foot bottom) (severe) + injury? (Plantar Fasciitis)	
	+ Hx of tick exp., Hx of recent camping? (Lyme Disease) (See Bites)	
	+ Swelling, warm, tenderness? (Bursitis, Tendinitis)	
Joint Pain (mild)	+ > Pain on movement, toes, wrist or fingers, chronic swelling, warmth, Hx of arthritis? (Rheumatoid Arthritis, Osteoarthritis)	
	+ Mild fever, generalized joint pain, URI Sx, ± rash? (Viral Syndrome)	
Limp	+ (24 hr, ± fever? (Infection Neoplastic Disease)	

Cross-References
Extremities Problem 4   Skin Problem: Bites/Stings

JOINT PROBLEM
Supplemental Information

Quick Reference: ► Ace Wrap Teaching

                                       ► Anterior Cruciate Ligament

                                       ► Arthritis

                                       ► Bursitis

                                       ► Dislocations (Subluxations)

                                             Dislocated Shoulder

                                       ► Gout

                                       ► Knee Arthroscopy

                                       ► Sprain

                                       ► Strain

                                       ► Tutorial

► **Ace Wrap Teaching**

     ® Wrap from bottom to top.

- Check circulation. If toes become cold, blue, or numb, then loosen the wrap.
- The bandage will help cut down on swelling, help to reduce pain, protect the injury, and help healing.
- Remove when sleeping.

► **Anterior Cruciate Ligament (ACL)**

- *Symptoms:* The symptoms include immediate and profound pain, aggravated with motion, and inability to walk or bear weight.
- *Occurrence:* Tears of the ACL are common and very serious knee injuries. Trauma to the knee is the second most common occupational accident.
- High-risk populations, age/gender.
  —Patients tend to be young males. Sports-related activities account for approximately 60% of knee injuries. Generally, knee dislocations arise from high-energy trauma, such as MVA.
  —Elderly patients may sustain fractures from minimal injuries that typically produce only soft-tissue injuries in younger patients.

► **Arthritis**

- Signs and symptoms: See Protocol.
- Risk Population: Common in females 30-50 yr.
- Causes: Unknown. Inflamed joint, aging, injury, infection.
- Complications: Joint that will not move. Disability.
- Arthritis, bursitis, tendinitis home Tx goals: Reduce pain, inflammation. Prevent increased symptoms.
  —Pain: Tylenol, Motrin
  —Use a heating pad x 15 min, or use cold pack (See Home Tx, Appendix A: Ice Pack).
  —Rest joint when pain is present.

—Do not do anything that makes pain worse.

—Do exercises that MD recommends after pain and swelling are reduced.

► Bursitis: Swelling of Sac or Area around Joint

® Signs and symptoms: See Protocol.

- Causes: Minor injury or repeated motion.
- Complications: Permanent injury, or limited ability to use joint.
- Prevention/Tx (See also Arthritis Tx):
  —Rest, ice, elevation
  —Pain meds: Tylenol, Motrin

► Dislocations (Subluxations)

® Subluxed radial head (nursemaid's elbow),

e Signs and symptoms: Pain w movement.

® Causes: Injury, e.g., lifting and/or jerking by the arm.

« Dislocations home Tx goals:

—Resume use of arm; pain greatly reduced.

—Educate parent or caretaker about cause of injuries.

Dislocated Shoulder

- Definition: The bones making up the shoulder joint become separated, so the joint cannot work.
- Cause: Dislocated shoulders are usually caused by fall onto outstretched arm or shoulder.

® Risk: This injury is most common in football, rugby, hockey, lacrosse, skiing, volleyball, soccer.

- Symptoms: Pain, tenderness, weakness in shoulder/upper arm, aggravated by any movement, numbness in shoulder, arm, hand, deformity.
- Diagnosis: Physical exam and x-ray.
- Tx: This injury needs immediate attention. First aid will include an ice pack (See Plome Tx SI, Appendix A: Ice Pack). The doctor may be able to put the head into the socket. If more than 15-30 min go by, you may need anesthesia, so the doctor can reposition the shoulder. Sometimes surgery is required to correct this injury. Healing may take 4-12 wk. Patients may return to activities after following the doctor's prescribed course of gradual exercise.

► Gout

- Definition: Recurrent, acute inflammation of peripheral joints. Starts with big toe, may involve other extremities, but usually common in lower extremities.

e Signs and symptoms: See Protocol.

- Cause: Too much uric acid starts an inflammatory process.
- Precipitating factors: Trauma, alcohol abuse, drugs, surgical stress, acute medical illness.
- Complications: Worsening of symptoms, recurrent attacks progressing to permanent joint damage.
- Prevention/Tx goal: Reduce pain, inflammation. Prevent recurrence.
  —Meds: Motrin, Tylenol. No aspirin.
  —Diet: Avoid rich foods or alcohol.
  —Rest.
  —Drink plenty of fluids.
  —Weight reduction.

► Knee Arthroscopy

What is a knee arthroscopy? This is a procedure involving an examination and repair of the knee. The doctor uses an instrument called an *arthroscope*. It is like a tube almost as thick as a pencil. The doctor inserts the tube into the knee to examine and repair the area. It has small instruments on the end.

Why is it done? Arthroscopy is used to diagnose and treat causes of pain, swelling, tenderness, and weakness in the knee.

How is it done? The doctor inserts the arthroscope. She/he injects saltwater fluid into the knee and looks at the area. She/he may remove pieces of cartilage or repair a tear. There will be a few stitches. If the problem cannot be fixed, it will need open-knee surgery. You will need local, regional, or general anesthesia for the arthroscopy.

What do I have to do? This procedure is minor surgery. It usually takes only a few hours. Before the surgery, if you have general anesthesia, you may not eat or drink anything after midnight or before the procedure. After the surgery, you will need someone to drive you home the day of the surgery. Plan to rest for several days. Keep the leg elevated on several pillows.

Are there any complications or side effects? Call the doctor if there is too much pain, drainage, swelling in the knee, calf, or thigh.

Are there alternatives to this procedure? Yes, alternatives can range from doing little or nothing to open-knee surgery. Limiting activity and taking NSAIDs sometimes help. Braces and physical therapy can help too.

► Sprain

® Definition: Stretching or tearing of muscles and tendons. More frequent on hip, knee, and ankle.

® Goal: Prevent swelling, pain, or complications.

® Assessment:

—First degree: Some fiber tear but no decreased strength. Mild point tenderness, no abnormal motion, minimal swelling

—Second degree: Partial tear with some loss of function, point tenderness, light to mod., abnormal motion, hemorrhage

—Third degree: Complete tear with total function loss, marked abnormal motion, possible deformity

® Signs and symptoms: Pain, swelling, difficult to use joint.

• Causes: Trauma, wrenching or twisting of joint w partial tear of its ligaments.

® Complications: Damage to adjacent muscles, blood vessels, tendons, and nerves.

• Tx goal: Prevent swelling pain. Prevent complications.

—Elevate the injured part to reduce swelling. Use pillows or blankets for comfort.

—Ice packs used intermittently help reduce swelling during the first 48 hr (See Home Tx SI, Appendix A: Ice Pack).

—Follow w heat to area (See Home Tx SI, Appendix A: Warm Compress).

—Tylenol as needed for discomfort.

—Limited activity until healing occurs.

—If you have an elastic bandage, don't wrap it too tightly. Always take it off when you sleep.

► Strain

• Definition: Injury to muscle, soft tissue between joints and tendon caused by overuse (chronic strain) or overstress (trauma). More frequent in muscles and feet.

° Assessment:

—First degree: Does not reduce strength. Local pain and tenderness increase w movement. Mild spasm and swelling may be present.

—Second degree: Partial decrease in strength, local pain, moderate spasm, swelling, bruising

—Third degree: Severe pain, swelling, hematoma, loss of muscle function

- Signs and symptoms: Pain w/o swelling.
- Causes: Overuse or overstretching of muscles around joint.
- Complications: Muscle, blood vessel, tendon, and nerve damage.
- Prevention/Tx: For mild strain.
  —Rest, or don't move area.
  —Ice Pack prn for spasm and swelling (See Home Tx SI, Appendix A: Ice Pack).
  —Analgesic as appropriate.

▶ Tutorial

Red Flags

Red flags are populations and symptoms that increase risk in orthopedic problems (SAVED: severe symptoms, high-risk populations: age, veracity, emotional distress, debilitation).

- Symptoms: Severe, sudden or suspicious pain. Beware of pain that is more severe than expected, unrelenting.
- Age: Very young and very old patients have increased risk of infection/fracture.
- Debilitation: Orthopedic problems occur more frequently in patients with diabetes, cardiac problems, or previous orthopedic problems.
- Pregnant: Postpartum: higher risk of deep vein thrombosis (DVT).
- Recent injury: Local joint trauma predisposes for infection.
- Illness/Infection: History of implants, chronic disease, IV drug abuse, local joint trauma, all immune deficiencies: AIDS/HIV, chemo, diabetes, cystic fibrosis, asthma, splenectomy, steroid therapy, transplants, cancer; frail elderly or children are high-risk populations for infection.

Rules of Thumb

- "5 P's" of compartment syndrome: Pain, Pallor, Paresthesia, Pulselessness, Paralysis.
- All severe pain must be seen within 8 hr or less.
- The open fracture has the greatest risk of infection.
- All orthopedics: Chronic diseases lengthen the healing process.
- The decision to apply a tourniquet is irreversible. (Use one only as last resort in life-threatening circumstances.)
- Always err on the side of caution.
- Beware the middle-of-the-night call.
- Beware of any pain that awakens patient or prevents sleep at night.
- Kids get sicker quicker.
- Minority callers may fail to recognize acute symptoms, report fewer symptoms, or attribute them to other causes.

Red Herrings

"Red herrings" are common distracters (symptoms or situations) that lead the nurse astray, away from the main problem.

- Remain vigilant to possible patient denial, minimization, and misinterpretation of symptoms.
- Regard with suspicion: All elderly callers and unusual sounding presentations, including symptoms described as "the flu," or new, sudden, or unexpected.
- Patients who have been "seen recently" may still need to be seen today.

- Do not be misled by concurrent complaints or patient self-explanation.
- Patients "on medication" may be on the wrong medication (antibiotics).
- Denial is the first symptom of abuse.
- Symptom presentation may be early, late, silent, atypical, or novel.
- Symptoms of two conditions may present concurrently, causing confusion or misinterpretation.

LIP/MOUTH; TEETH/GUMS; TONGUE PROBLEM
Pain with or without Trauma; Swelling; Laceration; Lesions

ASSESSMENT	ACUITY LEVEL	DISPOSITION/ADVICE
Key Questions	**Emergent Symptom Patterns**	**ED 0 min-1 hr**
Major Trauma	- ➤	Consider head/neck injury with face/mouth/tooth/trauma
Lip/Tongue Swelling	+ SOB, wheezing, stridor, difficulty swallowing, agitation, anxiety, rash (itchy, raised, "hive-like"), swelling of face/tongue, Hx of allergies or exp. to allergen [med., drug (esp. ACE inhibitors), food, chemical, substance, bite]? (Anaphylaxis)- - - - - - - - - - - - - ➤	Benadryl
Key Questions	**Urgent Symptom Patterns**	**ED/UCC/Office 1 -8 hr**
Laceration of Mouth, Lips, Tongue	+ Persistent bleeding, Hx of bleeding disorder, anticoagulants, liver/renal disorder? (> Risk Hemorrhage)- -	(See SI, First Aid)
Trauma to Tooth	+ Avulsed? (Head Injury).................................	(See Head Problem SI, First Aid)
Oral Lesion (any)	+ Difficulty swallowing, unable to eat or drink, dehydrated, decreased urine output? (Possible Dehydration)	
	+ Facial swelling, fever? (Abscess)	
Key Questions	**Acute/Nonacute Symptom Patterns**	**FA 8 + hr ± Home Tx**
Tooth Bleeding	+ Postop 24-48 hr? (See SI)	
Lesion/Pain (Mouth/Tongue)	+ Thick, white, patchy coating on tongue, sides of mouth, bleeds w attempts to wipe off, Hx of AIDS/immunosuppression, difficulty swallowing/ eating, Sx of mod. dehydration? (Thrush > Risk Dehydration)	
	+ Cluster of tiny clear blisters, begins w tingling, itching, pain, followed by yellow, crusty crater after 1-2 days; first time; w severe throat pain, poss. moderate dehydration? (Herpes)	

(continued)

Key Questions	Acute/Nonacute Symptom Patterns	FA 8 + hr ± Home Tx
Lesion/Pain (Mouth/Tongue) (continued)	+ Fistula drainage into gum from cheek? (Dental Root Abscess)	
	+ Ulcer, single, painless, doesn't bleed, Hx of STI exp.? (Syphilitic Chancres)	
Red Gums	+ Swelling, pain, bleeding, bad breath? (Gingivitis)	
Lesions (all)	+ Gum swelling, Hx of dilantin? (Gingival Hypertrophy)	
	+ Painless persistent sore, growth (floor of mouth, side of tongue)? (Carcinoma)	
	+ White plaque, persistent Hx of smoking? (Hairy Leukoplakia)	
Black Teeth	+ Broken, pain, soft, sticky sweets, poor dental hygiene? (Dental Caries)	

Cross-References

Face/Jaw Problem	Head Problem 1; 2	

LIP/MOUTH; TEETH/GUMS; TONGUE PROBLEM
Supplemental Information

Quick Reference:
- ▶ First Aid
  - Laceration
  - Tooth Transport
  - Cold Compress
- ▶ Canker Sore (Aphthous Ulcer)
- ▶ Dental Hygiene

- ▶ Herpes (Herpes Simplex)
- ▶ Lip/Mouth/Gum Lesions
- ▶ Smokers/Tobacco Chewers
- ▶ Stomatitis (Viral)
- ▶ Tooth Bleeding
- ▶ Tooth Pain

▶ **First Aid**
- Laceration
  - —Apply firm pressure w clean cloth until patient gets to ED.
  - —Do not stop pressure—bleeding will get worse.
- Tooth transport
  - —Save tooth! Place tooth in glass of milk or saline solution or in mouth between gum and teeth (See Home Tx SI, Appendix A: Tooth Transport).
- Cold compress

▶ **Canker Sore (Aphthous Ulcer)**
- Signs and symptoms: Inner lip and mucous membranes only: Single lesion usually. Painful, red sore, becomes ulcer w red base and whitish center and less tender. Resolves in 2 to 14 days.
- Causes: Many—Hypersensitivity, physical/emotional stress, chemical/food irritants, endocrine changes.
- Tx:
  - —Pain: Tylenol as appropriate.
  - —Pain: Orajel.
  - —Don't drink citrus juice (orange, grapefruit, lemonade).
- Prevention: Do not share glasses, food, drink, utensils, kisses w person who has mouth/lip lesion.

▶ **Dental Hygiene**
- Home Tx:
  - —Brush teeth/gums at least once a day.
  - —Eat hard fruits and vegetables (apple, carrot, celery, etc.).
  - —New toothbrush after infection.
  - —No fruit rollups if possible.

▶ **Herpes (Herpes Simplex) (Recurrent or primary)**
- Signs and symptoms: See Protocol.
- Causes: Herpes simplex virus I and II.

- Tx:

    —Pain and fever: Tylenol as appropriate

    —Pain: Orajel, cold drinks, popsicles (age appropriate)

    —Wash hands often w warm water and soap.

- Prevention: Do not share glasses, food, drink, utensils, kisses w person who has mouth/lip lesions.

► **Lip/Mouth/Gum Lesions**

- Age appropriate:

    —Swish and swallow antacid.

    —Orajel

    —Bland diet and soothing liquids (See Home Tx SI, Appendix A: "BRAT" Diet; Clear Liquids).

    —No citrus juice (orange, grapefruit, lemonade).

    —Analgesics.

- Prevention: Do not share glasses, food, drink, utensils, kisses w person who has mouth/lip lesions. Boil nipples and pacifier if infection diagnosed.

► **Smokers/Tobacco Chewers**

- Complications:

    —Increased risk of cancer in mouth/tongue.

► **Stomatitis (Viral)**

- Frequent cause of throat pain. Sx should go away after a few days of home Tx. If there are lesions, white patches, severe pain, or bright red throat, the pt needs to be seen.

► **Tooth Bleeding**

- Tooth bleeding Tx goal: Stop bleeding.

    —Bite firmly on gauze pad x 20 min, or bite firmly on nonherbal, cooled tea bag. Tannic acid reduces bleeding.

    —Do not rinse mouth! It may remove clots and start bleeding again.

    —Soft diet (See Home Tx SI, Appendix A: Soft Diet).

► **Tooth Pain**

- Tooth pain Tx goal: Relieve pain.

    —Pain: Tylenol, NSAIDs.

    —Avoid hot and cold drinks.

    —Ice pack/cold compress to jaw area that is painful (See Home Tx SI, Appendix A: Cold/Cool Compress/Ice Pack).

NECK PROBLEM
Pain with or without Trauma; Swelling; Lump

1 ASSESSMENT	ACUITY LEVEL	DISPOSITION/ADVICE
Key Questions	**Emergent Symptom Patterns**	**ED 0 min-1 hr**
Major Trauma	- ➤	+ Do not move patient! Consider head injury w face/jaw/neck trauma
	+ All penetrating wounds?...............-......................	(See Neck Problem SI, First Aid)
	+ Trouble breathing, severe pain or tenderness, crying w/o sound, can't talk, hoarseness, coughing up blood, extreme anxiety? (Tracheal Injury)	
	+ Weakness/numbness/tingling or inability to move one or more extremities, loss of bowel/bladder control, change in level of consciousness? (Cervical Spine Injury)	
Pain	+ Chest pain: ± exertion (dull ache, pressure, squeezing, crushing, radiates to neck/jaw/arms), SOB, sweating, dizziness, lightheadedness, N/V, pale, anxiety, sense of impending doom? (MI/Angina)	
	+ Headache, photophobia, fever/chills, N/V, ± confusion, restlessness, somnolence, ± Hx of HIV? (Meningitis/Encephalitis)-----------------------	SA: Pain when putting chin to chest + (inability to touch chin to chest = +) + Do not attempt if recent trauma.

Key Questions	**Urgent Symptom Patterns**	**ED/UCC/Office 1-8 hr**
Trauma	+ Hx of trauma within 2-3 days w/o emergent symptoms, increasing stiffness and/or pain, interfering w sleep? (Cervical Strain/Sprain)	
	+ Twitching of neck muscles (uncontrollable, painful, severe), Hx phenothiazine use? (Dystonic Reaction)	
Lump/Swelling	+ Redness, tenderness, warm to touch, fever? (Abscess, Cervical Lymphadenitis)	

Key Questions	Acute/Nonacute Symptom Patterns	ED/UCC/Office 1 -8 hr
Pain	+ Stiff neck from sleeping, repetitive motions, ± Hx recent MVA? (Cervical Strain, Torticollis)	
	+ Hx of arthritis, > pain w movement? (Arthritis)	
	+ Hx recent trauma, cancer, spinal surgery, rheumatoid arthritis, immunosuppression? (> Risk)	
Lump/Swelling	+ Progressive > in size, nontender, w/o Hx recent infection? (Mass: Benign/Neoplastic)	
	+ W/o redness/drainage, w Hx HRI or flu? (Lymphadenopathy)	
	+ Pain, ± fever, anorexia, malaise, pain on chewing/ swallowing acidic fluids, exp. to mumps? (Mumps)	
	+ Swollen glands, fever, fatigue, anorexia, N/V, sore throat? (Mononucleosis)	

Cross References
Respiratory Problem 2

NECK PROBLEM
Supplemental Information

Quick Reference:
- ► First Aid
  - Laceration/Penetrating Object
- ► General Advice
- ► Drug Side Effect (Dystonia)
- ► Mumps
- ► Neck Injury Instructions

► **First Aid**
- Laceration/Penetrating Object
  - —Do not remove penetrating object!
    - ° If bleeding, apply direct pressure.
    - o Never apply pressure to both sides of the neck at the same time.

► **General Advice**
- Lymph node swelling: Lymph nodes can double in size w minor throat or cold infections. Can take months to go down.
- Neck trauma: Stiffness and pain are worst on the day following injury.

► **Drug Side Effect: Dystonia**
- Signs and symptoms: Uncontrollable, painful, severe twitching of neck muscles
- Drugs and classes of drugs that may cause dystonia:
  - —Fluphenazine (Prolixin)
  - —Haloperidol (Haldol)
  - —Loxapine (Loxatine)
  - —Molindone (Moban)
  - —Perphenazine (Trilafon)
  - —Phenothiazines:
    - ° Chlorpromazine (Thorazine)
    - o Prochlorperazine (Compazine)
    - ° Thioridazine (Mellaril)
    - ° Trifluoperazine (Stelazine)
  - —Risperidone (Risperdal)
  - —Thiothixene (Navane)

► **Mumps**
- Signs and symptoms: See Protocol.
- Causes: Virus, contagious.
- Complications: May cause meningitis, pancreatitis, or inflammation of testicles and ovaries. Usually does not affect fertility.
- Tx: Soft diet (See Home Tx SI, Appendix A: Soft Diet), isolation; no acidic drinks
- Prevention: MMR immunization

▶ Neck Injury Instructions

- Goal: Relieve pain. Increase function.
- Pain: Tylenol.
- Use hot or cold compresses (See Home Tx SI, Appendix A: Cold/Cool Compress) on the injured area, whichever seems to help the most. Be careful not to burn yourself.
- Rest as much as possible until you feel better.
- Don't do anything that causes the pain. Do not drive if possible.
- Relax. Tension makes the problem worse.
- Take a hot shower; drink warm tea. Do whatever helps you to relax.
- Gentle but firm massage will relax the muscles and will help to get rid of the soreness.

NOSE/SINUS PROBLEM
Pain with or without Trauma; Foreign Body; Bleeding; Discharge; Congestion

1 ASSESSMENT	ACUITY LEVEL	DISPOSITION/ADVICE
Key Questions	**Emergent Symptom Patterns**	ED 0 Min-1 Hr
Major Trauma	+ All head trauma? (See Head Problem 1; 2)-------→	- Always consider head/neck injury with nose trauma
Key Questions	**Urgent Symptom Patterns**	ED/UCC/Office 1-8 hr
Trauma	+ Obvious deformity, blocked breathing (unilateral)? (Septal Hematoma/Nasal Fx)	
Bleeding ± Trauma	+ Uncontrolled w home Tx x 20 min, ± Hx anticoagulants, bleeding disorder, Hx of > BP, renal/liver disease, w/o symptom shock? (Epistaxis, > Risk Hemorrhage)	
Pain w/o Trauma	+ Acute facial sinus pain, ± high fever, redness, swelling, esp. near eye, abnormal vision, severe headache, weak immune system, recent chemotherapy, Hx steroid medication, diabetic, recently hospitalized, mental status change? (Acute Bacterial Sinusitis/Preseptal/Periorbital Cellulitis)	
Key Questions	**Acute/Nonacute Symptom Patterns**	FA 8+ hr ± Home Tx
Pain w/o Trauma	+ Facial/sinus pain, URI symptoms >7-10 days, yellow/green nasal discharge, postnasal discharge, cough, pressure in teeth, bad breath, ± fever, swollen glands? (Rhinosinusitis)	
Bleeding w/o Trauma	+ (Mild) ± Nose picking, recurrent, brief? (Simple Epistaxis)-----------------------------------	Humidify air; lubricate nostrils
	+ Cocaine Hx? (Mucosal Damage, Chronic Irritation)	
	+ Recurrent, frequent? (Leukemia Neoplasm)	

(continued)

Key Questions	Acute/Nonacute Symptom Patterns		FA 8+ hr ± Home Tx

Congestion	+ Discharge (watery), itchy, teary eyes, sneezing
	  + fatigue, pollen season? (Allergic Rhinitis)
	
	+ Discharge, cough, sputum, fever, achy, hoarseness?
	  (URI) (See Respiratory Problem 1)
	
	+ Stuffiness, Hx of nasal Rx or BP Rx?
	  (Chronic Rhinitis)		

Cross-References

Eye Problem 1; 2	Face/Jaw Problem	Head Problem 1; 2	Respiratory Problem 1; 2

NOSE/SINUS PROBLEM
Supplemental Information

Quick Reference:
- ▶ General Advice
- ▶ Allergies
- ▶ Drug Side Effect (Nasal Congestion)
- ▶ Nosebleed
- ▶ Sinus Infection
  - Rhinosinusitis

▶ General Advice
- Smoking: Increases risk for URI.
- Blowing nose too hard may lead to earache.
- Dairy products (cheese, milk, ice cream, yogurt) increase mucus. Avoid when you have a cold.

▶ Allergies
- Tx goal: Relieve symptoms. Prevent > exposure to allergen.
  - —Don't go outdoors on hot, windy days in pollen season.
  - —No indoor flowers, feather pillows, pets.
  - —Drink 8 glasses water, juice, soda daily.
  - —Nasal congestion: Saline nose drops (See Home Tx SI, Appendix A: Saline Nose Drops).
  - —Congestion: No OTC nasal sprays.
  - —Steam Tx (See Home Tx SI, Appendix A: Steam Treatment).

▶ Drug Side Effect: Nasal Congestion

Rules of Thumb
- Overuse of nasal meds can lead to chronic, stuffy, congested nose. Following are drugs or classes of drugs that cause nasal congestion:
  - —Amitriptyline
  - —Birth control pills
  - —Beta-blockers
  - —Chlordiazepoxide (Librium)
  - —Clonidine (Catapres)
  - —Estrogens
  - —Hydralazine (Apresoline)
  - —Methyldopa (Aldomet)
  - —Reserpine (Serpasil-Apresoline)

▶ Nosebleed
- Tx goal: Stop nosebleed. Prevent more nosebleeds.
  - —Sit up, lean forward.

- Adult Protocols

      —Don't swallow blood, spit it out.

      —Pinch soft part of nose x 10 min; if bleeding continues, call back.

      —Apply cold compress to bridge of nose (See Home Tx SI, Appendix A: Cold/Cool Compress).

      —Use steam to < dryness of air.

      —Put small amount of Vaseline inside nose.

- Prevention:

      —No hot beverages x 24 hr after nosebleed (may start bleeding).

      —No heavy lifting, straining x 24 hr.

      —No ASA, Motrin, Ibuprofen, Naprosyn, Advil (> Bleeding).

      —You may throw up from swallowing blood. It will look like coffee grounds.

      —After nosebleed stops, do not blow nose. It can cause bleeding to start again.

      —Always blow nose gently.

► Sinus Infection

There are four sinuses in the head. They help to warm and moisturize the air.

Rhinosinusitis

- Cause: Most sinus infections are caused by viruses, which are not treated with antibiotics. Some sinus infections become bacterial infections (Acute Bacterial Sinusitis).
- Prevention/Tx:

      —Antibiotics will be needed if the symptoms do not get better or if symptoms include high fever, acute facial pain, redness, or swelling.

      —Bacterial sinus infection may be serious if untreated, although this is rare.

      —Swimming allowed. Avoid jumping in water feet first.

      —No diving unless wearing nose plug—causes pressure on sinuses.

      —Warm washcloth over face, nose, TID.

      —Avoid smoking.

PENILE/SCROTAL/TESTICLE PROBLEM
Trauma; Foreign Body; Pain; Discharge; Lumps, Lesions; STI Exposure

ASSESSMENT	ACUITY LEVEL	DISPOSITION/ADVICE
Key Questions	Emergent Symptom Patterns	ED 0 min-1 hr
Major Trauma	+ Severe hemorrhage, refusal to urinate? (Urethral Rupture/Poss. pelvic Fx)	
Key Questions	Urgent Symptom Patterns	ED/UCC/Office 1-8 hr
Trauma	+ Straddle injury w or w/o bleeding at meatus, swelling? (Urethral Injury)	
	+ Zipper injury w glans or foreskin embedded in zipper?--Do not attempt to unzip	
	+ Scrotum pain/swelling? (Hematocele)	
	+ Recent circumcision, bleeding continuous? (> Risk Hemorrhage)	
Pain (Penile)	+ Continuous erection > 1 hr, Hx sickle cell disease/leukemia? ± Hx ED Rx: Viagra, shots, pellets (Priapism)	
Pain (Scrotal/Testicle)	+ (Sudden, severe, unilateral) Swelling, N/V ± Hx of similar pain, impotence (Testicular Torsion; Testicular Rupture)	
	+ Bulge at groin/scrotum, tender, N/V, uncomfortable? (Incarcerated Hernia) (See Abdomen Problem 2; SI)──▶	SA: Touch: Tense or
	+ Swelling, gradual, ± Hx of mumps, STI exp.? (Orchitis)	hand = +
	+ Fever frequency, urgency, painful urination swelling of scrotum? (Epididymitis)	
	+ Grossly bloody urine? (Kidney Stone)	
	+ Severe pain, ± rapid onset/red skin, recent cicumcision, ± streaking, swollen, tender, hot; ± discharge, often w fever, swollen nodes, + Hx of infection? (Cellulitis; Necrotizing Fasciitis)	
Discharge (Penile)	+ Uncircumcised, redness/swelling of glans, pus discharge? (Balanitis)	

Key Questions	Acute/Nonacute Symptom Patterns	FA 8+ hr ± Home Tx
Lump (Scrotal/ Testicular)?	+ Diffuse enlargement, unilateral, or hard/painless lump in testicle? (Testicular Tumor)	
Discharge (Penile)	+ Hx of unprotected intercourse 1-3 wk prior? (Gonorrhea, *Trichomonas, Chlamydia*)	
Lesion (Ulceration)	+ Cluster of tiny clear blisters, begins w tingling, itching, pain, followed by yellow, crusty crater after 1-2 days, watery discharge, dysuria; first time? (Herpes)	
	+ Painless, red papule, generalized rash? (Syphilitic Chancre)	
Scrotal Pain/Swelling	+ Inguinal swelling, bright, beefy red, lived in tropical area? (Lymphogranuloma Venereum)	
	+ Soft, moist, pink, cauliflowerlike (Venereal Warts)	
	+ Bulge at groin/scrotum, tender, no N/V & comfortable? (Inguinal Hernia) (See Abdomen Problem)	
	+ Painless dull ache; swelling, unilateral, ± feels like "bag of worms"? (Varicocele/Hydrocele)	
	+ Gradual onset, mild fever, no Hx mumps/MMR immz, swelling below ears on neck? (Orchitis)	
Lesion/Ulceration (Groin)	+ Inguinal swelling, abscess in groin w red shiny skin over abscess? (Chancroid)	
Irritation (Penile)	+ Sore glands/prepuce, penis after intercourse, white, cheesy discharge, Hx of partner w yeast infection? (*Candida*)	
Recent Vasectomy?	- -▶	Apply ice and elevate scrotum on towels until Rx can be obtained

Cross-References Abdomen Problem 1; 2	Urinary Problem	Vaginal Problem: STI SI

PENILE/SCROTAL/TESTICLE PROBLEM
Supplemental Information

Quick Reference:

- » Adhesions
- ► Circumcision
- ► Impotence
- ► Meatitis
- ► Mumps

- ► Penile Hygiene
- ► Postop Vasectomy
- ► Sexually Transmitted Infection
- ► Smegma
- ► Torsion

See also: Directory of Hotlines/Web Sites for Support Groups, Appendix E

► Adhesions

- Definition: Scar tissue, contracted tissue stuck to infection/trauma site/surface
- Causes: Infection, trauma, previous surgery, chronic manipulation of tissue
- Q Complications: Inability to retract tissue w > amount of adhesions (i.e., foreskin)
- 0 Prevention/Tx: Sitz bath (See Home Tx SI, Appendix A: Sitz Bath) to release adhesions to widen opening/ tissue ROM. Only pull foreskin if it pulls back easily. *Never force it back!* Clean w soap and water.

► Circumcision

- ® Definition: Surgical removal of the foreskin (prepuce) from the penis.
- Causes: Surgery is done for cultural or religious reasons, or because parents want it done.
- Complications: Hemorrhage, infection.
- Prevention/Tx: Cover glans after procedure w sterile gauze and petroleum jelly to prevent infection and irritation. Change dressing frequently. Watch for signs and Sx of bleeding, infection, urine output. Heals within 3-4 days.

► Impotence

- ® Definition: Inability to have an erection
- Causes: May be caused by systemic disease, alcoholism, drugs, thyroid problem, vascular problem, emotional problem, diabetes. Medical checkup recommended
- « Complications: Infection, abscess, depression, not able to function sexually

► Meatitis

- s Definition: Inflammation/infection of urethra at end of penis
- ® Causes: Mild phimosis, hypospadias, trauma, diaper rash
- « Complications: UTI, meatal ulcerations, meatal stenosis, septicemia
- o Prevention/Tx:
  - —Penile hygiene if uncircumcised; sitz bath (See Home Tx SI, Appendix A: Sitz Bath). Age > 4 yr: Only pull foreskin if it pulls back easily. *Never force it back!* Clean w soap and water.
  - —Systemic antibiotic therapy.

► **Mumps**

> (See Skin Problem Lesion/Lump/Swelling)

► **Penile Hygiene**

- Prevention/Tx: Sitz bath (See Home Tx, Appendix A: Sitz Bath)

► **Postop Vasectomy**

- Definition: Surgical sterilization of male
- Complications: Infection, bleeding
- Tx: Mild discomfort, bruising, swelling are to be expected; should improve each day

► **Sexually Transmitted Infection (STI)**

> (See Vaginal Problem: STI SI)

- Definition: Infection passed from person to person through genital, oral, rectal contact.
- Causes: Bacteria, virus, yeast.
- Complications: Sterility, severe illness affecting heart, brain, reproduction.
- Prevention: Condoms should be used during entire act of intercourse and should not break. Avoid intercourse, rectal, or oral contact until treated for lesions or discharge (any STIs).
- Additional teaching:

  —*Chlamydia* is now the most common bacterial cause of STI.

  —Best time for obtaining culture is early morning after awakening and before shower.

  —Never collect urine specimen before culture is taken from male.
- HIV Testing: Suggest testing for virus if Hx of unprotected sex.
- Patients using IV drugs or w Hx of exposure to HIV are at risk.

► **Smegma**

- Definition: Cheesy material in or around foreskin of penis; may smell bad
- Cause: Normal discharge
- Prevention/Tx: Sitz bath (See Home Tx SI, Appendix A: Sitz Bath)

► **Torsion**

- Definition: Twisting of testicle on its cord. This is an emergency.
- Causes: Strenuous activity, or development abnormality.
- Complications: Loss of testicle.
- Tx: Needs immediate surgical intervention.

RECTAL PROBLEM
Pain with or without Trauma; FB; Bleeding; Itching; Discharge; Lesion

ASSESSMENT	ACUITY LEVEL	DISPOSITION/ADVICE
Key Questions	Emergent Symptom Patterns	ED 0 min–1 hr
Major Trauma	+ Sx of shock: weak, dizzy, cold/mottled/pale skin, blue lips/nail beds, rapid/shallow breathing, unresponsive, loss of consciousness? (Shock) (See Shock)	
Key Questions	Urgent Symptom Patterns	EDU/UCC/Office 1–8 hr
Bleeding	+ Large amt. rectal bleeding, black, maroon or tarry stools? (GI Bleeding)	
	+ Throbbing (severe.), swelling, ± fever? (Anorectal Abscess)	
Key Questions	Acute/Nonacute Symptom Patterns	FA 8+ hr ± Home Tx
Pain	+ Itching, bleeding (mod. to sm.), burning, painful BM, purulent discharge, Hx of STI exp.? (Proctitis, STI)	
	+ Female age > 60 yr, new onset difficult bowel movements? (Rectocele)	
	+ Swelling, discharge in rectal/sacral area? (Pilonidal Cyst)	
	+ Prolapsed rectum, female > 60 yr? (Prolapsed Rectum)	
Lesion(s)	+ Painless, red papule in anus? (Syphilis) (See Vaginal Problem: STI)	
	+ Itchy Warts? (Condylomata, Syphilis) (See Vaginal Problem: STI SI)	
	+ Cluster of tiny clear blisters, begins w tingling, itching, pain, followed by yellow, crusty crater after 1-2 days; first time; w sev. pain? (Herpes) (See Vaginal Problem: STI SI)	

(continued)

Key Questions	Acute/Nonacute Symptom Patterns	FA 8+ hr ± Home Tx
Bleeding (w Mild Pain or w/o Pain)	+ Sm. amt., bright red, on outside of BM, on toilet tissue, or toilet bowl? (Hemorrhoids, Fissure, Polyp, Carcinoma)	
Discharge	+ Hx recurrent abscess? (Fistula)	
Itching	+ Excessive scratching? (Contact Dermatitis) (See Skin Problem: Rash)	
	+ Red, moist, perianal area, reddened patchy rash? (Candidiasis)	
	+ Hx of pinworm infestation in household? (Pinworms)	

Cross-References		
Bowel Problem 1; 2	Skin Problem: Rash	Vaginal Problem: STI SI

RECTAL PROBLEM
Supplemental Information

Quick Reference: ► Fissures

                     ► Hemorrhoids

► Fissures

- Definition/Cause: Cracks in rectal area caused by stretching and tearing of skin
- Complication: Constipation
- Prevention/Tx:
  —Sitz baths (See Home Tx SI, Appendix A: Sitz Bath)

► Hemorrhoids

- Definition: Enlarged blood vessels in the rectal area.
- Causes: Standing for prolonged periods, straining during bowel movement, pregnancy.
- Complications: Bleeding, pain, blood vessel sticks out, constipation.
- Prevention: Increase fiber and liquids (8 glasses/day) in diet. Avoid prolonged standing and sitting.
  —Eat more fruit and veg. (3 x day), prunes.
  —Drink 8 glasses water or juice daily.
  —Avoid standing and sitting for long periods of time.
- Home Tx goal: Relieve pain, itching. Prevent infection or complications.
  —Warm sitz baths. (See Home Tx SI, Appendix A: Sitz Bath)
  —Warm water bottle to rectal area.
  —OTC meds: Tucks, Preparation H.
  —Gently push hemorrhoid back up w finger.
  —Diet: Increase fiber; eat more fruits, vegetables, grains. (See Bowel Problem: Constipation)

RESPIRATORY PROBLEM 1: BREATHING PROBLEM/COUGH

Respiratory Distress; Choking; Shortness of Breath; Stridor; with or without Trauma

ASSESSMENT	ACUITY LEVEL	DISPOSITION/ADVICE
Key Questions	Emergent Symptom Patterns	ED 0 min-1 hr
Major Trauma	+ Respiratory distress?	
Severe Choking Episode w Anxiety/ Agitation	+ Assoc. w solid food/FB w color change, wheeze, unable to breathe/talk/cry, ± loss of consciousness? (FB aspiration)	
Stridor	+ Rapid onset high fever > 39.5°C or 103°F, muffled voice, throat pain, drooling, difficulty breathing/ swallowing, sits very still w jaw extended? (Epiglottitis)---	■*- Discourage opening mouth widely; nothing by mouth; do not use thermometer, or give food/drink + First Aid: keep patient sitting upright & calm until you reach ED
	+ SOB, wheezing, difficulty swallowing, agitation, anxiety, rash (itchy, raised, "hivelike"), swelling of face/tongue, Hx of allergies or exp. to allergen (med., drug, food, chemical, substance, bite)? (Anaphylaxis)--*	▶ Benadryl
Shortness of Breath	+ (Rapid, shallow) Fruity-smelling breath, recent Hx polyuria, polydipsia? (Diabetic Ketoacidosis)	
	+ Known asthmatic w failure to respond to 2-3 doses of Rx inhalant; resp. distress: Labored/rapid, wheezing; cyanosis; diaphoresis; agitation, confusion, lethargy? (Status Asthmaticus)	
	+ Steam, smoke, or toxic inhalant: Ammonia, fertilizers, chemical fumes? (Chemical/Thermal Burn)................	*- Bring substance to ED w you
	+ Acute onset: Frothy pink sputum, ± chest pain, unable to lie flat? (Pulmonary Edema)	
	+ Chest pain/SOB/cough; anxious, restless, sweating, faintness, Hx BCP/phlebitis/immobilization/ calf pain/surgery/postpartum? (Pulmonary Embolus)	

(continued)

Key Questions	Emergent Symptom Patterns	ED 0 min-1 hr
Shortness of Breath (continued)	+ Chest pain: ± exertion (dull ache, pressure, squeezing, crushing, radiates to neck/jaw/arms), SOB, sweating, dizziness, lightheaded, N/V, pale, anxiety, sense of impending doom? (MI/Angina)	
	+ ± Trauma, sharp, severe chest pain, ± referred to shoulder/abd., dry hacking cough, ± Hx of TB, cystic fibrosis (school age), COPD, pneumothorax? (Pneumothorax: Traumatic or Spontaneous)	
Decreased, Shallow Respirations (marked)	+ Confusion, lethargy, blue lips, ± OD/ingestion? (Respiratory Failure)	

Key Questions	Urgent Symptom Patterns	ED/UCC/Office 1 -8 hr
Cough ± SOB	+ Sudden or gradual SOB, chest tightness, wheezing, coughing? (Asthma)	
	+ Chest/back/abd. pain, + > w resp., fever/chills, cough ± productive difficult breathing, N/V, fatigue? (Pneumonia: Viral, Bacterial, Aspiration)	
	+ W SOB, inspiratory chest pain, fever/chills? (Pleuritis: Bacterial, Viral, Fungal)	
	+ Palpitations, racing pulse, dizzy, lightheaded, > respiration (rapid, shallow), ± chest pressure, choking sensation, gasping, numbness/tingling in face, fingers, toes? (Hyperventilation Syndrome)	
	+ Chronic, > w exertion, > sputum, hx smoking? (COPD)	
	+ Difficult breathing, > w exertion, ± pedal edema, Hx heart disease, > BP? (Congestive Heart Failure)	

Key Questions	Acute/Nonacute Symptom Patterns	FA 8+ hr ± Home Tx
Cough (gradual onset)	+ Change in pattern, ± blood in sputum, chest pain? (Tumor)	
	+ Hx of HIV, lung disease, chemotherapy, diabetes, lupus, autoimmune disease? (> Risk Infection)	
	+ ± Productive, ± dyspnea, ± smoking, ± fever? (Bronchitis)	
	+ x 2 wk, w/o other Sx? (FB, TB, Asthma, CF, GE reflux)	
	+ Made worse by exercise or cold air, ± Hx of asthma? (Exercise-Induced Asthma)	
SOB	+ Pregnancy? (See Pregnancy Problems)	
Cough/Congestion	+ Chronic w clearing, > AM, seasonal rhinitis + Hx of allergy? (Allergy, Postnasal Drip)	
	+ Productive, runny nose, + fever? (Upper Respiratory Infection)	

Cross-References
Abuse
Chest Pain

Pregnancy Problems (As Appropriate)

Respiratory Problem 2:
Throat Pain

RESPIRATORY PROBLEM 2: THROAT PAIN
Choking; Foreign Body/Trauma; Pain; Burn: Chemical/Thermal

ASSESSMENT ACUITY LEVEL		DISPOSITION/ADVICE
Key Questions	Emergent Symptom Patterns	ED 0 min-1 hr
Cough (sudden), w Anxiety/Agitation	+ Severe chocking episode assoc, w solid food/FB w color change, wheeze, unable to breathe, talk, cry, w or w/o loss of consciousness? (FB Aspiration)	
Trauma (major)	+ Penetrating object? (Laceration/Hemorrhage)--------- → Do not remove impaled object!	
	+ Resp. distress? (Tracheal Injury)	
Pain/Difficulty Swallowing	+ Rapid onset high fever > 39.5°C or 103°F, muffled voice, drooling, insp. stridor, difficulty breathing, sits very still w jaw extended? (Epiglottitis/ Peritonsillar Abscess)----------------------------------- →	Discourage opening mouth widely; nothing by mouth; do not use thermometer, or give food/drink + First Aid: Keep pt. sitting upright & calm until you reach ED
Sore Throat	+ Throat/neck swelling, fever, difficulty swallowing, drooling, Hx of OM, nasal/pharyngeal infection, stiff neck, neck pain w movement? (Retropharyngeal Abscess)	
	+ Hx of ingestion or inhalation of caustic substance, steam, smoke, or toxic inhalant: chemical/fertilizer/ ammonia? (Chemical/Thermal Burn)-------------------- → Bring substance to ED w you	
	+ SOB, wheezing, stridor, difficulty swallowing, agitation, anxiety, rash (itchy, raised, "hivelike"), swelling of face/tongue, Hx of allergies or exp. to allergen (med, drug, food, chemical, substance, bite?) (Anaphylaxis)----------------------------------- – → Benadryl	

Key Questions	Urgent Symptom Patterns	ED/UCC/Office 1-8 hr
Sore Throat	+ + Severe, redness, swelling, difficulty swallowing, ± fever, ± STI exp. (oral sex)? (Pharyngitis: Gonorrhea, Syphilis, Herpes, *Chlamydia*)	

Key Questions	Acute/Nonacute Symptom Patterns	FA 8+ hr ± Home Tx
Pain (± severe)	+ Lesion, thick, white, patchy, coating on tongue, sides of mouth, bleeds w attempts to wipe off, Hx of AIDS/immunosuppression, difficulty swallowing/ eating? (Candidiasis, > Risk Dehydration)	
Pain (± mild)	+ Fever, fatigue, anorexia, N/V, sore throat, swollen glands? (Mononucleosis)	
	+ Hx allergies? (Postnasal Drip) (See Nose/Sinus Problem)	
	+ Runny nose, hoarseness, cough, minor aches and pains, ± fever, *Strep* unlikely? (Upper Respiratory Infection) (See Respiratory Problem 1)	

Cross-References		
Nose/Sinus Problem	Respiratory Problem 1	Vaginal Problem: STI SI

RESPIRATORY PROBLEM
Supplemental Information

Quick Reference:

▶ Asthma
▶ Bronchitis
▶ Cough Treatment
▶ Epiglottitis
▶ Pneumonia

▶ Pneumothorax
▶ Sore Throat (Pharyngitis)
▶ *Strep* Pharyngitis
▶ Tuberculosis
▶ Upper Respiratory Infection

See also: Directory of Hotlines/Web Sites for Support Groups, Appendix E

▶ **Asthma**

Chronic Disease of Lung

- Signs and symptoms: See Protocol.
- Cause: Anxiety, allergies, and stress may be triggers.
- Complications: Severe, life-threatening asthma attack; death.
- Prevention/Tx:
    —Take Rx.
    —Avoid triggers: Exposure to cigarette smoke, pollen, dust, pets, sulfites, exercise, food allergies, strong fumes.
    —Avoid sudden change in temperature, altitude, humidity.
    —Avoid ASA; possible ASA-induced asthma.

▶ **Bronchitis**

Infection of Upper Breathing Tubes

® Signs and symptoms: See Protocol.
- Cause: Bacteria, virus, chemical.
- Complications: Pneumonia.
® Prevention: Take antibiotics until gone. Follow MD orders.

▶ **Cough Treatment**

- Cough Tx goal: Relieve Coughing. Prevent Complications.
    —Cough suppressant.
    —Steam Tx (See Home Tx SI, Appendix A: Steam Treatment).
    —Drink 2-3 extra glasses water or juice.

▶ **Epiglottitis**

- Signs and symptoms: See Protocol.
- Cause: Bacterial infection.
- Complications: Swelling blocks throat

>> Tx:

—Paramedic transport

—Antibiotics

—Hospitalization

• Prevention:

—Immunization

► Pneumonia

Infection of Lung (Contagious)

• Signs and symptoms: See Protocol.

• Cause: Bacteria, virus, or chemical; Aspiration.

• Complications: Lungs can be permanently damaged; death.

>> Prevention/Tx:

—Take all antibiotics. Follow MD orders.

—Pneumovax for splenectomy, sickle cell patients, elderly > 65, chronically ill, and all immunocompromised patients

► Pneumothorax

Collapsed Lung (Due to Break in Lung)

• Signs and symptoms: See Protocol

« Cause: Injury or disease such as TB

e Complications: Shock

► Sore Throat (Pharyngitis)

• Signs and symptoms: See Protocol

• Cause: Virus

• Complications: Tonsillitis

• Prevention/Tx:

—Soothe throat. Prevent others from getting infection.

—Rest. Drink 2-3 extra glasses of clear liquids—makes mucus easier to cough up.

—Steam treatment or humidifier at bedtime/nap time (See Home Tx SI, Appendix A: Steam Treatment).

—Throat pain: Tylenol; lozenges, Life-Savers, saline gargles, popsicles (See Home Tx SI, Appendix A: Popsicle; Saline Gargle/Mouthwash).

—Soft diet x days (bland, cooked, nonspicy foods).

—Don't eat ice cream, cheese, yogurt, milk (makes mucus).

—Stop smoking in house, reduces throat irritation.

—Avoid overheated rooms, esp. at night, reduces drying of throat.

—Antibiotics don't work. (Home Tx as above.) Most sore throats are viral.

► *Strep* Pharyngitis

Serious, Contagious Infection of Throat (Acute in onset, and lasts 3-4 days)

® Signs and symptoms: See Protocol.

® Cause: Bacteria. Streptococcal.

• Complications: Rheumatic fever, kidney disease, acute post-*Strep* glomerulonephritis.

℞ Prevention/Tx:

—Wash hands with soap frequently, esp. before meals.

—Do not share food, drinks, kisses.

—Do not go to work or school until 24 hr on antibiotics.

℞ Always take all Rx! Call back if no improvements within 48 hr.

—Throat pain: Tylenol; lozenges, Life-Savers, saline gargles, popsicles (See Home Tx SI, Appendix A: Popsicles; Saline Gargle/Mouthwash)

► Tuberculosis

Highly Contagious Lung Infection

o Signs and symptoms: See Protocol.

*   Cause: Bacteria.

*   Complications: May come back again and again. May affect bones, heart, kidneys.

0 Prevention:

—Always take all Rx. If you stop, the infection may come back stronger than before and may not respond to the medicine again.

—Family members and other contacts should have TB skin test.

► Upper Respiratory Infection (URI)

Affects lung, throat, nose—"cold"

℞ Causes: Virus, bacteria

o Complications: Bacterial infections; pneumonia

o Prevention:

—Avoid spreading germs by washing hands with soap + water frequently.

—Avoid kissing and sharing food.

—Antibiotics won't work on viruses, only bacteria. Discard unused or old antibiotics!

—Never use another person's Rx!

*   Tx:

—Comfort; relieve cough; liquefy secretions; < fever.

—Rest.

—Drink 8 or more glasses of clear liquids daily.

—Saline nose drops (See Home Tx SI, Appendix A).

—Steam treatment (See Home Tx SI, Appendix A).

—Pain/Fever: Tylenol (unless allergic).

—Cough: Robitussin.

—Congestion: Sudafed.

SEIZURES
With or without Trauma

ASSESSMENT ACUITY LEVEL		DISPOSITION/ADVICE
Key Questions	Emergent Symptom Patterns	ED 0 min-1 hr
Seizures (All)	+ Sudden falling, pale, loss of consciousness, twitching, jerking, stiffening, incontinence, eyes roll upward---	Rule of Thumb: All first-time seizures must come in
	+ Most often grand mal type; continuous seizure activity lasting > 20 min; also recurrent seizures (> 2) w/o regaining consciousness between seizures? (Status Epilepticus)----------------------------	*- (See Seizures SI, First Aid)
	+ Any first time seizure?	
	+ Trauma Hx?	
	+ Pregnancy? (Pregnancy-Induced Hypertension; Eclampsia)	
	+ Febrile, heat stroke? (Hyperpyrexic Seizure)------------	(See Heat Exposures SI, First Aid)
	+ Meningitis, encephalitis, abscess? (CNS Infection)	
	+ Skull Fx?	
	+ Hx exposure to street drugs/cocaine/alcohol, Rx, poisonous plant; inhalation/ingestion of toxic chemical, pesticide, carbon monoxide (Toxic Exposure)---	Contact poison center; bring substance w you
	+ Hypoglycemia, liver failure, inborn errors of metabolism? (Metabolic)	
	+ Alcohol, tranquilizers, hypnotics? (Withdrawal)	
	+ Hematoma, tumor (Brain Lesions)	
		(continued)

Key Questions	Urgent Symptom Patterns	ED/UCC/Office 1-8 hr
Seizures (All) (continued)	+ Known epileptic single episode < 20 min followed by deep sleep, memory loss, confusion? + Hx seizure disorder? (Subtherapeutic Anticonvulsant Level: Noncompliance, Lowered Seizure Threshold Due to Illness)--► + Brief lapses in awareness, w/o loss of consciousness, ± rhythmic blinking, staring, nodding? (Petit Mai Seizure)	SA: Are you taking your medicine? ("No" = Noncompliance) + May need to come in for blood test

SEIZURES
Supplemental Information

Quick Reference: ► First Aid for Seizures

                        Rules of Thumb

                  ► First Aid for Heat Exposure

► **First Aid for Seizures**

    ® Do not pry jaw open. Do not put anything in mouth!

    ® If vomiting, turn on side.

    ® Protect patient from injury (e.g., move furniture or objects).

    • Do not restrain patient but be ready to protect head and clear out mouth if pt. vomits.

    • Patient may sleep after seizure. You don't have to keep person awake.

Rules of Thumb

o Seizures in person > 35 may precede a cardiac arrest.

® Grand mal seizures typically last 1 min.

► **First Aid for Heat Exposure**

    • Move to shaded/cool area.

    • Remove clothing.

    • Cool off as rapidly as possible w cool water by sponging skin: Head, groin, armpits.

    • If pt. is conscious and awake, give frequent sips of cool fluids,

e Massage extremities to > peripheral blood flow.

» Do not give ASA or Tylenol.

SHOCK
Distributive; Cardiogenic; Hypovolemic

ASSESSMENT	ACUITY LEVEL	DISPOSITION/ADVICE
Key Questions	Emergent Symptom Patterns	ED 0 min-1 hr
Shock Symptoms	---Call 911	
	+ Progressive: anxious, weak, dizzy, thirsty, N/V. Skin: pale, blotchy/discolored/cool or cold, sweaty. Lips/Nail Bed: blue; Pulse: weak/fast; Breathing: rapid/shallow, unresponsive, loss of consciousness? (Shock)---	*- (See Shock SI, First Aid)
	+ Major trauma history: MVA, fall, possible head/ spine injury/paraplegia? (Neurogenic)........................	-*-SA: Spinal injury (if yes, don't move unless in danger) + Loss of feeling? + Unable to move hands, legs, feet? + Numbness, tingling of hands/feet? + Sore spine?
	+ SOB, wheezing, stridor, difficulty swallowing, N/V, abdomen pain, agitation/anxiety, rash (itching, raised, "hivelike"), swelling of face/tongue, allergy history or within minutes of exposure to allergens (med, drug, food, chemical, substance, bite)? (Anaphylaxis)........................	■► Epikitas appropriate + Benadryl in any available form + Dose: Age and weight dependent
	+ Headache, neck pain, photophobia, fever/chills, N/V, ± confusion, restlessness, somnolence, ± history of HIV? (Sepsis, Meningitis)	
	+ Chest pain: ± exertion (dull ache, pressure, squeezing, crushing, radiates to neck/jaw/arms), SOB, sweating, dizziness, lightheaded, N/V, pale, anxiety, (MI/Angina, Cardiogenic)	
	+ Drug ingestion: accidental/purposeful, street drugs/Rx: barbiturates, poisonous plant, toxic chemical or pesticide? (Toxic Exposure/Ingestion)--^-	Contact poison center; bring substance w you
		(continued)

Key Questions	Emergent Symptom Patterns	ED 0 min–1 hr
Shock Symptoms (continued)	+ Pelvic pain, sharp, progressive, unilateral, ± radiates to shoulder, pale, lightheaded, fainting, history of ST1, PID, tubal/any abdominal surgery, prior IUD use, missed period x 3-6 wk, spotting, painful intercourse? (Ectopic Pregnancy)	
	+ Nausea/vomiting, fever, severe intractable diarrhea, rash, muscle aches, headache, confusion, dizziness, fainting? (Sepsis Syndrome)	
Shock history	-- ■▶	(See Shock SI, First Aid)
	+ Heat/cold exposure? (See Cold Exposure, Heat Exposure)	
	+ Electric shock?--- ▶	Caution: May not be safe to touch victim to administer first aid
	+ Severe dehydration, dizziness, weakness, diarrhea, hyperthermia?	
	+ Severe trauma to lower extremity? (Femur Fracture, Two or more Long-Bone Fractures)	
	+ Abdominal trauma, abdominal pain, left shoulder pain? (Liver/Spleen Rupture, Internal Bleeding)	
	+ Severe bleeding/hemorrhage/laceration?---------------- ▶	See Shock SI, First Aid: Bleeding/Laceration)

SHOCK
Supplemental Information

Quick Reference   ▶ First Aid

                         ▶ Rule of Thumb

                         ▶ Aggravating Factors for Shock

▶   **First Aid**

Shock

- Keep victim calm, warm, and quiet.
- Cover w blanket, if cold.
- Make sure victim can breathe easily.
- If no back or neck trauma (See below):
  —Lay patient flat. Raise feet 8-12 in.
  —Loosen clothing, tight belts, collar.
- Do not give food or drink.
- Stay w victim; watch carefully for signs of worsening shock.

Bleeding/Laceration

- Lay patient down.
- Raise the extremity that is bleeding above heart to cut down on bleeding.
- Apply pressure with a clean folded cloth.
- Arm wound: Apply pressure (firm and continuous) to pulse point inside the upper arm.
- Use four fingers. Apply pressure firmly against the bone until you can no longer feel the pulse.
- Leg wound: Place the victim on their back. Feel for the pulse in the groin area—at the top of the leg where the leg bends. Use the heel/palm of your hand for pressure. Keep your arm straight; press the artery firmly against the bone. If you need to, use both hands.
- Keep pressure on until help arrives.

▶   **Rule of Thumb**

- Any accident or illness can lead to shock.

▶   **Aggravating Factors for Shock**

- Pain
- Temperature extremes: Heat/cold exposure
- Exhaustion caused by extreme physical exertion: lack of food intake or dehydration
- Chronic illness: Chronic disease such as heart disease or diabetes
- Individual response to injury, pain, or emotional stress
- Improper care: Rough handling; improper treatment

SKIN PROBLEM: BITES (HUMAN, ANIMAL)
Cat; Dog; Bat; Horse; Squirrel; Skunk; Raccoon; Fox

ASSESSMENT	ACUITY LEVEL	DISPOSITION/ADVICE
Key Questions	Emergent Symptom Patterns	ED 0 min-1 hr
All Bites (Animal)	+ Progressive: anxious, weak, dizzy, thirsty, N/V, Skin: pale, blotchy/discolored/cool or cold, sweaty. Lips/Nail Bed: blue. Pulse: weak/fast. Breathing: rapid/shallow, unresponsive, loss of consciousness? (Shock) (See Shock)	
Key Questions	Urgent Symptom Patterns	ED/UCC/Office 1-8 hr
Bite	+ Multiple or large wound, face, head, or neck laceration? (> Risk Infection, Hemorrhage)	
	+ Persistent bleeding, history of bleeding disorder, anticoagulants, kidney/liver disease, Hx cancer, chemotherapy radiation (> Risk Hemorrhage)	
	+ High-risk locations: hand, wrist, foot, over major joint, through cheek, face or scalp? (Infection, Fracture)	
	+ High-risk wounds: all punctures, crushing (horses, cows), over vital structure: nerve, joint, artery? (Infection, Fracture)	
	+ Unprovoked attack by sick, rabid cat, dog, or any wild animal: raccoons, squirrels, bats, foxes, skunks, rodents? (> Risk Rabies)	
	+ Over knuckles: "fight bite," abraded, lacerated, punctured skin from teeth of another human? (> Risk Infection)	
	+ Red ± streaking, swollen, tender, hot; ± discharge, often w fever, swollen nodes, history of trauma/ bite/local infection? (Cellulitis)	
	+ High-risk patients: > 50 yr, asplenic, diabetic, alcoholic, AIDS/HIV, history of chemotherapy, steroid therapy, cardiac valve disease? (> Risk Infection)	

(continued)

Key Questions	Urgent Symptom Patterns	ED/UCC/Office 1-8 hr
Bite (Human or Animal)	+ Any cat, human, primate, pig? (> Risk Infection High-Risk Species)	
	+ Tetanus immunization > 10 yr? (> Risk)	
Bite (Cat)	+ Hand: rapidly progressing redness/swelling *(Pasteurella Multicedens* Cellulitis)	

Cross-References
Skin Problem:
Laceration/Wound

SKIN PROBLEM: BUES/STINGS (REPTILE, MARINE)
Snake; Jellyfish; Sea Urchin; Stingray

ASSESSMENT	ACUITY LEVEL	DISPOSITION/ADVICE
Key Questions	**Emergent Symptom Patterns**	**Ed 0 min-1 hr**
Snake Bite	+ Progressive: anxious, weak, dizzy, thirsty, N/V. Skin: pale, blotchy/discolored/cool or cold, sweaty. Lips/Nail Bed: blue, Pulse: weak/fast, Breathing: rapid/shallow, unresponsive, loss of consciousness? (Shock) (See Shock)	
Marine Animal Sting	+ SOB, wheezing, stridor, difficulty swallowing, agitation, anxiety, rash (itchy, raised, "hivelike"), swelling of face/tongue, history of allergies or exp. to allergen (substance, bite)? (Anaphylaxis)	
Key Questions	**Urgent Symptom Patterns**	**ED/UCC/Office 1-8 hr**
Snake Bite	+ Rattlesnake?	(See Skin Problem: Bites/Stings, First Aid: Bites/Stings)
	+ Coral Snake?	
	+ Water moccasin/cottonmouth snake?	
	+ Copperhead snake?	
Jellyfish/Portuguese Man-of-War Sting? (Neurotoxicity)	.... ▶	(See Skin Problem: Bites/Stings, First Aid: Bites/Stings) Contact poison center.
Sea Urchin Spines? (toxicity)	_____ ■▶	(See Skin Problem: Bites/Stings, First Aid: Bites/Stings) Contact poison center
Stingray? (toxicity)	..............-.. ▶	(See Skin Problem: Bites/Stings, First Aid: Bites/Stings) Contact poison center
All Bites/Stings	+ Previous medical history: bleeding disorder, kidney/liver disease, anticoagulants? (> Risk Hemorrhage)	

(continued)

Key Questions	Urgent Symptom Patterns	ED/UCC/Office 1 -8 hr
All Bites/Stings (continued)	+ Previous medical history: asplenic, diabetic, alcoholic, AIDS/HIV, history of chemotherapy, steroid therapy, cardiac valve disease? (> Risk Infection) + Age: > 50 yr (> Risk Toxicity) + Red ± streaking, swollen, tender, hot; ± discharge, often w fever, swollen nodes, history of trauma/ bite/local infection? (Cellulitis/Infection)	
Cross-Reference Skin Problem SI: Bites/Stings		

SKIN PROBLEM: BITES/STINGS (INSECT)
Bee, Yellow Jacket, Hornet, Wasp Stings; Spiders; Scorpions; Fleas; Ticks

ASSESSMENT	ACUITY LEVEL	DISPOSITION/ADVICE
Key Questions	Emergent Symptom Patterns	ED 0 min-1 hr
Any Sting/Bite	+ SOB, wheezing, stridor, retractions, difficulty swallowing, agitation, anxiety, rash (itchy, raised, "hivelike"), swelling of face/tongue, history of allergies or exp. to allergen (med., drug, food, chemical, substance, bite)? (Anaphylaxis) (See Shock)--	▶ Epi kit as appropriate + Benadryl (in any form) immediately
	+ Progressive: anxious, weak, dizzy, thirsty, N/V. Skin: pale, blotchy/discolored/cool or cold, sweaty. Lips/Nail Bed: blue. Pulse: weak/fast. Breathing: rapid/shallow, unresponsive, loss of consciousness? (Shock) (See Shock)	
Scorpion Bite (small, silver white)	+ Pain at site, restlessness, roving eye movements, difficult speech, loss of bowel/bladder control, difficult breathing, shaking, resp. distress? (Neurotoxicity)---	▶ Contact poison center First Aid (scorpion/black widow): + Keep bite area below heart level + Wash bite w soap & Water + Keep patient sitting quietly + Remove all jewelry + Splint affected area + Place covered ice pack on bite
Black Widow Spider Bite	+ Cramps/pain, abdomen/chest/back, difficult breathing, N/V, SOB, weakness, headache, cardiac arrhythmias, boardlike rigidity, paralysis? (Neurotoxicity) (See Skin Problem: Bites/Stings SI: First Aid: Bites/Stings)................................	▶ Contact poison center (See First Aid above) + Rule of Thumb: Black widow bite symptoms may mimic MI or acute abdomen

Key Questions	Urgent Symptom Patterns	ED/UCC/Office 1 -8 hr
Brown Recluse Spider Bite	--	Contact poison center
	+ Painful, burning sensation within 10 min, "bull's eye" ulcer with rash, fever, N/V, jaundice (Neurotoxicity) --	*■ (See First Aid above)
Bee Stings	+ Multiple stings, near eyes, on face/genitals, generalized itching, raised reddened areas/hives, child or elderly? (> Risk Toxicity)	
All Bites (Insect)	+ Red ± streaking, swollen, tender, hot; + discharge, often w fever, swollen nodes, history of trauma/ bite/local infection? (Cellulitis/Infection)	

Key Questions	Acute/Nonacute Symptom Patterns	FA 8+ hr ± Home Tx
Spider/Scorpion Bites Tick Bite History	+ Present on skin x 24-36 hr? (> Risk Complications)	
	+ Parts of tick left in skin after removal? (Infection)	
	+ Red rash that looks like ring, 3-30 days after bite, ± flu symptoms, aching muscles, fatigue, headache? (Lyme Disease)	
Bee Sting	+ Moderate local swelling, pain, itching at the site? (Localized Reaction)	

Cross-Reference
Skin Problem: Rashes

SKIN PROBLEM: BITES/STINGS
Supplemental Information

Quick Reference:
▶ First Aid
 Bites/Stings (Reptile, Marine)
 Snake
 Jellyfish
 Stingray/Sea Urchin
▶ Rules of Thumb
 Human Bites
 Animal Bites
▶ Bites (All) Treatment
▶ Rabies
▶ Rules of Thumb
 Snakebite

▶ Community Alert: Snakebite
▶ Insect Bites and Stings
 Rule of Thumb
 Spider Bites
 Bee Stings
▶ Tick Bites
 Community Alert
 Lyme Disease
 Rocky Mountain Spotted Fever

▶ First Aid

Bites/Stings (Reptile, Marine)

- Snakebite
  - —Never "cut and suck." Apply ice, apply tourniquet or pressure bandage!
  - —Move patient 20 ft from snake.
  - —Keep patient calm, warm, and quiet.
  - —Gently wash wound w soap and water.
  - —Keep bite area *below* heart level.
  - —Remove all jewelry, tight clothes, shoes as needed.
  - —Splint area as for fracture.
- Jellyfish Sting
  - —Remove tentacles/stingers.
  - —Relieve pain.
  - —Pain: Soak w V_2 sea water + $'/_2$ vinegar x 30 min. Apply topical antihistamine (e.g., Calamine Lotion).
  - —Pour flour or baking powder on affected area, remove stingers.
  - —Do not rub the wound! It will make the stinging & pain worse!
  - —Jellyfish: No antivenin.
- Stingray/Sea Urchin
  - —Remove spines.
  - —Wash wound with any available water.
  - —Place injured part in nonscalding hot water

▶ **Rules of Thumb**

Human Bites

- All bites: Check tetanus status.
- + Lack of/outdated immunization = > risk tetanus.
- Beware of "fight bites"—human bites over knuckles. Because of its location, this type of injury is high risk for serious joint infections.
- Whether accidental or intentional, all breaks in skin caused by human teeth = human bite.
- All human bites are potentially serious.

Animal Bites

- Notify animal control.
- Report All animal bites, especially bats and skunks.
- Treat all wild animals as rabid: wolves, foxes, skunks, bats, coyotes, woodchucks, bobcats, squirrels, feral or stray cats and dogs.
- Cat bites: Up to 50% of all cat bites become infected. Cat bite of hand must be seen within 1 hr!!

▶ **Bites (All) Treatment**

- Goal: Prevent infection.
  - —Control bleeding by keeping bite area *above* heart (will decrease pain/swelling).
  - —Flush with clean water from tap.
  - —Wash with soap and water by filling large clean plastic bag with soap and water, poke hole in it with a knife or pin, and squirt directly into wound X 3 min.
  - —Cover with clean cloth or sterile dressing.
  - —Tetanus must be given within 72 hr.

▶ **Rabies**

- Signs and symptoms: Depression, restlessness, fever. Progresses to muscle spasm, drooling, fear of water, coma, death.
- Rabid wild animal behavior:
  - —Daytime activity of nocturnal bats, raccoons, skunks, and foxes.
  - —Wild animals who seem to lack normal fear of humans.
  - —Any animal with furious behavior (See below)
- Rabid domestic animals' and humans' behavior
  - —Furious rabies: Agitation and viciousness followed by paralysis and death within days.
- Cause: Virus. Incubation in humans 10 days-1 yr (usually 6 wk).
- Prevention:
  - —DO NOT GO NEAR ANY WILD ANIMALS! Even in parks or campsites, deer, raccoons, chipmunks, and skunks are still wild animals!
  - —Never pick up sick or injured animals.
  - —Never pet strange animals.
  - —Never disturb eating animals.
  - —Never stop animals from fighting.
  - —Report all strays to police or animal control.

► Rules of Thumb

Snakebite

- Treat all snakes as poisonous until proven otherwise.
- Bite victims are often young, intoxicated males who have been playing with snakes.

► Community Alert: Snakebites

- Most snakebites occur in July and August. Snakes are active, and people are interacting with the outdoors.
- Snakes are more active at night.
- Prevention:
  —Stay alert at all times: Watch where you walk or put your hands.
  —Wear high boots, carry long pole to poke areas you cannot see.
  —If you see a snake, stay 20-30 ft away. Maximum strike distance is a few feet.
  —When it is hot, snakes seek cool places: under rocks, logs, caves, crevices, pools, water.
  —When it is cold, snakes seek warm places: warm rocks, sleeping bags, boots.
  —Never handle "dead" snakes; even after the snake is dead, accidental snakebites can happen.

► Insect Bites and Stings

Rule of Thumb
Elderly are more sensitive to insect venom; therefore, are at greater risk for toxicity.

Spider Bites
- Black widow: Shiny black body w red hourglass figure on belly.
  —Found in damp, cool places (woodpiles).
- Brown recluse: Light brown color with violin-shaped marking on back.
  —Found in dark areas (basement, garage).

Bee Stings
- Goal: Remove stinger; relieve the pain.
- Tx:
  —Remove stinger: Scrape gently w fingernail or credit card. Touch w Scotch tape.
  —To reduce pain:
    ° Baking soda paste (See Home Treatment SI, Appendix A: Baking Soda Paste). Caution: Do not use baking soda or meat tenderizer near eyes or other sensitive skin,
    o *Cloth-covered* ice pack on affected area. (See Home Treatment SI, Appendix A: Ice Pack)
    ° Raise bite area above heart if possible.
    ° Remove all jewelry, including rings, on affected hand, arm, ankle, or foot as needed.
    ° Tylenol as appropriate.
    o Itching: Benadryl. (Dose: Age and wt. appropriate)
- Bee sting prevention:
  —Don't wear bright colors.
  —Wear shirt and shoes.

—Use care when drinking from cans (bees may go inside).

—Avoid using perfume when outdoors.

- Insect bite care:

—Wash with soap and water.

—Cover with clean bandage or Band-Aid.

—Don't scratch the bite—it can become infected.

—Cut nails; keep clean and short.

—Itching: Antihistamines, Calamine Lotion, hydrocortisone.

—Watch for signs of infection (review).

► Tick Bites

Community Alert

- General information about ticks:

—Tick season: December to June.

—In endemic areas, only 1%-2% of ticks are infected w Lyme disease. However, there are "pockets" where the rate is much higher.

- Tick bite care.
- Goal: remove tick. Prevent complications. Tick removal:

—Use tweezers (pointed are best).

—Grab tick's mouth as close to skin as possible.

—Gently but firmly pull tick straight out. Do not twist or jerk.

—Don't touch or squeeze the tick.

—Save tick whenever possible (See Lyme disease test below.)

—Mark date of bite on calendar. Mark a circle w ink around bite and check it daily x 3-4 days.

—Observe for complications.

Lyme Disease

Infection caused by bacteria, carried by ticks, and transmitted by tick bites.

- Signs and symptoms: See Skin Problem: Insect Bites/Stings.
- Complications:

—(Week to months) Heart rhythm problems, facial drooping, impaired walking, moving.

—(1 mo to 1-2 yr) Arthritis, joint swelling (knees).

- Prevention:

—Where found: Grasses and bushes in country and city.

—How they get to humans: Ticks climb to tips of weeds and plants. They wait for humans or animals to brush against the plants and jump on them. They do not fly.

—When walking in woods, tuck pants into boots or socks. Tuck shirt in.

—Wear light-colored clothes. You can see the tick better that way.

—Stay out of grassy areas.

—Stay on wide clear trails.

—Check your skin often. Look behind ears, in armpits, on back, neck, and in belly button.

—Shower or bathe with soap and washcloth after being in woods.

—Carry "needle-nosed" pointed tick tweezers on hikes.

—Mow grass along trails, buildings.

—Check pets for ticks. Use tick collar or Rx.

—Put special tick repellent on pants, socks, shoes.

- Treatment:

    —Antibiotics work well if they are taken when the rash is first seen.

    —If tick has Lyme disease, then antibiotics are given.

- Lyme disease test:

    —For humans: Most accurate if done 4-6 wk after tick bite.

    —For tick: Save tick: To save tick for future (when symptoms appear), put tick in wet paper towel in baggie, in glass jar in refrigerator. To get test results, mail tick in wet towel and baggie to local Public Health Department.

Rocky Mountain Spotted Fever

- Signs and symptoms: Resistant fever, headaches, fatigue, joint pain; red flat rash progressing to red/purple pinpoint, starts on wrist/ankles; periorbital edema w conjunctivis, meningism, coma.

- Incubation period: 2-14 days.

SKIN PROBLEM: BURNS 1
Electrical; Thermal; Chemical

ASSESSMENT	ACUITY LEVEL	DISPOSITION/ADVICE
Key Questions	Emergent Symptom Patterns	Ed 0 min-1 hr
All Electrical Burns	+ ± Chest pain, palpitations, > heart rate, fainting, Hx of lightning strike? (Cardiac Dysrhythmia)............►	All electrical burns have potential for progressive injury; may be worse than they look! Seconds count See Burns SI, First Aid
All Thermal Burns	- ►	(See Skin Problem: Burns SI, First Aid)
Burn w Decreased Consciousness	+ Weak, dizzy, cold/mottled/pale skin, blue lips/nail beds, rapid/shallow breathing, unresponsive, loss of consciousness? (Shock) (See Shock)	
Burn w Respiratory Symptoms	+ Hoarseness, cough, wheezing, SOB, singed/black nares, facial burn, smoke inhalation, black sputum? (Inhalation Injury)	
Burn (Deep)	+ White, dark, charred appearance, loss of skin, regardless of size? (3rd Degree)	
Burn (Over 9%)	+ Red, mottled, blisters, extreme pain? (2nd Degree, Major)	
Burn of Finger(s) (Circumferential)	+ Unable to remove rings? (> Risk Circ.)	
Facial/Neck Burn? (Retinal, Inhalation Burn)		
All Chemical Burns (Including Eyes)	- ►	All chemical burns have potential for progressive injury; may be worse than they look! Seconds count!

Key Questions	Urgent Symptom Patterns	ED/UCC/Office 1 -8 hr
Burn (Circumferential)	+ Face/neck/hands/feet/arms/legs/perineum/ any joint? (Circ. obstruction)- - - - - - - - - - - - - - - - -•►	(See Skin Problem: Burns SI, First Aid
Burn w Blisters	+ Red, mottled, extreme pain, 5%-9%? (2nd Degree)--►	(See Skin Problem: Burns SI, First Aid

Key Questions	Acute/Nonacute Symptom Patterns	FA 8+ hr ± Home Tx
Burn Hx	+ Foul smelling, purulent discharge, > swelling, > streaks and pain, fever? (Infection)---------------------▶	Check tetanus status (See Skin Problem: Burns SI, First Aid)
Burn (Moderate)	+ Tetanus immunization > 10 yr? (> Risk Infection) + Red, blisters, pain 1%-5%? (2nd Degree)	
Burn (Minor)	+ Reddened, mild, swelling, moderate pain, no blisters? (1st Degree) + Red, motded, blisters, pain, < the size of one hand (1%)? (2nd Degree)	
Cross-Reference Abuse		

SKIN PROBLEM: BURNS 2
Sunburn

1 ASSESSMENT	ACUITY LEVEL	DISPOSITION/ADVICE
Key Questions	**Emergent Symptom Patterns**	Ed 0 min-1 hr
Sunburn w < consciousness	+ Fever (high), sev. fatigue, confusion, fainting, hot, dry red skin, rapid shallow breathing? (See Heat Exposure)	
Key Questions	**Urgent Symptom Patterns**	ED/UCC/Office 1-8 hr
Sunburn	+ Eye pain, photophobia, < vision? (Retinal Involvement)	
	+ Extensive, deep sunburn, fever, pain (sev. to mod.), dehydration Sx, generalized swelling of burned area? (Sun Poisoning)	
Red, mottled, blisters + > 5%, Extreme pain? (2nd Degree)		
Sunburn Hx	+ Foul smelling, purulent discharge, worsening swelling or pain, streaks, fever? (Infection)	
Key Questions	**Acute/Nonacute Symptoms Patterns**	FA 8+ hr ± Home Tx
Sunburn w blisters	+ Red, mottled, tender, covering 5% of body? (> Risk Infection)	
Open blisters	± Discharge ± fever? (> Risk Infection)	
Sunburn	+ Pain/tenderness, deeply pigmented skin types? (1st Degree)	
	+ Red, mild swelling, moderate pain, no blisters? (1st Degree)	
Cross-References Abuse	Heat Exposure	

SKIN PROBLEM: BURNS
Supplemental Information

Quick Reference: ▶ First Aid   ▶ Burn Assessment ▶ Blister Care

                 Thermal Burn   Rule of Nines ▶ Burn Care

                 Chemical Burn

▶ **First Aid**

Thermal Burn

- If clothing sticks to skin, do not remove clothing! Immerse burned area for no more than 3 min in cool tap water.
- If clothing does not stick to skin, remove it.
  - —If > 5%, do not immerse. Cover with clean wet sheet + plastic wrap.
  - —If < 5%, immerse immediately in cool tap water x 10 min.
- Do not put butter, oil, or creams on burn!
- Do not put ice on burn: could lead to > skin damage, > shock.
  - —For transport: Wrap burn in clean plastic wrap to keep warm, clean, and reduce pain.

Chemical Burn

- Contact poison center immediately and quickly do the following:
  - —Wet Chemicals: Rinse skin/eyes w cool tap water.
  - —Dry Chemicals: Brush from skin/eyes.
  - —Bring substance to ED w you.

▶ **Burn Assessment**

Rule of Nines: A useful, quick method to estimate percentage of body surface areas that were burned.

Rule of Nines

Adult

- Palm of *victim's* hand, not including fingers = 1%
- Perineum = 1%
- Head/Neck = 9%
- Arm = 9%
- Leg =18%
- Ant. trunk = 18%
- Post, trunk = 18%

▶ **Burn Care**

Immediate Care

- Pain: Tylenol.
- Pain/Swelling: Cold compress QID. (See Home Tx SI, Appendix A: Cold/Cool Compress)

- Remove rings, bracelets, etc., only if you can do so easily. If not, you need to come in to have the items removed.
- Pain/Swelling: Raise the burn area above heart level.
- Don't use "Caines" or Benadryl sprays for burn—may cause a reaction.
- Check tetanus status. If you have a clean burn and your last tetanus shot was > 10 yr ago, you need a tetanus shot within 72 hr.

▶ Blister Care

- Don't break blisters. They are like "nature's Band-Aids" and will protect your skin from infection.
- If they break, leave them alone. Do not peel off skin from broken blisters.
- Cover w clean, dry dressing. Change as needed.
- Watch for signs and symptoms of infection. (See Burn Care above; Protocol.)

SKIN PROBLEM: DISCOLORATION
Bruise; Yellow; All Color Changes

ASSESSMENT	ACUITY LEVEL	DISPOSITION/ADVICE
Key Questions	Emergent Symptom Patterns	Ed 0 min-1 hr
Bruise w Trauma Hx	+ Weak, dizzy, cold/mottled/or pale skin, blue lips/ nail beds, rapid/shallow breathing, unresponsive, loss of consciousness? (Shock/Internal Hemorrhage) (See Shock)	
Bruise w/o Trauma	+ Fever, stiff neck, headache, N/V, extreme fatigue, pinpoint red purplish spots progressing to purple patches, extremely irritable or unresponsive, photophobia, ± seizure? (Meningococcal Meningitis)	
Key Questions	Urgent Symptom Patterns	ED/UCC/Office 1-8 hr
Bruise w Trauma	+ Multiple, unusual pattern, various stages of healing? (Abuse)	
	+ Quickly enlarging bruise, w swelling, unresponsive to first aid? (Hematoma)	
Bruise w/o Trauma	+ Spontaneous, frequent, recurrent Hx of anticoagulants, hemophilia, bleeding disorder, kidney/liver disease, Hx cancer, chemo, radiation? (Leukemia/Hemorrhage)	
Key Questions	Acute/Nonacute Symptoms Patterns	FA 8+ hr ± Home Tx
Yellow Skin	+ Fever, N/V, anorexia, yellow sclera, fatigue, swollen glands, day-colored stools, dark urine, ± exp. to hepatitis? (Hepatitis) (See Hepatitis SI, Appendix C)	
Pink/purple	+ Barely elevated, plaque, round or oval, upper body/mucosa? (Kaposi Sarcoma)	

(continued)

Key Questions	Acute/Nonacute Symptoms Patterns	FA 8+ hr ± Home Tx
Skin Color Change	+ White patches of skin, Hx of eczema, any Hx of skin problem (Vitiligo)	
	+ Silvery, white/pink or white, streaks on hips/thighs/abdomen? (Stretch Marks)	
	+ Yellow/orange color esp. on palms and soles of feet? (Carotenemia)	
	+ Hx Rx? (Drug Side Effect) (See Skin Problem: Discoloration SI)	

Cross-References
Hepatitis SI, Appendix C

SKIN PROBLEM: DISCOLORATION
Supplemental Information

Quick Reference:
- ▶ Disease Side Effect (Discoloration)
- ▶ Drug Side Effect (Color Change)
- ▶ Environmental Side Effect (White Patches)
- ▶ Hematoma
- ▶ Hepatitis
- ▶ Jaundice
- ▶ Petechiae
- ▶ Purpura

▶ Disease Side Effect: Discoloration

® Causes:
—Adrenal (tan)
—Blood disorders (pale)
—Liver (yellow)
—Porphyria (tan)
—Thyroid (vitiligo—white patches)
—Tinea (white patches)
—Vitiligo (white patches)

▶ Drug Side Effect: Color Change

a Causes:
—Antimalarials
—Birth control pills (brownish spots)
—Nicotinic acid (red)
—Stelazine
—Thorazine

▶ Environmental Side Effect: White Patches

a Causes: Repeated chemical/rubber contact

▶ Hematoma

® Tx goal: Reduce swelling, pain; provide comfort,

a Tx:
—Ice Pack QID x 48 hr (See Home Tx SI, Appendix A: Ice Pack)
—Raise injured part above heart level.
—Rest the part that was bruised.
—Do not rub or massage area.
—Mark the border of the bruise w pen.
—Watch to see if the bruise gets bigger.
—If it gets bigger, you will need to come in within 2 hr.

—Warm, moist compress QID after 48 hr.

—Bruise will change color and reabsorb over time. It may move down arm or leg.

► Hepatitis

(See Hepatitis, Appendix C)

► Jaundice

- Signs and symptoms: Yellow skin and whites of eyes
- Causes: Possible liver, gallbladder, or blood problem
- Complications: Could become a serious health problem

► Petechiae

- Signs and symptoms: Multiple, pinpoint, round, purplish red spots
- Cause: Bleeding under the skin caused by bacterial infection
- Complications: Serious symptoms of infection (Meningitis, Blood infection)

► Purpura

- Signs and symptoms: Large, purplish-red areas that look like flat bruises.
- Cause: Bleeding under skin as a result of bacterial infection
- Complications: Serious symptom of infection (Meningitis, Blood Infection, Bleeding Problem)

SKIN PROBLEM: LACERATION/WOUND
Amputations; Abrasions; Puncture Wounds

ASSESSMENT ACUITY LEVEL		DISPOSITION/ADVICE
Key Questions	Emergent Symptom Patterns	Ed 0 min-1 hr
Penetrating Wound	(Head/Chest/Abdomen/Throat)?------------------------- ▶	Never remove impaled object! (Unless it is penetrating the trachea)
Amputations (All)	-.. .... ■▶	(See Skin Problem: Laceration/ Wound SI, First Aid: Pressure Points) Save body part, wrap in clean cloth; place in plastic bag; pack in ice
Laceration/Stab Wound	(Trunk, Neck, Groin)------------------------------------- ▶	Stab wounds of chest/abd. may be worse than they first appear!
	+ Forceful, spurting, uncontrolled by direct pressure, bright red bleeding? (> Risk Hemorrhage, Shock)---▶	(See Skin Problem: Laceration/ Wound SI, First Aid: Pressure Points)
	+ Persistent bleeding, Hx of bleeding disorder, kidney/liver disease, Hx of anticoagulants? (> Risk Hemorrhage)..................-............................... ▶	(See Skin Problem: Laceration/ Wound SI, First Aid: Pressure Points)
	+ Blue, cold, pale extremity, numbness distal to wound? (> Risk of Loss of Limb)	

Key Questions	Urgent Symptom Patterns	ED/UCC/Office 1 -8 hr
Laceration	+ Able to see fat when separated slightly? (Needs Sutures)-- --▶	Come to ED now!
Imbedded Foreign Body (All)	+ (Nail, Glass, Other Object)? -- --■▶	First Aid: + Cover w clean, dry dressing + If blood saturates, reinforce w another dressing. DO NOT REMOVE!
Laceration Hx	+ (All skin) Red, ± streaking, swollen, tender, hot; + discharge, often w fever, swollen nodes, hx of trauma/bite/local infection? (Cellulitis)	
Puncture Wound	+ Rusty, dirty nail, gardening wounds, through rubber footwear? (> Risk Infection)------------------- --▶	First Aid: Scrub x 5 min., soak in soapy water x 15 min.

Key Questions	Acute/Nonacute Symptoms Patterns	FA 8+ hr ± Home Tx
Laceration(s)	+ (All) Immunizations not up-to-date?	
	+ (All) Dirty, puncture wound, last tetanus > 5 yr? (Immz)	
	+ Hx diabetes? (> Risk Infection)	
Abrasion (Severe)	+ "Road burn," heavily encrusted w dirt/foreign body, able to carry out first aid? (> Risk Infection)	
Laceration	+ (Minor) Abrasion, splinter, puncture wound (Clean)?	
Cat Scratch	+ Fever, fatigue, anorexia, headache, Pustule at site in 3-5 days, swollen tender lymph nodes? (Cat Scratch Fever)	

Cross-References
Skin Problem:
Bites/Stings

SKIN PROBLEM: LACERATION/WOUND
Supplemental Information

Quick Reference: ► First Aid: Pressure Points ► Puncture

► Abrasion Scrapes   ► Suture Removal Schedule

► Laceration and Wound Care ► Tetanus

► **First Aid: Pressure Points**
- Lay patient down.
- Raise extremity above heart to decrease bleeding.
- Apply pressure firmly with clean folded cloth.
- Arm wound: Apply pressure (firm and continuous) to pulse point inside the upper arm. Use four fingers. Apply pressure firmly against bone until you can no longer feel pulse.
- Leg wound: Place victim on back and feel for pulse in groin area—at top of leg where leg bends. Use the heel/palm of hand, keep arm straight, press artery against bone. If you need to, use both hands.
- Keep pressure on until help arrives.

► **Abrasion Scrapes**
- Cause: Scraping of skin or mucous membranes
- Complications: Infection
- First Aid:
  —Pain: Tylenol 1 hr prior to Tx
  —Flush/scrub w washcloth area w water x 5 min.
  —Use tweezers to remove large particles
  —Warm Soapy Soak (See Home Tx SI, Appendix A: Warm Soapy Soak)
- Prevention/Tx: Wash area w warm, soapy water 3 x day. Cover w dry, sterile dressing.

► **- Laceration and Wound Care (Cuts, Abrasions, Burns)**
- Check tetanus status.
- Tetanus must be given within 72 hr.
- Wash w warm soapy water. Remove all dirt. Cover w sterile dressing (See Home Tx SI, Appendix A: Warm Soapy Soak).
- If there is dirt in wound, remove all dirt by scrubbing gently.
- Keep cut clean and dry.
- Elevate the wound to help relieve soreness and speed wound healing.
- Watch for signs and symptoms of infection.
- Despite the greatest care, any cut can become infected. Return if any of the following develop:
  —Increasing pain or tenderness after the first 24 hr
  —Pus
  —Red streaks
  —Increasing swelling
  —Fever

▶ Puncture

Small cut or wound made by sharp, thin object (nail, needle)

• Rule of Thumb: Puncture wounds w rubber footwear always need antibiotics

® Signs and symptoms: Skin pierced w pointed object or instrument

® Cause: Penetration or piercing of skin w pointed object or instrument

® Complications: Infection, bleeding, tetanus

° Prevention/Tx:

—Wear shoes outside.

—Wear gloves when gardening.

▶ Suture Removal Schedule

Area	Days
Face	3-4
Neck	5
Scalp	7
Chest, abdomen	7
Arms	7
Legs	10
Back	12
Palms, soles, over joints	14

▶ Tetanus

® Definition: A serious, life-threatening bacterial infection.

° Signs and symptoms: Pain at wound site, muscle spasms, stiff jaw and neck, difficulty swallowing or opening mouth, irritability, convulsions.

® Cause: A germ enters the skin through a wound. The germ is often found in the soil or on sharp pieces of metal.

® Complication: The death rate is very high.

® Prevention:

—Tetanus is completely preventable by immunization. Get an immunization booster every 10 yr.

• Adults who have never been immunized require 2 doses of tetanus toxoid 1 mo apart, w booster dose 6-12 mo later, and booster every 10 yr thereafter.

® Tx:

—Anyone who has been immunized but has not had a booster within the past 5 yr and who has a puncture wound, dirty wound, burn, or frostbite should receive a tetanus booster.

—Any nonimmunized person w a puncture wound, dirty wound, burn, or frostbite should receive tetanus immune globulin IM (passive immunity) and antibiotics.

—Careful washing of cut w soap and water. (See Laceration and Wound Care above)

—Dirty wounds—Get booster every 5 yr.

SKIN PROBLEM: LESION/LUMP/SWELLING
With or without Trauma

ASSESSMENT	ACUITY LEVEL	DISPOSITION/ADVICE
Key Questions	Emergent Symptom Patterns	ED/UCC/Office 1 -8 hr
Trauma	+ Quickly enlarging/swelling/bruise, unresponsive to first aid, Hx cancer, chemo, radiation, anticoagulation? (Hematoma)----------------------------▶	Come to ED now!
Swelling	+ Hx pregnancy? (See Pregnancy Problem 2)	
	+ In extremities? (See Extremities Problem 1; 2; 3)	
	+ (All skin) red ± streaking, tender, hot; ± discharge, often w fever, swollen nodes, hx of trauma/bite/local infection, ± contact known MRSA? (Cellulitis)	
	+ Hx IV drug abuse ± fever, red, hot, ± soft/mushy, ± draining pus, immunocompromised, Hx diabetes ± contact known MRSA? (Abscess)	
Key Questions	Acute/Nonacute Symptom Patterns	FA 8+ hr ± Home Tx
Lesion(s)/Swelling	+ (Neck) Redness, tenderness, warm to touch, fever? (Cervical Adenitis)	
Lesion(s)	+ Cluster of tiny clear blisters, begins w tingling, itching, pain, followed by yellow, crusty crater after 1-2 days; first time; near eye; w sev. throat pain, poss. followed by sev./mod. dehydration; w sev. vaginal pain, difficulty urinating? (Herpes)	
	+ On mouth, rectum, or genitalia + poss. exp. to STI? (STI) (See Vaginal Problem: STI SI)	
	+ One or more, facial, red, hot, painful, thickened tissue; ± fever; pea-to walnut-sized, 3 or more, soft & mushy, draining pus > 7 days, ± contact known MRSA? (Abscess)	
	+ Pustules, around hair, painful, draining, ± contact known MRSA? (Folliculitis, Furunculosis, Carbuncles)	

(continued)

Key Questions	Acute/Nonacute Symptoms Patterns	FA 8+ hr ⁎ Home Tx
Lesion(s) (continued)	+ Redness, swelling, blisters, broken skin over pressure points, frail elderly, mentally challenged, cerebral palsy, or muscular dystrophy? (Pressure Sore/Decubitus Ulcer/Neglect)	
	+ Itchy, honey-colored, crusted, ± blisters/pustules? (Impetigo)	
	+ Papules, pustules, face/back/chest, young adult? (Acne)	
	+ Patches of cracked skin, dry, scaly, flaky, itchy areas, face, trunk, inner arm, ± Hx allergies? (Atopic Dermatitis)	
	+ Linear/painful, follows the path of nerve, unilateral, begins as cluster of bumps, becomes blisters, then dry crust, ± sev. itching? (Herpes Zoster/Shingles)	
	+ Pigmented mole, different colors (blue, purple, white, tan), irregular border, change in size, satellites? (Melanoma)	
	+ Fleshy, growing/red, scaling lesion in sun-exposed areas (Basal Cell Carcinoma/Squamous Cell Carcinoma)	
	+ Plaques, irregular, greasy surface, sun-exposed area, yellow, dark, tan, defined edge? (Seborrhea Dermatitis)	
	+ Small skin-colored bumps w rough surfaces? (Warts)	
Swelling/Lump	+ Small, not warm to touch, w/o fever or tenderness, may be felt in neck, behind ears, axilla, groin, base of skull? (Lymphadenopathy)	
	+ Face, scalp, trunk ± tenderness, does not move freely? (Sebaceous Cyst)	
	+ No change in size, appearance over years, moves freely? (Lipoma)	

Cross-References
Pregnancy Problem 2 Vaginal Problem: STI SI   Extremities Problem 2

SKIN PROBLEM: LESION/LUMP/SWELLING
Supplemental Information

Quick Reference:
- ► Acne
- ► Boil
- ► Cellulitis
- ► Herpes Simplex (Cold Sore, Fever Blister)
- ► Herpes (Zoster) (Shingles)

- ► Impetigo
- ► MRSA (Methicillin-Resistant Staph Aureus)
- ► Mumps
- ► Pitting Edema
- ► Tetanus

► Acne
- Home Tx: Prevent infection/scarring/pitting
  —Wash hands/face w soap and water.
  —Don't pick pimples.
  —Use moisturizer.

► Boil
- Definition: Pocket of pus.
- Cause: Infection caused by *Staph* germs.
- Complications: May come back for months or years.
- Prevention/Tx: Handle very gently.
  —Warm, moist soaks 4 x /day or more.
  —Clean w soap often.
  —Don't squeeze boil. Wait for it to "pop" and infection will come out.

► Cellulitis
- Signs and symptoms: See Protocol.
- Cause: Bacterial infection w streptococci, staphylococci, or other organisms.
- Complications: Infection in blood and skin. Potentially dangerous, esp. around face—can spread to brain.
- Prevention/Tx:
  —Keep skin clean.
  —Clean wounds immediately.

► Herpes Simplex (Cold Sore, Fever Blister)
  May appear anywhere on skin: Lips, eye, genitals, thumb (thumb suckers).
- Signs and symptoms: See Protocol.
- Cause: Contagious virus
- Complications: Usually heal by themselves in 1-2 wk
- Prevention/Tx:

• Adult Protocols

Oral (Herpes Simplex 1)

- OTC ointment, e.g., glyoxide
- Cool compresses (See Home Tx SI, Appendix A: Cold/Cool Compress)
- No kissing

Genital (Herpes Simplex 2)

- May need prescription.
- Keep sores clean and dry.
- Pain: Tylenol.
- Sitz baths (See Home Tx SI, Appendix A: Sitz Bath).

► ### Herpes (Zoster) (Shingles)

- Signs and symptoms: See Protocol.
- Causes: Virus; exposure to chickenpox; stress.
- Complications: Blindness; secondary infection.
- Prevention/Tx:
  —Calamine.
  —Keep sores clean and dry.
  —Pain: Tylenol.

► ### Impetigo

- Signs and symptoms: Sores w pus that break open and form yellow crusts
- Causes: Bacterial infection, Group A *Streptococcus* and *Staphylococcus* species, highly contagious
- Complications: Severe infection; kidney problems; can be fatal to newborns
- Prevention/Tx:
  —Wash w soap and water.
  —Keep open to air so it will dry out and heal.
  —Don't scratch. Isolation: Don't touch sores and pus. Wash hands after touching.
  —Needs antibiotics.

► ### MRSA (Methicillin-Resistant *Staph Aureus)*

- Definition: *"Staph"* is a very common kind of germ that one-half of all people carry on their skin. MRSA is a kind of *Staph* infection that many antibiotics cannot cure.
- Sign and symptoms: There may be no symptoms or it may cause boils, blisters, pustules or abscesses (See Protocol)
- Complications: Serious infections like pneumonia or sepsis shock
- Risk factors for MRSA include the 5 C's:
  —Contact: Avoid skin-to-skin contact with anyone with a skin infection.
  —Cuts/scrapes/scratches: Use extra care to clean and keep clean cuts, scratches, or scrapes on the skin.
  —Contamination: Only use clean towels or clothes from other people.
  —Crowding: Avoid sharing any clothes, equipment, or towels in places where many people use these items, or if someone in your family has a skin infection.

—Cleanliness:

° Wash your hands and bathe with soap and water often.

o Cover all cuts and scrapes with a Band-Aid.

° Don't share towels or razors.

<= See a doctor or nurse if you think you have an MRSA infection.

° Always take all of your antibiotics until they are gone.

► Mumps

- Sign and symptoms: See Protocol.
- Causes: Virus, contagious.
- Complications: May cause meningitis, encephalitis, pancreatitis, or inflammation of testicles and ovaries. Usually does not affect fertility. Males of childbearing age who have not been immunized may be at increased risk of infertility if they get the mumps.
- Tx: Soft diet (See Home Tx SI, Appendix A); isolation; no acidic drinks.
- Prevention: MMR immunization.

► Pitting Edema

- Signs and symptoms: Abnormal collection of fluid in legs and feet; when skin is pressed, it stays indented, like a valley.
- Causes: Failure of circulation; heart disease, kidney disease, liver disease.
- Complications: Dehydration; dizzy, faint.
- Prevention/Tx:

—Rest.

—Elevate limb on pillows.

—Decrease salt in diet.

—Do not wear tight stockings.

—Control cause.

► Tetanus

See Skin Problem: Laceration/Wound.

SKIN PROBLEM: RASHES
With or without Itching

ASSESSMENT	ACUITY LEVEL	DISPOSITION/ADVICE
Key Questions	**Emergent Symptom Patterns**	ED/UCC/Office 1-8 hr
Rash	+ "Hivelike," itchy, raised: SOB, wheezing, stridor, retractions, difficulty swallowing, agitation, anxiety, swelling of face/tongue, Hx of allergies or exp. to allergen (med., drug, food, chemical, substance, bite)? (Anaphylaxis)-------------------------- -▶ Benadryl	
	+ Fever, stiff neck, headache, N/V, extreme fatigue/ irritability/unresponsive, ± pinpoint red purplish spots progressing to purple patches, ± seizure? (Meningococcal Meningitis)	
	+ Painful, local redness, rapidly spreading, blisters, "looks like 2nd degree burn," peels in large sheets, fatigue, fever/chills, joint pain, ± Hx Rx? (Drug Side Effect: Toxic Epidermal Necrolysis)	
	+ Fever, N/V, severe intractable diarrhea, muscle aches, headache, confusion, dizziness, fainting? (Sepsis Syndrome)	
Rash w Fever	+ Small red or purple spots, linear red brown spots in nail bed, flat spots on hands and soles, Hx IV drug user/Hx heart murmur/Hx artificial heart valve? (Infective Endocarditis)	
Key Questions	**Urgent Symptom Patterns**	ED/UCC/Office 1-8 hr
Rash w Fever	+ Fine rash on ankles/wrists moving to palms/soles, Fix fever, headache, muscle aches, Hx tick bite, more common: spring & summer months/southeastern or south central states? (Rocky Mountain Spotted Fever)	
	+ Preceded by cough, ± fever, pink > red, flat, w or w/o itching, face to trunk & extremities, red eyes, small white/grey/blue spots in mouth, no MMR Hx? (Measles)	
	+ Few pustular or blister-like lesions, joint pain/ swelling, swelling in tendons of wrist/fingers/ ankles/toes, STI exposure? (Disseminated Gonorrhea)	
	+ Immunocompromised: Hx chemotherapy or AIDS (> Risk Serious Infections)	

(continued

Key Questions	Urgent Symptom Patterns	ED/UCC/Office 1-8 hr
Rash w fever (continued)	+ Hx of recent travel, "ill appearing"? (> Risk Infection Depending upon Travel Area)	
	+ Red rash, slightly raised or flat, face to trunk/ extremities, swollen glands behind ears/+ neck, joint pain, no MMR Hx, not very sick, low grade fever? (German Measles/Rubella)------------------------4 ▶	Avoid contact with pregnant women
Rash w/o Itching	+ Round, red, target-like lesions ± blisters, fatigue, joint pain, ± fever, ± Hx infection, ± Hx meds? (Erythema Multiforme) + Sandpaper-like rash (most intense on neck, axilla, groin, behind knees, may cover entire body), lasts 7 days ± then peels; ± Hx of sore throat/fever? (Scarlet Fever)	
Rash w Itching	+ Itchy, w red, weepy, oozing blisters on face/near eyes/or on genitals? (Poison Oak > Risk)	

Key Questions	Acute/Nonacute Symptoms Patterns	FA 8+ hr± HomeTx
Rash w Itching	+ Intense itching at night, tiny blisters in "tracks," fingers, webs of fingers, toes, heels, wrists, elbows, armpits, breast, crease of buttocks, ± Hx of contact? (Scabies)	
	+ Cluster of red bumps, becomes blisters, painful, follows nerve, one-sided, then dry crust, ± burning/ itching? (Herpes Zoster/Shingles)	
	+ Patches of cracked skin, dry, scaly, flaky, itchy areas, face, trunk, inner arm, ± Hx allergies? (Atopic Dermatitis)	
	+ Redness, swelling on area of skin in contact w irritants (e.g., plants, chem., fabric softener, soaps, cosmetic)? (Contact Dermatitis)	
	+ Red, dry, scaly, excoriated, extreme itching? (Eczema)	
	+ Red, moist, peeling skin in groin area or between toes? ("Jock Itch," Athlete's Foot)	
	+ Eyelids/scalp, skin breakdown, gray-white lice eggs attached to eyelashes, eyebrows, or hair shaft, Hx of contact? (Head/Body Lice)	

(continued)

Key Questions	Acute/Nonacute Symptoms Patterns	FA 8+ hr.* Home Tx
Rash w Itching (continued)	+ Pubic area, skin breakdown, gray-white lice eggs attached to hair shaft, Hx of sexual contact? (Pubic Lice) (See Vaginal Problem: STI SI)	
	+ Fever, red rash (dewdrop on rose petal appearance), starts on trunk/face, intensely itchy, turns to crusts when blisters break, w/o resp. Sx? (Chickenpox)	
	+ ± Itching, Hx Rx or OTC drug 2 wk? (Drug Side Effect/Allergy)	
Rash w/o Itching	+ Round, red, scaly, on trunk, preceded by single lesion, young adult? (Pityriasis Rosea)	
	+ Growing red rash, ± clearing in the center, under arms, in groin, behind knees or beltline, ± fatigue, headaches, muscle aches, Hx tick bite in Lyme disease region? (Erythema Migrans of Lyme Disease)	
	+ Small skin-colored bumps w rough surfaces? (Warts)	
	+ Rough, pinhead-sized lumps on knees/back of arms/buttocks? (Keratosis Pilaris)	
	+ Chronic, gradual onset, raised, silvery, scaly patches, worse in winter? (Psoriasis)	

Cross-References
Skin Problem: Lesion/ Vaginal Problem: STI SI
Lump/Swelling

SKIN PROBLEM: RASHES WITH OR WITHOUT ITCHING

Supplemental Information

Quick Reference ► Infectious Rashes

Rules of Thumb	
Isolation Procedure	
Chickenpox	
German Measles	
(Rubella)	
Red or Seven-Day Measles	
(Rubeola)	
Roseola	
Scarlet Fever	

► Other Rashes

Contact Dermatitis
Drug Side Effect (Rash)
Eczema
Hives
Lice (Head and Body)
Poison Oak
Scabies
Tinea (Athlete's Foot, Jock
Itch, Ringworm)

► **Infectious Rashes**

Rules of Thumb

- For all appointments review isolation procedure.
- Treat all rashes as contagious until proven differently.

Isolation Procedure

- Isolation procedure when coming to clinic or hospital.
  - —Avoid contact with people who are pregnant, have been on cancer drugs, or who have AIDS. They are very susceptible to contagious infections.
  - —If you follow these instructions, you will not expose others to infection.
- Do not let infected person go outside or be with anyone in high-risk group (See Rules of Thumb above).
- Wash hands in warm soapy water every time you eat.
- Prevent infection of the sores by washing hands with soap and water at least four times a day.
- Do not share food, spoons, forks, towels, handkerchiefs, bath, or kisses with infected person.

Chickenpox

- Cause: Virus—antibiotics will not work.
  - —Exp. to chickenpox, measles, + Hx splenectomy or immunocompromised person (See above)? (> Risk)
- Treatment/course: Chickenpox lasts about 10-14 days. Chickenpox should be treated at home unless the person becomes very sick. Complications are rare.
- For Itching:
  - —Cut fingernails and try not to scratch.
  - —Baking soda baths (See Home Tx SI, Appendix A: Baking Soda Bath).
  - —Benadryl.

- Sores in mouth:

  —Pain: Tylenol; cold nonacid drinks

- Prevention: Chickenpox is very contagious, spread by coughing, sneezing, kissing, or sharing food. It is contagious from one day before the rash appears to 6 days after the rash appears. Most brothers and sisters of children who have it will get it, too. Once someone has had chickenpox, he or she rarely ever gets it again. But sometimes people who have had chickenpox get shingles later on.

German Measles (Rubella)

- Cause/Course: Mild virus. Antibiotics will not work. It is not as contagious as measles or chickenpox. Spread by coughing, sneezing, kissing, sharing food. The rash lasts for 2-4 days.

- Prevention: German measles is very dangerous to pregnant women who have not had their vaccination (MMR). If it happens in the first 3 mo of pregnancy, the child may be born deaf, have serious eye or heart problems, or brain damage. Do not let pt. have contact with or go near anyone who could possibly be pregnant.

- Treatment: Treat at home.

  —Fever: Tylenol

Red or Seven-Day Measles (Rubeola)

- Cause/Course: Highly contagious viral illness. No antibiotics are needed. The red measles last 4-7 days.

- Prevention: Spread through the air or by coughing, sneezing, kissing, sharing food, or used Kleenex. Not contagious after the rash is gone. All children who have been near the person with measles should come in immediately to get their immunizations (MMR).

- Treatment: Do not let children visit.

  —Fever: Tylenol.

  —Cough: Vaporizer.

  —Eye sensitivity to light: Darken the room; sunglasses when outside.

Roseola

- Cause/Course: Virus. Antibiotics won't work. Rash lasts 1-2 days. Usually found in children under the age of 3 yr but may occur at any age.

- Prevention/Tx:

  —Do not let other children visit. Watch for complications.

  —Should not last more than 4-5 days.

  —Fever: Tylenol as appropriate.

Scarlet Fever

- Cause/Course: *Streptococcus* bacteria. Needs antibiotics. Rash lasts 5-7 days.

- Treatment:

  —Fever: Tylenol

  —Sore throat: Cold clear liquids (See Home Tx SI, Appendix A: Clear Liquids)

► Other Rashes

Contact Dermatitis

- Causes: Exposure to things your body is extra sensitive to, like metal

- Complications: Itching, discomfort

- Prevention/Tx:
  —Wash exposed area well. Also wash contaminated clothing with soap and water.
  —Avoid exposure in future by wearing protective clothing, gloves, etc.
  —Always wash hands after contact with any skin rash.
  —Avoid scratching (will spread if contagious).
  —Avoid sun exposure; keep as cool as possible.
  —Avoid powders/cornstarch: They can cake in skin folds and increase irritation.

Drug Side Effect: Rash

Rule of Thumb: All drugs have the potential to cause a rash at any time. The drugs and classes of drugs below are related to a serious drug reaction, toxic epidermal necrolysis.

- Antibiotics (many)
- Allopurinol (Zyloprim)
- Barbiturates
- Lithium
- Nonsteroidal anti-inflammatory drugs
  —Advil
  —Ibuprofen
  —Midol 200
  —Motrin
  —Nuprin
- Penicillin
- Phenytoin (Dilantin)
- Sulfas

Eczema

- Cause: Skin sensitivity
- Complication: Infection
- Prevention/Tx:
  —Avoid rough clothing, wool, overheating.
  —Use Lowilla soap, Cetaphil, Keri, Nivea Lotion. Use after bath and 4-6 x day.
  —Hydrocortisone cream 0.5% to itching areas.
  —Bathe 3 x wk.

Hives

- Signs and symptoms: Itching, raised, pink rash. Hives may come and go for 3-4 days, then disappear.
- Causes: Your body reacts in a bad way to something that you come into contact with, such as too much cold, heat, stress, tension, or allergies to Rx, food, plant, chemical, or insect bite/sting.
- Complications: Itching, swelling, discomfort.
- Prevention/Tx:
  —Take medicine for itching. Don't wait for hives to disappear. Continue until hives are gone x 24 hr.
  —Cool baiting soda bath (See Home Tx SI, Appendix A: Baking Soda Bath).
  —Stay out of sun—makes itching worse.
  —Stop the Rx that caused rash. Talk w MD immediately.

—Be careful about eating foods such as shellfish, nuts, etc.

—Benadryl, Chlor-Trimeton.

—Calamine Lotion, not Caladryl.

—Try to discover and avoid whatever makes you itch or causes hives/rash.

Lice (Head and Body)

- Signs and symptoms: Itching; tiny white lumps on hair strands.
- Cause: Parasites. Lice may be spread by linens, toilet seats, and sexual contact.
- Complications: Discomfort; spreading lice to others
- Prevention: Do not share combs, brushes, hats, clothing.
- Tx goal: Remove parasites. Prevent others from getting them. Prevent parasites from coming back.
    —RID: Follow directions on medication package.

    —Wash all clothes/bedding.

    —You may put bedding in plastic bags for 10-14 days instead of sending them to the dry cleaners.

    —It is important to treat everyone in the family and clean everything the same day. Otherwise the lice may come back.

    —Med for lice is not recommended for pregnant women or very young children.

Poison Oak (Three-Leaf Low-Growing Shrub)

- Signs and symptoms: Severe itching, rash; red swelling, weeping, oozing blisters
- Causes: Oil from plant forms an invisible coating on the skin. Smoke from burning bush can also cause rash or severe allergic reaction.
- Complications: Rash may spread to eyes. Infection could develop.
- Prevention/Tx:
    —Shower and wash well w strong soap (Dial) as soon as possible after touching plant. Wash clothes. Do not put them back on until they have been washed with soap and water.

    —If it becomes worse, or fever develops, see MD.

    —Avoid exposure in future.

    —Avoid sun exposure; keep as cool as possible.

    —Avoid powders/cornstarch: They can cake in skin folds and increase irritation.
- Itching:
    —Benadryl.

    —Dress cool, bathe cool, sleep cool.

    —Cool compresses every 2 hr (See Home Tx SI, Appendix A: Cold/Cool Compress).

    —Cool baking soda and Aveeno baths (1/2 cup baking soda/tub) (See Home Tx SI, Appendix A: Baking Soda Bath).

    —Calamine Lotion (not Caladryl).

    —Hydrocortisone cream 1%.

    —Tylenol.

Scabies

* Signs and symptoms: See Protocol.
* Cause: Parasites lay eggs under skin.
* Prevention/Tx:
    —Needs appt. and Tx with prescription meds.
    —Scabies is highly contagious. All family members and close contacts need to be notified and treated. Incubation period is 2-6 wk. Bedding needs to be washed in hot, soapy water. Dry in dryer x 20 min or more; or put in double plastic bag x 7 days.

Tinea (Athlete's Foot, Jock Itch, Ringworm)

Contagious Fungal Infections

* Athlete's Foot
    —Signs and symptoms: See Protocol.
    —Complication: Infection.
    —Prevention/Tx:
        o Clean feet carefully w soap and water. Dry carefully,
        o Wear shoes that are made of canvas, or sandals,
        o Wear cotton socks, change often if possible,
        o Lotrimin

* Jock Itch
    —Signs and symptoms: See Protocol.
    —Complication: Infection.
    —Prevention/Tx:
        o Wear boxer shorts, decreases friction and moisture.
        ° Dry area well after bathing. Apply powder to help keep dry.
        o Tinactin powder.

* Ringworm
    —Signs and symptoms: See Protocol.
    —Cause: Fungus living on dead skin.
    —Complication: Secondary infection.
    —Prevention/Tx: Use topical antifungal cream 2-3 x day. If it doesn't clear up in 3 days, make an appt.
        ° Lotrimin
        ° Micatin
        ° Tinactin

SUBSTANCE ABUSE
Drugs; Alcohol; Prescription Drugs/Inhalants

ASSESSMENT	ACUITY LEVEL	DISPOSITION/ADVICE
Key Questions	Emergent Symptom Patterns	Ed 0 min-1 hr
Substance Abuse (Any)	+ Suicidal or homicidal ideation/threat or attempt? (See Emotional Problem 1)	
Inhalants	+ Respiratory arrest, asphyxia?	
Alcohol	+ Severe agitation, panic/anxiety, confusion, severe sweating? (DTs)	
	+ Seizures, coma, respiratory arrest, ± aspiration?	
Amphetamines ("Speed," "Ice")	+ Anxiety, restlessness, > heart rate, chest pain, muscle rigidity/twitching, seizures, fever?	
Cocaine	+ Anxiety, agitation, delirium, muscle rigidity, hyperactivity, seizures, fever, chest, pain, irregular heartbeat?	
Ecstasy	+ Muscle tension, teeth clenching, nausea, blurred vision, fainting, fever, chills, sweating,? (Malignant Hyperthermia)	
Opiates	+ Coma, respiratory arrest?	
PCP	+ Rigidity, fever, sweating, constricted pupils, seizures?	
Sedatives/Hypnotics	+ Hypothermia, coma, respiratory arrest?	
Hallucinogenics	+ Dilated pupils, red eyes, trembling, hallucinations, unpredictable behavior?	

Key Questions	Urgent Symptom Patterns	ED/UCC/Office 1-8 hr
IV, IM, SQ use Hx	+ Gradual onset: fever, chills/night sweats, fatigue, weight loss, joint pain? (Subacute Bacterial Endocarditis)	
	+ (All skin) Red ± streaking, swollen, tender, hot; ± discharge, often w fever, swollen nodes, ± Hx of trauma/bite/local infection? (Cellulitis, Lymphangitis, Abscess)	
Opiates	+ Sweating, N/V, abd. cramps, hot/cold flashes, fast breathing, inability to sleep, runny nose, sweating, tearing, shaky, rapid heartbeat, breathing? (Opiate Withdrawal)	
Snorting/Sniffing	+ Heroin w cocaine? (> Risk Hepatitis C)	

Key Questions	Acute/Nonacute Symptom Patterns	FA 8+ hr ± Home Tx
Substance Abuse (Any)	+ Pregnancy, breastfeeding (> Risk)	
	+ Patient requests information/test for HIV/hepatitis?	
	+ Patient/family requests drug or alcohol Tx program information?	

Cross-References

Confusion	Emotional Problems 1,2	Hepatitis, Appendix C Seizure	Shock

SUBSTANCE ABUSE
Supplemental Information

Quick Reference:
- ► FAQs: Drug Abuse
- ► Signs and Symptoms of Use/Abuse
  - CNS Depressants
  - Stimulants
  - Hallucinogens (Marijuana, LSD)
  - Inhalants
- ► Teens and Drug Abuse
- ► Senior Drinking and Prescription Drug Abuse
- ► Pregnancy and Drug Abuse
- ► Tutorial

See also: Directory of Hotlines/Web Sites for Support Groups, Appendix E

► FAQs: Drug Abuse
- How can you tell if someone is using drugs? (See Also Signs and Symptoms of Use/Abuse section below)
  - —Fall in grades (teen)
  - —Fall in extracurricular activities (teen)
  - —Family conflict/peer conflict
  - —Family Hx of drug abuse
  - —Drug paraphernalia: pipes, papers, roach clips
  - —Increased time spent in room or out of house
  - —Mood swings
- Why do people abuse drugs?
  - —Self-medication of emotional pain
  - —Experimentation
  - —Peer/family use
  - —Stress/anxiety
- How can drug abuse be prevented?
  - —Develop better ways of relieving stress, depression, and loneliness, such as exercise, friendships, and meditation or prayer
  - —Seek help from support groups (as detailed in the following questions)
  - —Use painkillers, tranquilizers, and sleeping pills cautiously. Don't take more than prescribed.
  - —Use meds for sleep or weight loss only under MD's supervision.
  - —Avoid taking alcohol when taking other meds to avoid reactions.
  - —Avoid stopping long-term meds w/o checking w MD.
- What is problem drinking?
  - —Woman who drinks > 7 drinks per week or > 3 drinks per occasion
  - —Man who drinks > 14 drinks per week or > 4 drinks per occasion
  - —Anyone > age 65 who drinks > 7 drinks per week or > 3 drinks per occasion
- How should someone be treated for withdrawal from drugs or alcohol?
  - —Patients who are withdrawing from alcohol or drugs need to be in the hospital.
  - —Withdrawal can last as long as 7-10 days.

—You need to be seen by an MD after withdrawal for blood tests and evaluation.

—Use support groups such as Alcoholics Anonymous, Cocaine Anonymous, or Narcotics Anonymous (See Substance Abuse: Drug/Alcohol, Appendix E).

▶ Signs and Symptoms of Use/Abuse

The following substances include common CNS depressants, alcohol, opiates, synthetic narcotics (e.g., Demerol, methadone), barbiturates: amobarbital, secobarbital (Seconal), and phenobarbital.

CNS Depressants

- Alcohol: Intoxication; euphoria; slurred speech; unsteady gait; breath smells of alcohol; decreased inhibition; decreased alertness; unusual inactivity, extreme apathy; nausea, hangover
- Opiates (OxyContin, Vicodin, Darvon, Dilaudid, Demerol, codeine, heroin, methadone, morphine, opium): "Pinpoint" constricted pupils; mood swings; slurred speech; sore eyes; weight loss; sweating; euphoria; flushing; itching; drowsiness; decreased respirations; nausea/vomiting
- Sedatives/hypnotics/tranquilizers [Valium (Diazepam), Librium (chlordiazepoxide), Dalmane (flurazepam), Ativan (lorazepam), Halcion (triazolam), Klonopin (clonazepam), alprazolam (Xanax), "date-rape drugs"—Rohypnol, GHB, ketamine]: drowsiness; rapid, jerky eye movements; staggering, unsteady gait; slurred, confused speech; poor memory; faulty judgment; mood swings; disrupted sleep pattern

Stimulants

- Cocaine/crack: Dilated pupils; constant sniffing; hallucinations/delusions; "coke fever" assoc, w muscle rigidity; trembling; nasal ulcers; itching all over body, ± open sores; chronic use: insomnia, weight loss, paranoia, intense craving
- Amphetamines ["speed," "crank," PCP ("angel dust"), club drugs, "ecstasy," Dexedrine, Ritalin—may be taken IV, snorted, smoked, via suppository, or ingested orally]: Dilated pupils; wakefulness; decreased sense of fatigue; elevated mood; increased self-confidence; increased motor activity; delusions; talkative; insomnia; trembling; w prolonged use: depression, fatigue, violent behavior, paranoia, intense craving
  —PCP ("angel dust"): rapid, jerky eye movements; dilated pupils; hallucinations (pleasant or frightening); trembling; chills; staggering; slurred speech

Hallucinogens (Marijuana, LSD)

- Marijuana: Red eyes; feeling of well-being; relaxation; inner joyfulness; heightened perception; altered sense of timing; unusual inactivity, extreme apathy; fatigue; decreased coordination
- LSD, mescaline: Dilated pupils, fever/chills, trembling, hallucinations, "flashbacks," unpredictable behavior

Inhalants

- Inhalants include, solvents, and aerosol sprays: air fresheners; butane; gasoline; glues and adhesives; hairsprays; nail polish removers; paints and paint thinners; pressurized aerosol sprays; refrigerants (freon); rust removers; spray paints; spray deodorants.
- Signs and symptoms of inhalant abuse are dilated pupils, flushed face, confusion, dizziness, euphoria, hallucinations, lightheadedness, slurred speech, unsteady gait.
- Inhalants can be extremely deadly. They can cause
  —Suffocation
  —Choking on one's own vomit

—Accidents and injuries from motor vehicle accidents or accidental injuries

—Burns if using butane, gasoline, or other flammable substances

—Suicide attempts

—Heart attacks

► **Teens and Drug Abuse**

- Most common reasons for teens to visit ED:

—Acute intoxication

—Associated trauma

—Frightening reaction to drug

—Drug-seeking behavior

—Parental request for drug screen

► **Senior Drinking and Prescription Drug Abuse**

- Approximately 17% of Americans age 55 or older have alcohol or drug problems.
- Out of the older Americans admitted to hospitals, 6%-11% have symptoms of alcoholism.
- Out of the elderly patients in psychiatric wards, 20% have symptoms of alcoholism.
- Out of the elderly patients in emergency rooms, 14% have symptoms of alcoholism.
- The most common addiction among the elderly is to benzodiazepines.

► **Pregnancy and Drug Abuse**

- Marijuana

—Babies more likely to have health problems

- Cocaine or Heroin

—Women may have severe bleeding in pregnancy.

—Premature birth.

—The baby or mother may die.

—The baby may be born addicted.

- PCP, Ketamine, LSD

—Mother may become violent.

—Baby may be smaller than normal.

—Learning, behavioral problems.

—Birth defects.

- Inhalants

—Birth defects: small head, joint problems, heart problems

- Amphetamines

—Premature birth

—Death of baby

—Inadequate growth

- Ecstasy

—Long-term learning and memory problems

► Tutorial

Assessment Tips

- Inhalant abuse clues for parents:
  —Teens may spray the substance into a bag, can, or other container and breathe the fumes.
  —They may spray or pour the substance onto a cloth or piece of clothing and inhale the fumes.
- Drug abuse may lead to increased accidents and falls.

Red Flags

Populations and symptoms that increase risk for substance abuse (SAVED: Severe symptoms, high-risk populations—age, veracity, emotional distress, debilitation)

- Symptoms:
  —Severe, sudden, or suspicious pain.
  —Beware of pain that is more severe than expected or unrelenting.
  —Beware of any pain that awakens patient or keeps him or her awake at night.
- Age/gender:
  —Adolescents, seniors, and women have increased potential for drug and alcohol abuse.
  —Women are more likely than men to be prescribed abusable prescription drugs.
- Occupation:
  —Health care professionals: MDs, nurses, pharmacists, veterinarians, dentists, and anesthesiologists are high risk due to ease of access and self-prescribing.
- Emotion:
  —Substance abuse carries serious short- and long-term risk for suicide. In general, alcohol and substance abuse is a predisposing risk for suicide.
  —Short-term substance abuse may precipitate a suicide attempt, as a result of increased impulsivity and acute stress related to self-medicating, depression, and anxiety with street drugs, alcohol, and prescription medications.
- Veracity:
  —Remain alert for possible denial.
  —All second-party calls regarding substance abuse or alcohol ingestion should raise suspicions.
- Debilitation:
  —Chronic disease, IV drug abuse, ALL immune deficiencies: AIDS/HIV. Frail elderly are high-risk populations for concurrent infection. Note: With the elderly, there is always the potential for Adverse Drug Reactions.
  —Recent injury: Remain alert for possible abuse.

Rules of Thumb

- Beware of the tendency to under-triage "frequent flyers" (drug seekers).
- Drug abuse often leads to domestic violence, date rape, emotional problems, and motor vehicle accidents.
- Minority callers may fail to recognize acute symptoms, report fewer symptoms, or attribute them to other causes.
- Drug/alcohol abuse is a key risk factor in suicide.

URINARY PROBLEM
Pain with or without Trauma; Frequency; Urgency; Change in Output/Color; Bloody Urine

ASSESSMENT	ACUITY LEVEL	DISPOSITION/ADVICE
Key Questions	Emergent Symptom Patterns	ED 0 min-1 hr
Major Trauma	+ (Urethral/flank/ribs abdomen/pelvis) weak, dizzy, cold/mottled/pale skin, bloody urine, bruise on flank, blue lips/nail beds, rapid/shallow breathing, unresponsive, loss of consciousness? (See Shock)	
Key Questions	Urgent Symptom Patterns	ED/UCC/Office 1-8 hr
Trauma	+ (Flank/back) Bloody urine, ± N/V, ± abd. pain? (Renal Contusion)	
Discharge (All)	+ Sexual intercourse w/o condom? (STI urethritis)	
Pain/Burning/Difficult/ Bloody Urination	+ (Sev. to mod.), Radiating from abd./flank/back to groin, colicky then constant & severe, fever/chills, N/V, dysuria, ± hematuria, frequency/urgency? (Pyelonephritis)	
	+ Male, fever/chills, malaise, muscle aches, painful urination, pelvic/perineal pain, cloudy urine, dribbling, hesitancy, decreased urine output, ± vague/flulike symptoms? (Acute Prostatitis)	
	+ Frequency, urgency, ± blood-tinged urine, bladder/suprapubic pain, ± nocturia, ± cloudy, foul or strong-smelling urine, + fever? (UTI)	
	+ Lower abd. pain, < urine output x 8 hr anesthesia, Hx recent urologic procedure? (Urinary Retention)	
Bloody Urine	+ Back/flank/groin pain (sev.)? (Kidney Stone)	
	+ Bloody urine, ± < urine output, ± N/V? (Hemorrhagic Cystitis)	
	+ Bloody urine, painless, w/o infection Sx/dizziness/weakness? (Hematuria)	
Difficult Urination	+ (Male) + Fever, ± backache? (Prostatitis)	

Key Questions	Acute/Nonacute Symptom Patterns	FA 8+ hr ± Home Tx
Output Change	+ Decreased (progressive), generalized edema, ± SOB, < stream? (Acute Renal Failure)	
	+ Increased (extreme), dilute urine, ± trauma? (Diabetes Insipidus)	
	+ Increased, weight loss, thirst, > hunger? (Diabetes Mellitus)	
Nocturia/Frequency	+ Male, < force, dribbling, hesitancy, straining, leaking, ± fever, Hx enlarged prostate? (Prostatic Enlargement, Chronic Prostatitis)	
	+ Increased voiding at night (3-5 x)? (Diabetes, HTN, CHF)	
Color Change	+ Dark urine, fever, N/V, anorexia, yellow skin, yellow sclera, fatigue, swollen glands, clay-colored stools, ±exp. to hepatitis? (Hepatitis) (See Appendix C)	
Incontinence	+ Sm. amt, gradual onset, assoc, w cough, sneezing, lifting, running, laughing, Hx multipara, menopausal woman? (Stress Incontinence)	
	+ Large quantity, recent loss of control, frail elderly? (UTI)	
Unusual Color of Urine	+ > 24 hr? (See Urinary Problem SI)	

Cross-References

Abdomen Problem	Hepatitis SI, Appendix C Vaginal Problem	Vaginal Problem: STI SI

URINARY PROBLEM
Supplemental Information

Quick Reference:
- ► Rules of Thumb
- ► Bladder Infection
- ► Drug Side Effect
  - Urinary Color Change
  - Urine, Bloody
  - Urinary Incontinence
  - Urinary Retention
- ► Food Side Effect—Urinary Color Change
- ► Stress Incontinence

See also: Directory of Hotlines/Web Sites for Support Groups, Appendix E

► **Rules of Thumb**
- Low urine output: 2 tbsp/hr minimum.
- UTIs are 10 x more common in women. Female urethra is 1-2 in; male is 7-8 in.
- UTIs are common during pregnancy.
- Voiding dysfunction is rule rather than exception in elderly men.

► **Bladder Infection**
- Definition: Having a lot of germs, bacteria in any part of bladder or kidneys
- Signs and symptoms: See Protocol.
- Complications: Kidney infection symptoms: Flank side pain, severe shaking, chills, and fever.
- Prevention goal: Comfort; prevent infection.
  - —Drink 4-6 glasses of water/day, esp. in warm weather.
  - —Don't put off going to bathroom. Go when you feel the need to urinate.
  - —Take all antibiotics until they are gone. Call if no improvement after 48 hr or 8 doses.
  - —Avoid ASA, Advil, Motrin, antihistamines, decongestants—may cause constriction of ureters.
  - —Travel: Drink water often. Go to bathroom often.
  - —If unable to start stream, sit in warm bath, and urinate into tub.
  - —Females:
    - ° Always wipe from front to back to avoid bacteria from rectum,
    - o Urinate right after sex to clear out germs.
    - ° Avoid bubble bath—irritates skin in genital area.
    - ° Wear cotton underwear.
    - ° Avoid tight-fitting underwear, pantyhose, jeans.

►   Drug Side Effect

Urinary Color Change

Drugs and classes of drugs that may cause urinary color change:

- Metronidazole (Flagyl): yellow
- Nitrofurantoin (Furadantin, Macrodantin): Yellow, brown, or darker
- Phenazopyridine (Pyridium): orange/red
- Rifampin (Rifadin): Red/orange
- Sulfonamides: Yellow
- Vitamins: orange/yellow
- Vitamin B complex: Green

Urine, Bloody

Drugs and classes of drugs that may cause hematuria:

- Anticoagulants
- Aspirin
- Methenamine (Azo-mandelamine)
- Methotrexate (Folex, Mexate)
- Sulfonamides

Urinary Incontinence

Drugs and classes of drugs that may cause incontinence:

- Diuretics
- Methyldopa (Aldomet)
- Phenothiazines
  —Chlorpromazine (Thorazine)
  —Prochlorperazine (Compazine)
  —Thioridazine (Mellaril)
  —Trifluoperazine (Stelazine)

Urinary Retention

Drugs and classes of drugs that may cause retention:

- Alpha-adrenergic agents
- Anticholinergics
  —Atropine
  —Belladonna
  —Scopolamine
- Ephedrine
- Pseudoephedrine (Actifed, Chlor-Trimeton, Pediacare, Sudafed)
- Phenylpropanolamine (Acutrim, Allerest, Contac, Dexatrim, Dimetapp, Ornade, Triaminic)

►   Food Side Effect: Urinary Color Change

- Beets (orange)
- Rhubarb (brown)

► Stress Incontinence

- Definition: Loss of urine
- Signs and symptoms: Urine loss w coughing, sneezing, laughing, running, or lifting
- Causes: In women, cystocele as a result of aging or stretching of pelvic floor muscles during childbirth; in men, may follow removal of prostate or trauma to urethra
- Complications: Inconvenient, embarrassing
- Prevention/Tx:
  —Kegel exercises
  —Drug therapy
  —Surgical correction

VOMITING/NAUSEA

Bloody; Excessive; Projectile; Toxin; Headache; Abdominal Pain

ASSESSMENT	ACUITY LEVEL	DISPOSITION/ADVICE
Key Questions	Emergent Symptom Patterns	ED 0 min-1 hr
Nausea/Vomiting	+ Bright red blood/coffee ground, ± abd. pain? (Upper GI Bleed)	
	+ Fever, stiff neck, headache, extreme fatigue, ± pinpoint red purplish spots progressing to purple patches, extremely irritable, ± neck pain, photophobia, fever/chills, Hx HIV, confusion/restless/extremely sleepy ± seizure? (Meningococcal Meningitis)	
	+ Hx head trauma, ± projective vomiting, irritable, lethargic, ± loss of consciousness? (> Intracranial Pressure)	
	+ Hx of accidental/purposeful exp. to: street drugs/Rx, poisonous plant or wild mushroom or inhalation/ ingestion of toxic chemical or pesticide? (Toxic Exposure)--►Contact poison center and bring substance to ED w you.	
	+ Chest pain: ± exertion (dull ache, pressure, squeezing, crushing, radiates to neck/jaw/arms), SOB, sweating, dizziness, lightheaded, N/V, pale, severe anxiety? (MI/Angina)	
	+ Dehydration Sx., + confused, -t-altered level of consciousness, cold/clammy skin, ± decreased urine output? (Complicated Nausea/Vomiting requiring Correction of Fluids, Electrolytes, Acid/Base Status)	
	+ Ingestion of home-canned or Alaska native foods (fermented fish, seal, beaver, whale), blurred/double vision, drooping eyelids, trouble swallowing/talking/ breathing, muscle weakness, abd. pain, diarrhea? (Botulism)	

Key Questions	Urgent Symptom Patterns	ED/UCC/Office 1 -8 hr
Nausea/Vomiting	+ Projectile or head trauma? (> Intracranial Pressure)	
	+ Persistent vomiting (> 12-24 hr)? (Severe Symptom)	
	+ Low or no intake, ± diarrhea, ± urine output 8 hr, weak, dizzy, dry mouth, sunken eyes, extreme thirst, confusion, fatigue? (> Risk Dehydration)--------------•▶	+ SA: Pinch skin briefly and release; describe; if skin stays pinched looking = tenting or + for dehydration
	+ High-risk groups: frail elderly > 60 yr. all: immunocompromised, AIDS/HIV, chemotherapy, diabetes, bedridden, ileostomy Hx, temp. > 38.3°C or > 101°F? (> Risk Dehydration)	
	+ Abdominal pain, ± fever? (Appendicitis/Diverticulitis/ Peritonitis, Pyelonephritis, Cholecystitis, Infectious Diarrhea) (Pancreatitis, Hepatitis, Incarcerated Hernia, Food Poisoning) (See also Abdomen Problem 1; 2 SI).	
	+ Colicky, abd. distention, Hx of major change in bowel habits, not passing gas? (Bowel Obstruction)	
	+ Crampy abd. pain w dehydration symptoms, ± fever, ± joint pain, + headache, unable to hold down fluids x 6-8 hr? (Gastroenteritis)	
	+ Pregnant, unable to hold down food/fluids x 6-8 hr? (Hyperemesis Gravidarum) (See Pregnancy Problems)	
	+ Headache, dizziness/staggering (sudden onset), jerky eye movement, ± Hx URI, + hearing loss? (Labyrinthitis, Vestibular Neuronitis)	
	+ Headache (sev. to mod.), throbbing, ± unilateral, > sensitivity to light & noise, Hx similar headaches, female, ± triggers, ± preceded by aura (Migraine) (See Head Problem 2)	

Key Questions	Acute/Nonacute Symptom Patterns	FA 8+ hr ± Home Tx
Nausea/Vomiting	+ Sexually active, breast tenderness, late or missed period? (Rule Out Pregnancy, Poss. Morning Sickness)	
	+ Fever, anorexia, yellow skin, yellow sciera, fatigue, swollen glands, clay-colored stools, dark urine, ± exp. to hepatitis? (Hepatitis) (See Hepatitis SI, Appendix C)	
	+ Self-induced vomiting, ± extreme weight loss, laxative/diuretic/enema abuse, evidence of purging in bathroom, overstrict dieting, using bathroom frequently after meals, dental problems, sore throat, weakness/exhaustion, bloodshot eyes? (Bulimia Nervosa Risk Metabolic Electrolyte Disturbance Poss. Upgrade)	
	+ Hx effortless vomiting w/o pain following meal, acid taste in mouth (Gastroesophageal Reflux)	
	+ Following antibiotics? (Drug Reaction)	
	+ Following meds for chronic condition (i.e., seizure chemotherapy med)? (> Risk Seizures or Disease)	
	+ Crampy abd. pain w/o dehydration symptoms, diarrhea, ± fever, ± joint pain, ± headache? (Gastroenteritis)---	-^-Upgrade if symptoms of sev. to mod. dehydration.
	+ Coughing spasm leading to vomiting, worse at night? (Paroxysmal Coughing Posttussive Emesis)	

Cross-References
Abdomen Problem

Head Problem 1; 2		Pregnancy Problem 1
Hepatitis SI, Appendix C Urinary Problem		

VOMITING/NAUSEA
Supplemental Information

Quick Reference:
- ▶ Bulimia Nervosa
- ▶ Dehydration Treatment
- ▶ Drug Side Effect:
  Nausea/Vomiting
- ▶ HIV/AIDS and Vomiting
- ▶ Infectious Diarrhea
  ("Food Poisoning")
- ▶ Motion Sickness
- ▶ Nausea/Vomiting
- * Oncology
- ▶ Projectile Vomiting
- »- Surgical: Postoperative
  Nausea and Vomiting
- ▶ Tutorial

See also: Directory of Hotlines/Web Sites for Support Groups, Appendix E

▶ Bulimia Nervosa

® Signs and symptoms: See Protocol.

® Causes: Bulimia nervosa is a psychological disorder in which sufferers eat large amounts of food at once. They then cause themselves to vomit or use laxatives and/or diuretics. They might use intense exercise, fasting, and suffer extreme guilt and shame. The bulimic may be overweight or underweight.

- Risk groups: Up to 5% of college women in the United States are bulimic.

- Complications: Dehydration, damage to bowels, liver and kidney, chemical imbalance, which leads to irregular heartbeat, and in some cases, cardiac arrest.

- Prevention/Tx: It is important for a physician familiar with eating disorders to examine the patient. Counseling by a physician or a nutrition therapist, a psychologist, psychiatrist, or group therapy is needed. Inpatient treatment or residential treatment centers from 2 weeks to months with family involvement may be necessary.

▶ Dehydration Treatment

• Signs and symptoms: See Protocol.

e Causes: Loss of water because of vomiting, diarrhea, extreme heat or sweating, or not drinking enough water. Dehydration is a very serious condition and can lead to death, especially in the elderly and infants or those with chronic illness.

® Complications: Kidney problems, shock or death.

® Prevention/Tx: (See also Home Treatment)

—If you are having symptoms of dehydration, over a period of hours, drink enough water to make urine pale yellow or clear.

—You may buy oral rehydration solution.

—Drink extra water before exercising and in hot weather.

▶ Drug Side Effect: Nausea/Vomiting

Drugs and classes of drugs that may cause nausea and vomiting

® Antibiotics (many)

- Antihypertensives

- Antiretrovirals

- Codeine
- Cytotoxic drugs
- Digoxin (Lanoxin)
- Drugs for opportunistic infections
- Iron preparations
- Nicotine and nicotine gum
  —Nicoderm
  —Habitrol
  —Nicorette
- Nonsteroidal anti-inflammatory drugs
  —Advil
  —Aleve
  —Ibuprofen
  —Midol 200
  —Motrin
  —Nuprin
- Quinidine
- Salicylates
  —Aspirin
  —Bismuth subsalicylate (Pepto Bismol)
- Xanthine bronchodilators (Theophylline, Aminophylline)

► **HIV/AIDS and Vomiting**
- Some antiretroviral medications have a side effect of nausea. Don't alter your dose schedule until you have checked with MD. You may then try the following:
  —Splitting doses of medications may lessen nausea.
- Taking meds with food. (Check to see which can be taken with your medication.)
  —Try antinausea medication (OTC or Rx).
  —Take pills a few at a time, rather than a handful.
  —See Nausea/Vomiting: Prevention/Tx below.

► **Infectious Diarrhea ("Food Poisoning")**
- Signs and symptoms: See Protocol.
- Cause: Bacteria, toxins.
- Complications: Shock, dehydration. Rare fatalities in very young and the elderly or those w chronic illness.
- Prevention:
  —Never eat home-preserved meat, fish, poultry, or milk products that have been unrefrigerated or left in sun for any length of time.
  —Wash hands before preparing foods.
  —Cover and refrigerate foods quickly.
  —Boil home-canned foods 30 min.

- Tx:

    —Bed rest.

    —Convenient access to a bathroom.

    —See Dehydration Assessment/Home Treatment SI, Appendix A: Rehydration Guidelines.

► Motion Sickness

- Signs and symptoms: Pale, cold, sweating, fast breathing, nausea, and vomiting
- Causes: > Activity of the middle ear caused by > motion
- Prevention:

    —Don't eat large meals before traveling by car, boat, air.

    —In airplane: Sit by window near wing.

    —In car: Sit in front seat near window. Leave window open.

    —Don't read while in motion; it will make it worse.

- Tx:

    —< The problem by being where least motion is in airplanes, on ships.

    —Take Rx 1 hr before going on the ship, driving, or flying.

► Nausea/Vomiting

- Goal: Keep clear liquids down. Increase fluid intake. Prevent dehydration.
- Definition:

    —Severe = Unable to hold down food/fluid > 24 hr

    —Moderate = Unable to hold down food/fluid x 12-24 hr

    —Mild = Unable to hold down food/fluid x 3-12 hr

- Causes: Illness, obstruction, trauma, food poisoning, medications, and poisonous ingestion, motion.
- Complication: Dehydration.
- Prevention/Tx:

    —Nothing by mouth for 2 hr after vomiting.

    —When nauseated or vomiting: Rest quietly and avoid movement; it can trigger nausea and vomiting.

    —Rest the stomach. Try small sips of water, or ice chips.

    —If even sips of water will not stay down, call the doctor.

    —Next 2 hr: Sip clear liquids q 20-30 min. (See Home Tx SI, Appendix A: Clear Liquids)

    —If sips of water will stay down, take bigger amounts, little by little.

    —Next 2 hr: Increase amt. liquid q 20-30 min.

    —Next 8 hr: No solids. Take needed medications only.

    —Slowly start on a bland or "BRAT" diet x 24 hr. ("BRAT" diet: Bananas, rice, and applesauce, white toast, or crackers, cereal, pasta, mashed potato, and soup.)

    —As you are able, resume regular diet.

Do

- Eat small meals 5 to 7 times a day, rather than 3 large meals.
- Eat salty foods such as crackers, which can sometimes help nausea.
- Try foods that are cold or at room temperature; hot food may worsen nausea.
- Try herbal tea (e.g., peppermint or chamomile) or ginger tea.

Don'ts

- Don't drink milk, milk products, or carbonated drinks.
- Don't eat solids and liquids at the same time—space them 1 hr apart.
- Avoid greasy, spicy, fried or fatty foods; avoid solid and heavy food.
- Don't lie flat for at least 1 hr after you eat.

► Oncology

- Signs and symptoms: See Protocol.
- Causes: Cytotoxic treatments create high risk for vomiting and nausea.
- Complications: Dehydration. Constipation, abdominal cramps and swelling might indicate bowel obstruction.
- Prevention/Tx: Try to drink 6-8 glasses of water/day. See treatment for nausea and vomiting (above.)

► Projectile Vomiting

- Signs and symptoms: Sudden forceful vomiting, without nausea first (a very serious symptom).
- Causes: Blockage of the intestines, head injuries, and pyloric stenosis (in infants).

► Surgical: Postoperative Nausea and Vomiting (PONV)

Common side effect following surgery: 30% of all adults have PONV, and nearly 50% of all patients for both in- and outpatient surgery. Severe and persistent vomiting following surgery can cause postoperative bleeding, wound and esophageal tears and rupture, rib fractures, muscular fatigue, aspiration and dehydration, particularly in children.

At-Risk Groups for PONV

Age/Gender—High Risk

- Children are twice as likely as adults to experience PONV; children 6-16 yr of age are at highest risk.
- Adult women have more episodes and they are usually more severe than men.

Age/Gender—Low Risk

- PONV is less frequent in elderly patients and men.

Predisposing Factors

- PONV is more likely in patients with past history of PONV or motion sickness.
- Anxiety, body weight, and PONV are positively related.
- Postoperative: pain, movement, premature intake of fluids and food increase risk.
- Agents such as opioids, nitrous oxide, intravenous anesthetics, and volatile anesthetic
- High-risk surgery site: Abdominal, vaginal, laparoscopic, orthopedic, and ENT surgeries
- The longer the operation, the greater risk for PONV.

Diminishing Factors

- Lowest incidence: Peripheral and superficial extremity surgeries
- Spinal anesthesia is generally associated with less PONV.

► Tutorial

Red Flags (Remain Alert to Red Flags)

- Severe, sudden, or suspicious or intractable vomiting
- Severity and sudden onset of symptoms tends to be an indicator of high acuity.

- Remain suspicious: Beware of atypical presentations, especially in elderly. What appear as "flu symptoms" (i.e., nausea/vomiting), may be cardiac, infection-based, or covert suicidal ingestion.
- Nausea and vomiting are associated with "flu" symptoms and always considered suspicious.
- Age: Elderly are more susceptible to dehydration.
- Debilitation/chronic disease/pregnancy are often risk factors when nausea and vomiting occur.
- Medications (See Drug Side Effect: Nausea/Vomiting above).
- Recent Injury, esp. abdomen and head.
- Recent Surgery (See Surgical: Postoperative Nausea and Vomiting above).
- Recent Infection or Ingestion.

Rules of Thumb

- Minority callers often fail to recognize acute symptoms, report fewer symptoms, or attribute them to other causes.
- Beware of any symptom that awakens patient or keeps him or her awake at night.
- With elderly always rule out toxicity and dehydration.
- Assess all elderly with unexplained symptoms for possible unintentional or purposeful ingestion/exposure to toxins, inhalants, street or prescription drugs.

Red Herrings

- Remain vigilant to possible patient denial, minimization or misinterpretation of symptoms.
- Regard with suspicion: Elderly callers and unusual sounding presentations or described as the "flu," or new, sudden, or unexpected, onset.
- Patients who have been "seen recently" may still need to be seen today.
- Don't be misled by concurrent complaints or patient self-explanation.
- Symptom presentation may be early, late, silent, atypical, or novel.
- Symptoms of two conditions may present concurrently, thereby causing confusion or misinterpretation.
- Illness rarely presents as a single symptom.
- Patients often misinterpret or stereotype their symptoms.

BIRTH CONTROL OPTIONS, CONCERNS, AND FREQUENTLY ASKED QUESTIONS
Supplemental Information

Quick Reference:
- ▶ Signs and Symptoms of Pregnancy
- ▶ Emergency Contraception: Emergency Contraceptive Pill
- ▶ Birth Control Options
  - Abstinence
  - Chemical Barriers: Spermicides
  - Physical Barriers: Cervical Cap, Condoms (Male and Female), Diaphragm

- Hormonal: Birth Control Pills Depo-Provera; Implants
- IUD: Copper T, Copper 7, Progestesert
- ▶ Rhythm (Natural Family Planning/Fertility Awareness)
- ▶ Sterilization (Male and Female)
- ▶ Withdrawal
- ▶ Birth Control Tutorial

See also Abdomen Problem 1, 2; Vaginal Bleedings: Vaginal Problems, Directory of Hotlines/Web Sites for Support Groups, Appendix E

▶ Signs and Symptoms of Pregnancy

Caution: Always elicit and rule out symptoms related to abdominal pain/problem, vaginal discharge, and sexual abuse.

Am I Pregnant?

- Signs and symptoms: Missed period; nausea; swollen, tender breasts; fatigue; urinary frequency/urgency. It is possible to be pregnant and still have a period.

Always contact the MD/nurse about any abnormal bleeding, with or without sharp, progressive, unilateral pelvic pain, that radiates to shoulder, symptoms of lightheadedness or fainting and/or pallor. Always tell the nurse if you have a history of STIs (Sexually Transmitted Infections), PID (Pelvic Inflammatory Disease), any abdominal/tubal surgery, prior IUD use, spotting, or have missed a period for 3-6 wk, or painful intercourse (this may indicate an ectopic pregnancy). *Ectopic pregnancy* is a serious, life-threatening condition. So, if you have *any* abnormal bleeding, it is best to get a pregnancy test.

- Follow-up: If your period is more than one day late or if you have abnormal bleeding, you may get a pregnancy test. Make an appointment for contraceptive/sexual on-site counseling regarding pregnancy, cervical cancer, STIs, and HIV infections.

What Choices Do I Have about Birth Control (BC)?

- ® In an emergency, such as unprotected sexual intercourse, you can use emergency contraception. [See Emergency Contraceptive Pill (ECP)]
- For long-term temporary birth control, you may use abstinence, barriers (chemical/physical), hormone, IUD, rhythm, and withdrawal.
- If you want a permanent form of birth control, you or your partner can use sterilization.

What Are Common Causes for BC Failure?

- Condom broke, came off, got lost, couple got drunk/high and failed to use protection, etc.
- "Forgot to use" (condom, diaphragm, gel, etc.).
- Withdrawal may not have been in time.

► **Emergency Contraception: Emergency Contraceptive Pill (ECP)**

RN: This treatment does not require MD/NP authorization and an Rx before implementing if you are 18 yr of age or older.

How Does It Work?

- ECP is simply a very large dose of hormones or birth control pills.
- It works by preventing pregnancy from taking place.
- This treatment works *only* if taken within 72 hr after unprotected intercourse.

How Effective Is It in Preventing Pregnancy?

- 75%-80% effective if used correctly.

What Things Can Make This Method Less Effective in Preventing Pregnancy?

- ECP will not work at all if taken after 72 hr.

What Are the Side Effects?

- Nausea/vomiting, breast tenderness, headache, fatigue, dizziness.

Follow-up

- Routine follow-up is not required.
- A pregnancy test should be done if bleeding has not happened within 3-4 wk after ECP.

Other FAQs

What Can I Do for the Nausea?

- Take Dramamine 11 or Benadryl 1 hr before first dose. If no relief, call for prescription medication.

How Will I Know It Worked?

- If you get your period within 7-20 days, it worked. But you should always get a pregnancy test anyway.
- If you don't have a period within 21 days, you must get a pregnancy test.

► **Birth Control Options**

Abstinence

- Strictly speaking, abstinence means not having sexual intercourse. The penis may not come near or enter the vagina *at all* or you can get pregnant.

How Effective Is It in Preventing Pregnancy?

- 100% effective if used 100% of the time.

What Things Can Make This Method Less Effective in Preventing Pregnancy?

- Use of recreational drugs or alcohol may lead to unprotected intercourse.
- If you fail to practice it 100% of the time, it can result in getting pregnant.

What Are the Side Effects?

- None

What Are the Risks? (Life-Threatening or Serious Health Hazards)

- None

What Are the Benefits? (Enhance Quality of Life, Cost, Convenience, Decrease Stress)

- No cost; decreased stress related to anxiety about pregnancy, STIs, and AIDS.

Chemical Barriers: Spermicides

- Cream, foam, gel
- Suppositories
- Vaginal contraceptive film (VCF)

How Do They Work?

- Spermicides in all forms act by paralyzing sperm. They must be inserted into vagina before sexual intercourse. (See manufacturer's instructions about exactly when they must be inserted. If you don't do it at the right time, *it may not work!)*

How Effective Are They in Preventing Pregnancy?

- Spermicides are more effective (80%-85%) if used with condom, diaphragm.
- By itself, a spermicide prevents pregnancy < 50% of the time if used correctly.

What Can Make These Methods Less Effective in Preventing Pregnancy?

- Use of recreational drugs or alcohol may lead to unprotected intercourse.
- If you are not using them according to instructions and *every* time, you can become pregnant.

What Are the Side Effects?

- Some people are allergic to chemicals in spermicides. They might have symptoms such as rash, irritation, or burning on vagina or penis.

What Are the Risks? (Life-Threatening or Serious Health Hazards)

- None

What Are the Benefits? (Enhance Quality of Life, Cost, Convenience, Decrease Stress)

- Readily accessible; inexpensive

Follow-up

- Make an appointment for contraception/sexual counseling regarding pregnancy, cervical cancer, STIs, and HIV infections.

Other FAQs

- How do I use them?

  —See manufacturers' instructions, which are usually very clear and complete.

  —You must follow instructions about when to insert spermicide before having sex. It is important that you do it at the right time or it may not work.

- Are they harmful if swallowed?

  —No. They might taste funny but they're harmless. If you want to have oral sex, use a type of spermicide that can be inserted right before intercourse. (*Always Check Manufacturer's Instructions.)*

Physical Barrier: Cervical Cap

How Does It Work?

- A cervical cap is a small 2-in, thimblelike latex cap that fits over cervix. It is used with a spermicide. It acts as a physical barrier to block sperm from the uterus and holds spermicide in place to paralyze sperm.

How Effective Is It in Preventing Pregnancy?

- 60%-80% effective if used correctly and *every* time you have sex.
- May be inserted up to 2 hr before sexual intercourse and may be left in for up to 2 days after insertion.

What Can Make This Method Less Effective in Preventing Pregnancy?

- Use of recreational drugs or alcohol may lead to unprotected intercourse.
- Cervical cap may fall off the cervix. Sometimes it is difficult to position it properly, leading to the risk of pregnancy.
- Never use oil-based lubricants like mineral oil, Vaseline, hand or massage lotion, vegetable oil, or cold cream. These can damage the cap, causing it to lose its effectiveness. Use only with spermicide. You may use the spermicide as a lubricant.

What Are the Side Effects?

- Some people are allergic to latex or chemicals in spermicides. They might have symptoms such as rash, irritation, or burning in vagina or on penis.

What Are the Risks? (Life-Threatening or Serious Health Hazards)

- There is an extremely low risk for toxic shock: 1 per 100,000 women. This can happen when women using this device are having their period.

What Are the Benefits? (Enhance Quality of Life, Cost, Convenience, Decrease Stress)

- This method decreases risk of bladder infections, unlike the diaphragm.
- You may leave it in for up to 2 days.

Follow-up

- Make an appointment for contraceptive/sexual on-site counseling regarding pregnancy, cervical cancer, STIs, and HIV infections.

Other FAQs

- How do I know the cervical cap is in right?

    —You need an appointment to learn how to insert it correctly. You will also need a prescription.

Physical Barrier: Condoms (Male and Female)

How Does It Work?

- The condom works by physically blocking sperm from entering the uterus.
- If you are not sure how to use a condom, come in for an appointment to learn how to use one. In an emergency, buy brands that have instructions.

How Effective Is It in Preventing Pregnancy?

- Male condom with spermicide = 85% effective if used correctly and *every* time.
- Female condom with spermicide = 80% effective if used correctly and *every* time.

What Can Make This Method Less Effective in Preventing Pregnancy?

- Use of recreational drugs or alcohol may lead to unprotected intercourse.
- If condom is not used correctly or every time, pregnancy can happen.
- Condoms sometimes break or come off too soon and are left in vagina.

What Are the Side Effects?

- Some people are allergic to latex and to chemicals in spermicides. They might have symptoms such as rash, irritation, or burning in vagina or on penis.

What Are the Risks? (Life-Threatening or Serious Health Hazards)

- Failure to use condoms properly may result in pregnancy, STIs, or HIV.

What Are the Benefits? (Enhance Quality of Life, Cost, Convenience, Decrease Stress)

- Condoms are the best protection against STIs.

Follow-up

- Make an appointment for contraception/sexual on-site counseling regarding pregnancy, cervical cancer, STIs, and HIV infections.

Other FAQs

a What are the most reliable type of condoms?

—Latex and polyurethane condoms are the strongest and most resistant to damage/breakage.

Physical Barrier: Diaphragm

How Does It Work?

- A diaphragm is a latex dishlike bowl, approximately 2 in wide, that fits into the vagina to cover the cervix. It is usually used with a spermicide. It blocks sperm from getting into the uterus. The diaphragm holds spermicide against cervix to paralyze sperm.

How Effective Is It in Preventing Pregnancy?

a Diaphragm with spermicide = 80% effective if used correctly and *every* time.

What Can Make This Method Less Effective in Preventing Pregnancy?

- Use of recreational drugs or alcohol may lead to unprotected intercourse.
- Diaphragm sometimes gets tears or holes. This happens when it is not well cared for, or if it is too old (more than 1 yr).
- Never use oil-based lubricants like mineral oil, Vaseline, hand or massage lotion, vegetable oil or cold cream. These can damage the diaphragm, causing it. Use only with spermicide. You may use the spermicide as a lubricant.

What Are the Side Effects?

- Allergies to latex and to chemicals in spermicides can cause symptoms such as rash, irritation, or burning in vagina or on penis.
- Bladder infections may occur, because of pressure of diaphragm.
- Backache or abdominal pain may occur if there is a poor fit.

a You may have a foul vaginal discharge odor if you leave it in too long.

What Are the Risks? (Life-Threatening or Serious Health Hazards)

- There is an extremely low risk for toxic shock: 1 per 100,000 women. This can happen when women using this device are having their period.

What Are the Benefits? (Enhance Quality of Life, Cost, Convenience, Decrease Stress)

- You may insert it up to 4 hr before intercourse.

a Diaphragms offer some protection from STIs and HIV.

Follow-up

- Make an appointment for contraception/sexual on-site counseling regarding pregnancy, cervical cancer, STIs, and HIV infections.

Other FAQs

a How do I know diaphragm is in right?

—You need to be "fitted" for diaphragm. Make an appointment for prescription and instruction.

- How do I help prevent bladder infection?

—Go to bathroom before intercourse and right after, to decrease risk of bladder infection.

—Drink two to three glasses of water daily to flush out bladder.

- Can my partner feel it?

—Most of the time, no.

- Can I "change sizes" of diaphragm?

—Yes. For example, your body could need a larger or smaller size after gaining or losing 5-10 lb, after having a baby, or after pelvic surgery.

Hormonal: Birth Control Pills (BCPs)

- Synthetic hormones: a combination of estrogen and progestin or progestin alone.

How Do They Work?

- Hormones prevent eggs from being released.

How Effective Are they in Preventing Pregnancy?

- Combination of estrogen and progestin: 95%-99.6% effective if used as directed.
- Progestin: 95%-97% effective if used as directed.

What Can Make This Method Less Effective in Preventing Pregnancy?

- Failure to take BCP every day at the same time.
- Use of recreational drugs or alcohol with BCP may lead to failure to take pills on time, leading to unprotected intercourse.
- Use of the following medications with BCP may cause possible decreased contraceptive effect:
  —Antibiotics (penicillins, tetracycline, others)
  —Anticonvulsants [phenytoin (Dilantin), mephenytoin, ethotoin, carbamazepine (Tegretol), others]
  —Antifungals [griseofulvin (Fulvicin, Grifulvin V) others]
  —Anti-infectives (Septra, Bactrim, rifampicin, others)
  —Barbiturates (phenobarbital, primidone, ethosuximide, others)

What Are the "Absolute" Contraindications? (May Not Take BCPs)

- Hx of estrogen-dependent tumor
- Deep vein thrombosis
- Heart attack or history of heart attack
- Pulmonary embolus or history of pulmonary embolus
- Stroke or history of stroke
- Liver disease
- Undiagnosed abnormal vaginal bleeding
- > 35-yr-old smoker

What are the "relative" contraindications? (May Take BCPs with Caution)

- Breast-cancer history, no evidence x 5 yr
- Medications use (See BCPs Affected by Drugs; Drugs Affected by BCPs below)
- Migraine headaches
- Poorly controlled high blood pressure
- Postpartum <21 days
- Vaginal bleeding, undiagnosed

What Are the Side Effects?

- Abdominal bloating
- Breast tenderness or enlargement, discharge
- Dizziness
- Emotional changes: depression, irritability
- Headache
- Increased/decreased appetite
- Nausea
- Sex drive changes: > or <
- Skin changes, a spotty darkening of the skin on the face, acne, oiliness, hair growth

- Vaginal bleeding changes: irregular/scant/breakthrough, missed period (get pregnancy test)
- Vaginal discharge changes
- Weight changes, gain or loss

What Are the Risks? (Life-Threatening or Serious Health Hazards)

Come in immediately if these symptoms occur:

- Any leg/groin/calf pain
- Chest pain
- Coughing up blood
- Dizziness
- Faintness
- Headache: sudden or severe
- Loss of coordination
- Any respiratory problems or shortness of breath
- Slurred speech
- Visual changes

Call for immediate appointment for following symptoms:

- Abdominal pain, swelling, or tenderness
- Breast lumps
- Jaundice (yellowing skin/eyes)
- Vaginal bleeding, abnormal

What Are the Benefits? (Enhance Quality of Life, Cost, Convenience, Decrease Stress)

- Convenient daily pill
- Inexpensive
- Do not interfere with sexual intercourse, increase spontaneity

Follow-up

- Make appointment for counseling and examination. Always have a yearly check-up to re-evaluate overall health and risks/benefits of this form of birth control.
- Re-evaluate whether you still want to use this form of birth control at least every 6 months with your healthcare provider.

Other FAQs

- Will I get cancer from BCPs?
  —No, there is very little risk.
- How long can I take BCPs?
  —As long as you need, if you have no problems or side effects.
- Does taking BCPs affect my fertility?
  —There is no evidence that BCPs decrease fertility.
- Can I smoke and use BCPs?
  —Smoking is not advised; it may be dangerous to health in combination with BCPs.
- How expensive are BCPs?
  —$ 1 per day; cheaper through Planned Parenthood (Teens: Ask boyfriend to help pay one-half.)
- Why are my periods so light and short on BCPs?
  —This is normal; hormones *may* reduce growth of lining of uterus.

- Will I get cramps on BCPs?

  —It will help reduce cramps.

- Will my periods get lighter?

  —Yes, usually.

- What if I get pregnant while on BCPs?

  —It is not harmful to baby. Call and get pregnancy test if you are worried. Do *not* stop taking the pills until after getting results of pregnancy test.

- Will BCPs protect me against STIs and AIDS?

  —No. They only protect against pregnancy. Only the use of condoms, abstinence, or mutually monogamous relationship will protect against AIDS and STIs.

- What if I need to take a drug that decreases the effectiveness of BCPs?

  —You must use a backup form of birth control (condom, diaphragm with spermicide), or you *can get pregnant* if you are using these classes of medications or substances:

  o Antibiotics (penicillins, tetracycline, others)

  ° Anticonvulsants [phenytoin (Dilantin), mephenytoin, ethotoin, carbamazepine (Tegretol), others)

  ° Antifungals [griseofulvin (Fulvicin, Grifulvin V), others]

  ° Anti-infectives (Septra, Bactrim, rifampicin, others)

  ° Barbiturates (phenobarbital, primidone, ethosuximide, others)

- Which drugs are affected by taking BCPs?

  —Use of BCPs may cause possible increased or decreased effect of these drugs:

  ° Alcohol (increased effect of alcohol)

  ° Analgesics and antipyretics (acetaminophen, aspirin, meperidine, antipyrine) (decreased pain relief)

  ° Anticoagulants (oral) (decreased anticoagulant effect)

  ° Antidepressants (Elavil, Norpramin, Tofranil, others) (increased toxicity of antidepressant)

  ° Antidiabetics: unpredictable > or < in blood sugar

  o Antihypertensives (guanethidine, Esimil, Ismelin, Aldoclor, Aldomet, etc.) (decreased antihypertensive effect)

  ° Benzodiazepine tranquilizers (Ativan, Librium, Serax, Tranxene, Valium, Xanax, Centrax) (increased or decreased tranquilizer effect)

  o Beta-blockers (Corgard, Inderal, Lopressor, Tenormin) (increased blocker effect)

  o Corticosteroids (cortisone, prednisone) (increased corticosteroid effect)

  ° Hypoglycemics (tolbutamide, Diabinese, Orinase, Tolinase) (possible decreased hypoglycemic effect)

  ° Theophyllines (Bronkotabs, Marax, Primatene, Quibron, Tedral, Theo-Dur, others) (increased theophylline effect)

  ° Troleandomycin (TAO) (jaundice—additive)

  ° Vitamins, B_1, B_2, B_6, B_{12}, C, folic acid, calcium, magnesium, zinc (decreased serum concentration)

  ° Vitamin A, copper, iron (decreased serum concentration)

- How do I take BCPs?

  —Take the BCP at *exactly* the same time every day. This is very important. If you don't, you might have > risk of pregnancy and breakthrough bleeding. The first time you take the BCP as a new prescription, start on the first day of your period.

- When will BCPs be effective?

  —BCPs are effective after taking them for 2 wk. You must use a condom or a diaphragm with spermicide until then or you could get pregnant.

- Why do I have irregular bleeding and spotting while on BCP?
  —It takes three months to adjust to BCP. Sometimes people have "breakthrough" bleeding.
  —Causes of breakthrough bleeding:
    o Illness
    ° Increased physical activity or exercise
    o Missing pills
    o Stress
    ° Taking BCP at irregular times of day
  —If it lasts more than 3 months, make appointment with MD/NP.
- What do I do if I miss taking one or more pills?
  —If you miss one pill: As soon as you remember, take the pill. Take the next one at your regular time. Use condoms or diaphragm with spermicide until your next period.
  —If you miss two pills: Take two pills per day for two days. Use condoms or diaphragm with spermicide until your next period.
  —If you miss three or more pills: Stop taking BCP completely. Use condoms or diaphragm with spermicide until your next period. At beginning of period, start new pack of BCP. (You may have to "adjust" to taking BCP again.) Call your MD/NP if no period comes. Make appointment for pregnancy test.
- What does it mean if I miss my period while on BCPs?
  —It is not unusual to miss a period when taking BCP. If you did not miss any pills and did not take any medications or substances that decrease the effectiveness of BCPs, start with the next package of BCPs and take as prescribed. If you believe you may be pregnant, schedule an appointment for a pregnancy test.
- When can I get pregnant after I stop taking BCP?
  —If you wish to get pregnant, stop taking pills and wait three months until the medication is gone from your system. During that time, use spermicide with condoms or diaphragm.
- What can I do for side effects of BCPs?
  —Nausea: Take pills with food.
  —Breast changes: Decrease intake of caffeine (contained in chocolate, cola, coffee, tea). Take 200-400 mg vitamin E every day. Symptoms should go away within a few months.

Hormonal: Birth Control Options

Other combined hormonal options:

Transdermal contraception: The transdermal patch (Ortho Evra) is another option for delivering hormonal contraception. The risks, benefits, and contraindications are similar to those for combined oral contraceptives. *However*, the patch delivers a higher level of estrogen as compared to the pill. It is possible that this higher dose of estrogen is associated with a higher risk of venous thromboembolism or blood clots. The January 2008 product labeling reflects this concern. The patch is worn on the skin for three weeks out of each month.

Contraceptive vaginal ring: The vaginal ring (NuvaRing) is another option for delivering hormonal contraception. The risks, benefits and contraindications, are similar to those for combined oral contraceptives. The ring is placed inside the vagina for 3 wk out of each month.

Hormonal: Depo-Provera

How Does It Work?

® Depo-Provera is a form of progesterone that is given by injection every 3 months.

- It causes changes to uterus, tubes, cervix, and ovaries to decrease possibility of pregnancy.

How Effective Is It in Preventing Pregnancy?

- 99.7% effective if injections are taken as scheduled.

What Can Make This Method Less Effective in Preventing Pregnancy?

- If you don't get your injections on time (every 3 months).

What Are the Absolute Contraindications? (May Not Take Depo-Provera)

- Breast cancer, known or suspected
- Pregnancy, known or suspected
- Vaginal bleeding, undiagnosed

What Are the Relative Contraindications? (Caution in Taking Depo-Provera)

- Breast cancer (5 yr disease free)
- Cardiovascular disease: hypertension, stroke, ischemic heart disease
- Diabetes with neuropathy, retinopathy, nephropathy
- Liver conditions: cirrhosis, adenoma, cancer, hepatitis
- Medications (See above.)

What Are the Side Effects?

- Abdominal cramps/bloating
- Breast tenderness/swelling
- Decreased sex drive
- Depression
- Dizziness
- Fertility delayed, periods may not return for up to 1 yr or more
- Hair growth: excessive or loss of
- Headache
- Hot flashes
- Leg cramps, joint pain
- Nausea
- Nervousness
- Skin: rash
- Vaginal bleeding: irregular, unpredictable, increased, decreased, or absence of
- Vaginal discharge, irritation
- Weakness, fatigue
- Weight gain, typically 4 lb per year

What Are the Risks? (Life-Threatening or Serious Health Hazards)

- Increased risk of osteoporosis

What Are the Benefits? (Enhance Quality of Life, Cost, Convenience, Decrease Stress)

- Effective form of birth control
- Peace of mind
- Convenience
- Does not interfere with sexual intercourse

Follow-up

- Make an appointment for contraception/sexual on-site counseling regarding pregnancy, cervical cancer, STIs, and HIV infections.

Other FAQs

- Will this affect my ability to get pregnant?

    —It may take a while to get pregnant, maybe as long as 1 year.

- Why haven't I gotten my period?

    —Many people don't bleed at all while on this hormone.

- Why am I bleeding so much?

    —Many people have increased bleeding in first 3 months.

- When do I get my first Depo-Provera shot?

    —It must be given on day 1-5 of period.

- When do I get my next shot?

    —It must be given 3 months after first shot. Better early than late.

- When does it begin to be effective?

    —It is effective within 24 hr after first shot. Use a condom or diaphragm with spermicide in first 24 hr.

Hormonal: Implant

How Does It Work?

- The implant is a single tube filled with synthetic progestin. It is placed under the skin on the inside of the upper arm. It releases hormone for 3 yr. The hormone prevents eggs from being released.

How Effective Is It in Preventing Pregnancy?

- It is 95% effective for approximately 3 yr. The effectiveness decreases significantly after that.

What Can Make This Method Less Effective in Preventing Pregnancy?

- Some drugs may interact with the hormone. Always check with a pharmacist if you are taking any medication.

What Are the Side Effects?

- Acne
- Appetite changes, increased or decreased
- Breast tenderness, nipple discharge
- Dizziness
- Hair growth or loss
- Headaches
- Nausea
- Abnormal bleeding patterns
- Nervousness
- Weight gain

What Are the Absolute Contraindications? (May Not Use Norplant)

- Active thromboembolic episode
- Breast cancer, known or suspected
- Liver disease
- Pregnancy, known or suspected
- Vaginal bleeding, undiagnosed

What Are the Relative Contraindications? (Caution in Using Norplant)

- Allergy to local anesthetic
- Angina Hx

- Breast lumps upon examination or mammogram
- Bleeding disorder, clotting disorder history
- Depression, severe
- Ectopic pregnancy Hx
- Hyperlipidemia
- Hypertension
- Migraine headache Hx
- Myocardial infarction Hx
- Seizures, on anticonvulsant
- Stroke Hx
- BMI > 30

What Are the Risks? (Life-Threatening or Serious Health Hazards)

- Expulsion of implant
- Heavy vaginal bleeding, delayed period
- Infection: arm pain, swelling, redness, pus at site, fever, chills and "flu" symptoms
- Migraine headaches
- No protection from STIs or HIV
- Pregnancy

What Are the Benefits? (Enhance Quality of Life, Cost, Convenience, Decrease Stress)

- Decreased risk

  —Anemia

  —Bleeding/ cramping

  —Ectopic pregnancy

  —Endometrial cancer

  —Pelvic infection

- Other benefits

  —Long-term protection x 5 yr

  —Cost effective

  —Convenient

  —Does not interfere with sexual intercourse; spontaneity

Follow-up

- Make appointment 2 wk after insertion for checkup. Then see the MD/NP every 3 mo after that. Always get an annual examination.

Other FAQs

- How long after removal can I get pregnant?

  —Wait until you have had at least three periods, or at a minimum, one, before getting pregnant. You will have improved outcome if you wait until your hormones have returned to a normal balance.

IUD: Copper T, Copper 7, Progestasert

How Does It Work?

- The IUD is a small piece of plastic with copper or plastic with hormone. The IUD is inserted into the uterus.

How Effective Is It in Preventing Pregnancy?
- 90%-96% effective

What Can Make This Method Less Effective in Preventing Pregnancy?
- IUD can dislodge and fall out, or become embedded in uterus.

What Are the Side Effects?
- Painful, heavy, prolonged periods with cramps
- Anemia
- IUD may fall out or become embedded
- Irregular or breakthrough bleeding or missed/delayed period(s)

What Are the Risks? (Life-Threatening or Serious Health Hazards)
- Allergic reaction to materials
- Ectopic pregnancy
- Pelvic inflammatory disease (PID) if patient gets STI—increased risk
- Perforation of uterine wall or cervix—increased risk
- Pregnancy, with or without IUD in place

What Are the Benefits? (Enhance Quality of Life, Cost, Convenience, Decrease Stress)
- IUDs are an effective method.
- They last 8 to 10 years.
- IUDs are good for women who can't use hormones.
- A major advantage is that IUDs don't interfere with breastfeeding like hormones do.
- Progesterone may decrease blood flow and cramps/pain.

Follow-up
- Some IUDs may cause heavier periods, leading to anemia. If anemia develops, consider removal of IUD.

Other FAQs
- Who can have an IUD?

    —Not everyone is eligible for an IUD. You must have *all* of the following:

    ° You should have at least one child.
- Who is not eligible for IUD?

    —Allergic to copper

    —Ectopic pregnancy history

    —Multiple sexual partners or partner with multiple partners

    —PID: active, recurrent, or recent

    —Pregnant, known or suspected

    —Vaginal bleeding, undiagnosed
- When should IUD be inserted?

    —During your period or after you have given birth (4-8 wk).

    —For cesarean sections, you may have one inserted after 8 wk after delivery.
- What are signs of complications from IUD?

    —Complications IUD include pregnancy, ectopic pregnancy, infection. You may still get pregnant with an IUD. Always contact the MD/nurse about any abnormal bleeding, with or without sharp, progressive, unilateral pelvic pain, that radiates to shoulder, symptoms of lightheadedness or fainting and/or pallor. Always tell the nurse if you have a history of STIs (sexually transmitted infections),

PID, any abdominal/tubal surgery, prior IUD use, spotting, or have missed a period for 3-6 wk, or painful intercourse. (This may indicate an ectopic pregnancy.) *Ectopic pregnancy* is a serious, life-threatening condition. So, if you have *any* abnormal bleeding, it is best to get a pregnancy test.

° Abdominal pain, severe, lower

° Absence of strings or strings feel longer or are felt by partner during sex

° Fever, fever of unknown origin, fever/chills, "flu" symptoms, aching joints, fatigue

° Vaginal bleeding: Between periods, heavy bleeding, and/or severe cramping

° Vaginal discharge that is unusual, smells bad, different color

- What if pregnancy occurs with the IUD in place?

—If you get pregnant with an IUD in place, it should be removed. Do not try to remove IUD at home; it may result in a spontaneous abortion, or cause damage.

—If pregnancy progresses with IUD in place, there is an increased risk of infection, abortion, or premature delivery/birth.

▶ Rhythm (Natural Family Planning/Fertility Awareness)

How Does It Work?

- Natural family planning is a way of avoiding pregnancy by knowing when you are fertile by the signs and symptoms of ovulation. It requires careful recording of periods and time of fertility. You must not have sexual intercourse during the fertile period, which is about 7 days long.

How Effective Is It in Preventing Pregnancy?

- 75% effective

What Can Make This Method Less Effective in Preventing Pregnancy?

- BCPs, recently discontinued use.
- Breastfeeding.
- Childbirth.
- Medications (any).
- Menopause, approaching—Perimenopausal phase may begin as early as age 30.
- Menarche—periods started recently for first time.
- Periods that are irregular, or inability to keep accurate temperature charts and records.
- Stress recently increased.
- Travel.
- Use of recreational drugs or alcohol can lead to unprotected intercourse.

What Are the Side Effects?

- None

What Are the Risks? (Life-Threatening or Serious Health Hazards)

- Pregnancy
- Offers no protection against STIs or HIV

What Are the Benefits? (Enhance Quality of Life, Cost, Convenience, Decrease Stress)

- Low cost except for cost of barrier methods (condoms, diaphragms, spermicide) used to prevent pregnancy during fertile periods.

Follow-up

- You will need special training in the method and follow-up as needed.

Other FAQs

- Can this method be used to conceive?

—Yes, this method is used to avoid pregnancy as well as to become pregnant.

- Is there a home test kit for ovulation prediction and testing?

  —"Oviquick" Ovulation Predictor Kits may be bought without prescription over the counter in 5- or 9-day (two cycles) packages.

► Sterilization (Male and Female)

How Does It Work?

- The tubes that carry sperm or eggs are cut and tied off through surgery.

How Effective Is It in Preventing Pregnancy?

- Female: 95% effective
- Male: 99.8% effective

What Can Make This Method Less Effective in Preventing Pregnancy?

- Equipment failure (clip falls off)
- Fistula formation
- Pregnancy at time of sterilization
- Surgery error can lead to failure (30%-50%).

What Are the Side Effects?

- Regret of decision

What Are the Risks? (Life-Threatening or Serious Health Hazards)

- Male: Potential long-term effects unproven for increased risk of prostate cancer
- Female: Increased risk of ectopic pregnancy

What Are the Benefits? (Enhance Quality of Life, Cost, Convenience, Decrease Stress)

- Permanent, effective
- Convenient
- < Stress
- Cost effective
- No significant long-term effects

Follow-up

- Postop checkup for any surgical procedure

Other FAQs

- Why do people regret having had sterilization?

  —People who have unstable marriages, or who are young in age, recently divorced, living at the poverty level, or whose religion or culture does not commonly embrace this method (e.g., Hispanic, Catholic) often regret having had sterilization.

- Is sterilization reversible?

  —Yes, it can be reversed.

  —For males: Reversal rates of 16%-79%.

  —For females: reversal rates range from 43% for coagulation to 88% for clip-type sterilization.

► Withdrawal

How Does It Work?

- Male stops sexual intercourse, withdraws penis before ejaculation.

How Effective Is It in Preventing Pregnancy?

- 80% effective

What Can Make This Method Less Effective in Preventing Pregnancy?
- Use of recreational drugs or alcohol may lead to unprotected intercourse.
- Failure to withdraw in time.

What Are the Side Effects?
- Disrupts sexual enjoyment.

What Are the Risks? (Life-Threatening or Serious Health Hazards)
- Pregnancy
- > Risk of exposure to STIs and HIV

What Are the Benefits? (Enhance Quality of Life, Cost, Convenience, Decrease Stress)
- No cost
- No equipment

Follow-up
- None

▶ Birth Control Tutorial

Red Flags

Ectopic pregnancy: Missed period, nausea, swollen tender breasts, fatigue, urinary frequency/urgency. Any abnormal bleeding, with or without sharp, progressive, unilateral pelvic pain that radiates to shoulder, symptoms of lightheadedness or fainting and/or pallor. History of STIs, PID, any abdominal/tubal surgery, prior IUD use, spotting or have missed a period for 3-6 wk, or painful intercourse.

Rules of Thumb

- Once an ectopic, always an ectopic.
- Any woman of childbearing age with abdominal pain and/or unusual bleeding is treated as an ectopic pregnancy until proven otherwise.

Red Herrings

- Never assume a female is of pre-or postchildbearing years without asking first!
- No matter how reliable the form of contraception, always consider pregnancy (ectopic, early miscarriage).

Assessment Tips

- Number of pads per hour:
    —Severe = one large pad (saturated) per hour x 3 hr.
    —Moderate = one pad every 2 hr.
    —Light = one pad every 3-4 hr.
    —Weight gain or loss affects period. Extreme weight loss can lead to < vaginal bleeding or complete absence of period.

BREAST PROBLEM (FEMALE/MALE)
Pain with or without Trauma, Discharge; Lump; Lesions (Nonbreastfeeding; Nonpostpartum)

ASSESSMENT	ACUITY LEVEL	DISPOSITION/ADVICE
Key Questions	Emergent Symptom Patterns	ED 0 min–1 hr
Major Trauma	+ Severe pain, swelling, bruising, laceration? (Hematoma, Laceration)	
Key Questions	Urgent Symptom Patterns	ED/UCC/Office 1–8 hr
Pain	+ Hx of surgery/trauma? (Fat Necrosis/Postop Complication)	
	+ Sudden onset, localized redness, swelling, fever (chills, weakness, achy joints, N/V)? (Mastitis, Abscess)	
	+ Recent Hx of Surgery, Fever, Drainage? (Postop Complication/Infection)	
	+ (All Skin) Red ± streaking, swollen, tender, hot; ± discharge, often w fever, swollen nodes, hx of trauma/bite/local infection? (Cellulitis, Abscess)	
Key Questions	Acute/Nonacute Symptom Patterns	ED/UCC/Office 1–8 hr
Lump	+ Female or Male with Hx of *any* cancer, particularly breast? (Metastasis, Recurrence, or Secondary Tumor)	
	+ W or w/o nipple skin retraction, asymmetrical appearance breast/nipples, discoloration (bruiselike), dimpling, orange peel appearance, hardened, enlarged pores, thickening of skin of breast, ulcerations? (Carcinoma)	
	+ Round, soft/firm, moves freely, ± single/multiple, sudden onset, or cyclical? (Fibroadenoma, Fibrocystic Change)	

(continued)

Key Questions	Acute/Nonacute Symptom Patterns	ED/UCC/Office 1-8 hr
Breast Enlargement (Male Only)	+ All males? (Gynecomastia, Drug Side Effects)	
	± Tenderness? (Hyperthyroidism, Estrogen-Producing Cancer)	
	± Testicular mass? (Age 18-35 = > Risk Testicular Cancer)	
	+ Hx of alcoholism? (Liver Disease)	
Discharge: Nipple	+ (Female) milky/bilateral, Hx of amenorrhea? (Pituitary Tumor, Hypothyroidism, Drug/Med Use)	
	+ (Male/Female) bloody/watery pus, unilateral? (Carcinoma/Intraductal Papilloma, Hormones, Drug Side Effect)	
Lesion	+ Excoriation, pain involving nipple, skin under breast moist, foul-smelling? (Dermatitis, Infection, Paget Disease of Breast)	
Pain/Tenderness	+ W or w/o breast enlargement? (Premenstrual, Hormonal Meds, Possible Pregnancy)	
Cross-Reference Breastfeeding Problem	Pregnancy Problem (as Appropriate)	Skin Problem (as Appropriate)

BREAST PROBLEM (FEMALE/MALE)
Supplemental Information

Quick Reference:
- ▶ Breast Calcium Deposits
- ▶ Breast Pain
- ▶ Drug Side Effect
    - Breast Swelling
    - Nipple Discharge

- ▶ Fibrocystic Breast
- ▶ Galactorrhea
- ▶ Men and Breast Cancer
- ▶ FAQs regarding Breast Cancer
- ▶ Tutorial

See also: Directory of Hotlines/Web Sites for Support Groups, Appendix E

▶ Breast Calcium Deposits
- Definition: A small lump of calcium in the breast
- Cause: Previous injury to the breast; inflammation (mastitis); radiation therapy for breast cancer; cancer
- Complications: If you have a calcium deposit, it does not mean you have breast cancer.
- Tx: A doctor should evaluate any lump in the breast. Some calcium deposits can be a sign of breast cancer.

▶ Breast Pain
- Definition: Pain may be described as tender, swollen, or sore. It may also be described as a throbbing, burning, stabbing, or sharp pain that comes and goes. Most pain in the breast is normal. Sometimes, breast pain is a warning sign of disease.
- Causes: Hormone changes can cause swelling in the breasts and breast pain.
    - —The pain usually comes during the 2 wk before a woman's period begins.
    - —Fibrocystic changes in breast tissue. The breasts will feel lumpy and tender.
    - —Hormone replacement or birth control pills can cause tenderness and swelling. This side effect may go away after 3 to 4 mo.
    - —An infection in the milk ducts (mastitis) can cause pain.
    - —Any injury to your breast may cause pain.
- Goal: Relieve pain. Prevent pain, swelling.
- Prevention/Tx:
    - —*Over-the-counter medications:* Ibuprofen, Advil, Motrin, Aleve, Anaprox, Actron, or Orudis may help. Try each of them to see which one works the best.
    - —*Prescription medications:* If the over-the-counter medications don't work, and you are in a lot of discomfort, the doctor will need to write a prescription for either danazol (Danocrine) or bromocriptine. Danazol may cause irregular periods, weight gain, acne, headaches, or nausea. Bromocriptine may cause mild side effects—nausea, headaches, or constipation.
    - —*Caffeine:* Do not drink coffee or any sodas with caffeine.
    - —*Salt:* Cut down on salt the week before your period is due. It can lead to more swelling.
    - —*Vitamins:* Your doctor will advise what dose you need to take of the following vitamin: supplements or herbal.
- Vitamin E may help. It has minimal side effects.
- Evening primrose may help. It has few side effects.

> —*Hormone therapy changes:* If you are on birth control pills or hormones for menopause, the doctor may want you to stop the hormones for a short time. You might need to change your dosage or change the type of hormones you are taking. These changes may help to reduce breast discomfort.
>
> —Avoid foods associated with breast tenderness: Coffee, cola w caffeine, nonherbal teas, chocolate, some kinds of pain meds w caffeine (e.g., Excedrin).
>
> —Wear supportive bra.
>
> —Use ice packs (See Home Tx SI, Appendix A: Ice Pack).
>
> —Drugs Tx: Ibuprofen, Pamprin, Tylenol
>
> —Don't take OTC diet pills (e.g., Dexatrim), OTC stimulants (e.g., Vivarin).

► Drug Side Effect

Breast Swelling

- If drug-related, will resolve when drug Rx completed. Common drugs and classes of drugs causing breast swelling are:
  - —anticancer drugs
  - —calcium channel blockers or blocking agents
  - —cimetidine (Tagamet)
  - —digitalis (Digitoxin, Digoxin)
  - —estrogen (oral and topical)
  - —ketoconazole (Nizoral)
  - —methadone
  - —methyldopa (Aldomet)
  - —metronidazole (Flagyl)
  - —phenytoin (Dilantin)
  - —spironolactone
  - —theophylline
- Street drugs
  - —marijuana

Nipple Discharge

- If drug-related, will resolve when drug Rx is completed.
  - —imipramine
  - —isoniazid (INH)
  - —methyldopa (Aldomet)
  - —birth control pills
  - —reserpine
  - —tranquilizers
- Street drugs
  - —heroin

► Fibrocystic Breast

- Definition: "Lumpy breasts" that are tender and swollen are called fibrocystic breasts. These changes are not serious and do not increase the risk of cancer.
- Causes: These changes can happen during the years of childbearing or after menopause. These changes are common.

- Tx: See Breast Pain (above) for home care.

  —Monthly breast self-exam

  —Regular mammograms for ages > 40 or older or high-risk patients

► Galactorrhea

® Definition: A milky discharge from the nipple in anyone who is not breastfeeding an infant. It may occur in males and females. This is a symptom that should be evaluated by a doctor.

- Causes: It may be related to hormonal imbalances such as hypothyroidism. This discharge is more common in females. It happens when the female stops having periods. In males, it might be related to impotence. Some medications, like tranquilizers, antidepressants, and blood pressure-lowering drugs cause this discharge. It is a serious symptom that the doctor needs to evaluate.

® Tx: The doctor needs to do blood tests or a CAT scan to discover the reason for the symptom.

► Men and Breast Cancer

[3] Men who have large breasts will not get breast cancer.

- Men do not usually get screened for breast cancer if they have no symptoms, because breast cancer is so rare in men.

- Risk Factors: Hx of testicular cancer, breast cancer, and family history of female relatives with breast cancer, Jewish ancestry, and *BRCA2* gene abnormalities.

► FAQs Regarding Breast Cancer

What are breast cancer risk factors? No one knows the exact causes of breast cancer, but we do know many of the risks that may lead to breast cancer. Some risk factors like age, gender, or race can't be changed. Some personal choices such as smoking, drinking, and diet can change the level of risk. Some risks are more serious than others, and the risks can change over time. Simply aging or having a relative who develops breast cancer can change a person's risk. Most women who develop breast cancer have none of the *risk factors* listed below, other than growing older. Gender, race, and age are not alterable risk factors.

® Gender: Simply being a woman is the main risk factor for developing breast cancer. Men can develop breast cancer, but it is 100 times more common among women than men.

- Aging: Your risk of developing breast cancer increases as you get older. About 18% of breast cancer diagnoses are among women in their 40s, while about 77% of women with breast cancer are older than 50 when they are diagnosed. The risk of developing breast cancer between ages 30 to 40 is 1 out of 252, whereas between ages 60 to 70, it is 1 out of 27. A woman's risk of ever developing breast cancer in her lifetime is 1 out of 8.

- Previous history of breast cancer: Having cancer in one breast increases the risk 3 to 4 times of developing a new cancer in the other breast.

- Family history (mother, sister, aunt, grandmother, or daughter had breast cancer)

  —Female relatives with either or both breast or ovarian cancer

  —Male relatives with breast cancer

  —A family history of hereditary breast cancer

  —Any history of breast cancer before age 50 in a relative (mother, sister, grandmother, or aunt) on either side of the family

- Previous breast biopsy: A diagnosis of *atypical hyperplasia* increases a women's breast cancer risk by 4 to 5 times.

- Breast density: Breasts that are made up of more dense tissue than of fatty tissue are more likely to develop cancers. Dense tissue makes it more difficult to see abnormal areas on a mammogram.

- Genetic history: A blood test that shows you have a genetic risk

- Race:
  —White women have a higher risk of *developing* breast cancer than African-American women do.
  —African-American women *are more likely to die* of breast cancer because of late diagnosis when cancer is harder to treat and cure.
  —Asian, Hispanic, and native American women have a lower risk of breast cancer.
- Medically underserved: Any women of any race who are under- or uninsured or have poor access to health care have poor breast cancer survival rates.
- DES (diethylstilbestrol): Mothers who took DES during pregnancy to prevent complications have a higher risk.

What are some of the lifestyle risk factors associated with breast cancer?
Some factors related to lifestyle and lifestyle choices are breast cancer risk factors, and some of these risks may be lowered (see below).

- Alcohol: There is a risk of breast cancer among women who drink alcohol. Women who have 2 to 5 drinks daily have about 1.5 times the risk of women who drink no alcohol.
- Obesity and high-fat diets: Obesity (being overweight) is associated with an increased risk of developing breast cancer, especially for women after menopause (which usually occurs at age 50).
- Reproductive history and estrogen exposure: The longer a woman is exposed to estrogen (which includes one's own natural estrogen or any form of prescription), the higher the risk for breast cancer. Each factor listed below increases the amount of time a woman's body is exposed to estrogen.
  —*Early menstruation:* Having the first period before age 12 may increase risk.
  —*Late menopause:* Having one's last period after age 55 may increase risk.
  —*Never having children or having children late in life:* Women who have had no children or who had their first child after age 30 have a slightly higher breast cancer risk.
- Hormone replacement therapy: Most studies suggest that long-term use (several years or more) of hormone replacement therapy (HRT) after menopause may slightly increase the risk of breast cancer.
- Radiation therapy: Includes radiation therapy to the breasts before age 30 and radiation for Hodgkin disease.

What can I do to reduce the risk of breast cancer?
- Physical activity: Studies show that strenuous exercise in your youth might provide life-long protection against breast cancer and that even moderate to strenuous physical activity as an adult can lower breast cancer risk.
- Lifestyle changes:
  —Alcohol reduction
  —Lowering weight to normal and reducing intake of fat
  —Monitoring BCP and HRT carefully
- Pregnancy and breastfeeding factors
  —Pregnancy: Having more children can reduce the risk of breast cancer.
  —Breastfeeding longer (continued for 1.5 to 2 years) could reduce the risk of breast cancer by half.

i- Tutorial

Red Flags

Populations and symptoms which increase risk (SAVED): Severe symptoms, (high-risk populations: Age, Veracity, Emotional Distress, Debilitation)

• Symptoms:
  —Beware of pain that is more severe than expected or unrelenting.
  —Beware of any pain that awakens patient or keeps him or her awake at night.

® Age: 77% of women with breast cancer are > age 50 when diagnosed.

- Emotional: Denial may be associated with breast problems.
- Debilitation: Previous history or family history of cancer, diabetes

Rules of Thumb

® The younger the age of exposure to radiation therapy (of chest area), the higher the risk for developing breast cancer later.

- The older the woman, the higher the risk for breast cancer.

® Any nipple discharge, itching, scaling, or weeping of nipple in older patient is a concern.

- Remain vigilant to possible patient, parent, or caretaker denial, minimization, and misinterpretation of symptoms.
- Regard with suspicion: All unusual sounding presentations, including symptoms described as the "flu," or symptoms described as "new," "sudden," or "unexpected."

® Patients who have been "seen recently" may still need to be seen today.

® Don't be misled by concurrent complaints or patient self-explanation.

- Patients "on medication" may be on the wrong medication (antibiotics).
- Abuse is usually associated with denial.
- Symptom presentation may be early, late, silent, atypical, or novel.

® All severe pain must be seen within 8 hr or less.

® Minority callers may fail to recognize acute symptoms, report fewer symptoms, or attribute them to other causes.

- Symptoms of two conditions may present concurrently, causing confusion or misinterpretation.

Red Herrings

"Red herrings" are common distractions (symptoms or situations) that lead the nurse astray, away from the main problem.

- Remain vigilant to possible patient denial, minimization, and misinterpretation of symptoms.
- Previous history of fibrocystic breasts.

® Male gender.

BREASTFEEDING PROBLEM
Pain with or without Fever: Sore Nipples; Painful Breasts

ASSESSMENT	ACUITY LEVEL	DISPOSITION/ADVICE
Key Questions	Emergent Symptom Patterns	ED 0 min-1 hr
Any Breastfeeding Problem	--▶	See Initial Assessment Questions
Key Questions	Urgent Symptom Patterns	ED/UCC/Office 1-8 hr
Pain w Fever	+ Sudden onset: fever > 38.5°C or 101.3°F, localized red, hot, swollen area on breast, usually unilateral, intense pain, flulike Sx? (Mastitis)	
	+ Red, swollen, tender area, ± fever, nausea, dizziness, aching muscles, fatigue? (Abscess)	
Key Questions	Acute/Nonacute Symptom Patterns	FA 8+ hr ± Home Tx
Pain w/o Fever	+ Burning during breastfeeding, red or pink nipples/-areola, Hx of mom/baby on antibiotics or C-section, ± baby w thrush? (Thrush)	
	+ Feeling of fullness, ± swelling, ± hard, ± tender, warm? (Engorgement)	
Lump in Breast	+ Plug or white bump on nipple, + tenderness, + pressure around plug, no fever/flulike Sx? (Plugged Duct)	
Sore Nipples	+ Pain in nipples while breastfeeding, ± cracks on nipples? (Fissures)	
	+ Blisters on the nipple? (Nipple Trauma)---------------▶	Apply very warm compresses before feeding to soften blister + Review latch-on technique (See Breastfeeding Problem SI).
	+ Nipples tender, achy, red, abrasions, pain throughout feeding? (Poss. Improper Latch-on)------▶	Review latch-on technique (See Breastfeeding Problem SI).
	+ Nipples sting, more painful between feedings, in shower, when exposed to air immediately following feeding? (Dermatitis)	

(continued)

Key Questions	Acute/Nonacute Symptom Patterns	FA 8+ hr ± Home Tx
Sore Nipples (continued)	+ Blanched nipple tips 5-10 min after feeding/between feeding, worse w contact to cold air, better in warm shower or while baby nursing? (Vasospasm)---------- ■►	Home Tx: + Apply warm compress to nipple (See Home Tx SI, Appendix A: Warm Compress) + Take ibuprofen + Close bra flaps immediately after feeding

Cross-References

Breastfeeding Problem SI	Postpartum Concerns	Postpartum Emotional Problem SI

BREASTFEEDING INITIAL ASSESSMENT QUESTIONS

Quick Reference: ▶ Rules of Thumb   Urine Output   ▶ Red Flags

▶ infant Assessment   Stools   ▶ Cross-Reference

Intake

▶ Rules of Thumb

- Assess all new mothers for possible depression.
- Assess all infants for possible dehydration or toxicity.

▶ Infant Assessment

- If infant exhibits any of the following symptoms, bring baby in now.
    - Age < 3 mo: Fever (> 38°C or 100.4°F)?
    - Is baby jaundiced/yellow?
    - Weak cry?
    - "Floppy" baby?
    - Lethargic?
    - "Shriveled" appearance "like old man"?

Intake

- Breast only? How often? Number of min/feeding? Both breasts offered?
- Who initiates feeding? Who ends feeding?
- Mom's perception of baby's suck: Strong? Weak?
- Flow long does baby sleep at one time?

Urine Output

- Age > 3 days: When mother's milk is in, baby should have 6-8 wet diapers/24 hr. Urine should be pale with minimal odor.
- Number of soaked, heavy wet diapers/past 24 hr? Color: Dark? Pale?
- Type of diaper: Cloth? Disposable? Caution: Difficult to assess with disposable diapers.
- Red Flag: Orange-looking urine/crystals in diaper = possible dehydration.

Stools

- Number and characteristics of stools/past 24 hr
- Normals
    - First few days after birth: Dark, tarry stool (meconium)?
    - 24-48 hr after milk "comes in": Loose, wet, yellow, yellow-green, or tan? (2-5 stools/24 hr is normal.)
    - Green stool? (Occasional green stool is also normal.)
    - Red Flag: Continually green or brown stool = possible dehydration.

► **Red Flags**

Assess all mothers calling with breastfeeding problems for depression and domestic violence (See Post-partum Emotional Problem SI).

- How are you feeling? (Does tone of voice and affect match self-description?)
- Are you able to take care of yourself (i.e., sleeping, eating, drinking when thirsty, showering)?
- Is someone available to help you? (Assess support systems.)
- How are you feeling about the baby?

► **Cross-Reference**

Postpartum Emotional Problem SI

BREASTFEEDING PROBLEM
Supplemental Information

Quick Reference:	▶ Abscess	▶ Mastitis
	▶ Engorgement	▶ Mother Care
	▶ Feeding Problems	▶ Plugged Duct
	▶ Inadequate Milk Supply	▶ Sore Nipples
	▶ Lactation Suppression	▶ Thrush
	▶ Latch-on Technique	▶ Weaning from Breast

See also: Directory of Hotlines/Web Sites for Support Groups, Appendix E

▶ **Abscess**

e Definition: Infection. A collection of pus w nowhere to drain

e Signs and symptoms: Fever, flulike symptoms (nausea, dizziness, aching muscles, fatigue); red, swollen, and tender area

® Causes: Mastitis that has gone untreated or has not responded to antibiotics

® Prevention/Tx:

—May require surgical drainage.

—Antibiotics.

—Rest.

—Warm soaks.

—Complete emptying of breast every 2-4 hr.

—Breastfeeding can continue if the incision/drain is far enough from the areola.

—If breastfeeding is not temporarily stopped, watch the baby closely for signs of infection.

▶ **Engorgement**

• Definition: Swelling and fullness of the breasts because of blood vessels dilating and the milk ducts filling w milk

® Signs and symptoms: Moderately severe: Breasts feel full, hard, and tender. Severe: Hard, tense, and warm, generalized aching and/or throbbing pain. Both breasts are usually affected.

® Causes: Infrequent or missed breastfeedings. Inadequate letdown. Hard, overfull, heavy breasts as a result of short feedings or "sleepy baby." Breast makes more milk than baby is taking, causing swelling of breast tissue.

—Usually happens when you first begin breastfeeding new baby. Usually lessens in 24-48 hr.

—Swelling and discomfort may get worse if you don't nurse often or long enough.

[9] Complications:

—Slow infant weight gain if unable to latch on to breast

—Sore nipples if breast too firm to grasp

—Mastitis because of poor milk flow

—Decreased milk supply

- Tx goal: Reduce engorgement and pain. Prevent complications.
  —Breastfeed often around the clock. Feed baby as often as possible.
  —Apply cold, fresh *green* cabbage leaf to breast.
  —Take Tylenol as appropriate for pain relief.
- Before feeding:
  —Before feeding, put a warm cloth on breasts or take hot shower.
  —Baby must be positioned and latched on well (See Latch-On Technique below).
  —Hold breast between palms and gently squeeze breast while moving hands toward nipple to express small amount of milk. This softens breast and makes it easier for baby to latch on.
  —Massage breasts prior to and during breastfeeding.
- After feeding:
  —Apply Cold compresses between feedings to reduce pain and swelling.
  —Wear a well-fitting and supportive bra.
  —Do not pump breasts.

► Feeding Problems

- Foods causing fussiness: Keep a 2-7 day diary of food and drinks and dates/times of infant fussiness. Call back to discuss.
- "Fussy about breast": Some newborns are "disorganized" nursers—slow to latch on, frantic, or agitated. Start baby off sucking on your little finger. Then, when sucking is strong and consistent, transfer to breast.

»- Inadequate Milk Supply ("Not Enough Milk")

- How do I know I'm producing enough milk?
  —The amount of milk you produce depends on how often you breastfeed and how effectively your baby sucks.
  —When the baby is born, you produce colostrum. This is a very thick, concentrated liquid that the baby gets the first 3-5 days of life.
  —Three to five days after giving birth, your milk will begin to "come in."
  —During the first few weeks, breastfeed at least 8-12 x a day. Nurse for at least 10-15 min on each breast.
  —Your baby should have 6-8 wet diapers/day after your milk has come in (day 3-4); the urine should be pale yellow in color.
  —Your baby's stool after day 2-3 should be loose and seedy; and may be yellow to yellowish green to tan in color.
  —In first month of life, your baby should have at least 2 stools each day.

► Lactation Suppression

- Tx goal: To reduce swelling/pain of breasts when a mother does not wish to breastfeed or must stop quickly for some reason.
- Do the following for 1-2 days:
  —Fold large bath towel or sheet in half lengthwise.
  —Wrap snugly around breasts, pinning in front.
  —Tuck ice pack or cold pack (See Home Tx SI, Appendix A: Cold Pack, Ice Pack) between layers of towel or sheet against breasts for 24-48 hr.

—Change ice packs every hr.

—Don't nurse, touch, or wash breasts in warm water.

► Latch-on Technique

- Baby's tummy is turned toward mother's tummy.
- Baby's legs even with rest of body and baby held snugly against mother.
- Mother supporting breast with free hand. Her hand or fingers should not cover any part of the areola.
- Stroke baby's lower lip with nipple to encourage baby to open mouth, like a yawn.
- Mother quickly brings the baby onto her breast pulling baby in close.
- Baby takes breast 1 -1 'A in back from nipple.
- Baby's lips are rolled out and relaxed against breast.
- Baby's jaw movement is visible with little or no cheek movement.

» Mother can hear swallowing (clicking sound-not smacking of lips).

- Baby's chin and the top of his or her nose touch the breast during the entire nursing.
- Nipples should not be sore. If they are, you need to check for proper positioning.

► Mastitis

- Definition: A serious infection of the whole breast.

   —Mastitis: Can turn into an abscess if you don't take antibiotics.

   —Abscess: Pus collects in a pocket with nowhere to drain.

® Signs and symptoms: Fatigue, localized breast tenderness, flulike symptoms, fever, appearance of a hot, reddened, and tender area on breast (usually unilateral and in upper outer breast quadrant).

- Causes: Can occur as a result of an untreated plugged duct, cracked or fissured nipple, constriction caused by tight bra, engorgement, stress, or abrupt change in feeding pattern.
- Complication: Abscess.
- Prevention/Tx:

   —Bed rest

   —Antibiotics

   —Increased fluid intake

   —Moist heat applications

   —Breastfeed frequently on the affected side

   —Loosen constrictive clothing/bra

   —Nurse the baby in different positions (cradle hold, football hold, lying down)

   —Check for proper latch-on technique (make sure the baby has part of or the whole areola in his/her mouth)

   —Tylenol as appropriate for fever

► Mother Care

- Continue to take prenatal vitamins until baby has stopped breastfeeding.
- Eat more foods w calcium: Milk, yogurt, cheese, ice cream, carrots.
- Water is very important when breastfeeding. Drink 6-8 glasses of water, juice, milk, or decaf herbal tea every day.
- Eat a lot of fruits, vegetables, meat, eggs, fish, poultry.
- Rest when baby rests. Ask friends/family to help w housework, cooking, care of older children. Mother should care for baby and self.

▶ Plugged Duct

- Definition: Milk forms a plug; new milk backs up behind it.
- Signs and symptoms: A plug or "white head" on nipple; feeling of tenderness and pressure around the plug; no fever or flulike symptoms.
- Causes: Missed or shortened feedings leaving the breast overfull; poor positioning during feeding; lack of rest; breasts are too full; pressure on breast; infection from cracked nipple.
- Complications: Mastitis, serious infection, and abscess.
- Tx goal: Comfort. Unplug duct. Prevent Mastitis.
  —Put warm, damp cloths to area 5 min before feeding and while nursing to > milk flow and drainage.
  —Nurse on side w plug. Begin each feeding w side that is affected.
  —Massage area in gentle but firm circular motion before and during feeding.
  —Increase fluid intake.
  —Do not use underwire or tight-fitting bra.
  —Bed rest.
- Prevention: Adequate rest; nurse often; let baby finish feeding; wear supportive bra; avoid tight bra or clothes.
- Pain/Fever: Tylenol as appropriate.

▶ Sore Nipples

- Definition: Tenderness and pain while nursing
- Causes: Poor positioning and latch on; infrequent feedings; baby chewing or sucking on nipple; taking nipple out of the baby's mouth w/o breaking suction first; engorgement
- Prevention before nursing:
  —Make sure you are in a comfortable position before breastfeeding.
  —Check baby's position before putting to breast.
  —Make sure baby's mouth is open wide and mom's breast is put in the center of baby's mouth. Make sure baby gets as much of the areola as possible.
  —Breastfeed frequently to avoid engorgement.
  —When changing breasts, place little finger between baby's gums to break suction.
  —For painful breastfeeding, recheck positioning and latch-on technique.
- Prevention after nursing: Nipple care Tx:
  —Expose breast to air after feedings and keep it dry.
  —Air will toughen your nipples so they will be less sore. Use hair dryer to blow dry nipples after feeding to promote healing, or "go topless" without a bra when possible.
  —Put a few drops of breast milk on nipple and let dry after feeding. This keeps the skin healthy and strong.

▶ Thrush

- Signs and symptoms: Suspect thrush infection of nipples if the following symptoms occur:
  —Nipple soreness or pain throughout feeding session
  —Shooting pain/burning pain in the breast during or after feedings
  —Nipples appear pink, flaky, and itchy or may be red and burning
  —Baby has white patches on his/her tongue or inside cheeks
- Causes: Fungus infection of baby's mouth/diaper area and/or mother's breasts

- Prevention/Tx:
  —Call for appt.
  —Breastfeed for shorter periods of time but more often while pain is still present.

» Weaning from Breast

- Start by substituting bottle/cup feeding for one breast feeding.
- Wait until breasts adjust (not engorged), then substitute bottle/cup feeding for an additional breast-feeding.
- Continue until baby is entirely on bottle/cup feeding.
- If engorgement occurs, express only enough milk to relieve pressure (See Lactation Suppression above).

MENOPAUSE OPTIONS, CONCERNS, AND FREQUENTLY ASKED QUESTIONS
Supplemental Information

Quick Reference:
- ► Definition of Menopause
- ► Signs and Symptoms of Menopause
  - Emotional Changes
  - Hot Flashes/Night Sweats
  - Sleep Disorder
  - Sexual Difficulties: Painful Intercourse/Vaginal Dryness
  - Decreased Sex Drive
  - Urinary Problems
- ► Best Books/Resources
- ► Health Risks of Menopause
  - Cardiac Disease
  - Osteoporosis

- ► Treatments Associated with Menopause
  - Hormone Replacement Therapy Management
  - FAQs
- ► HRT Treatments
  - Creams (Estrogen, Vaginal Creams)
  - Patch (Estrogen)
  - Pills (Estrogen, Progesterone, or Combination)
  - Testosterone (Cream, Oral)

See also: Directory of Hotlines/Web Sites for Support Groups, Appendix E

► **Definition of Menopause**
- Menopause: When a woman has not had a period for 1 yr, she has reached menopause. The ovaries have stopped making eggs and are making less estrogen, progesterone, and testosterone. Menopause is often treated as if it were a single event. In fact, menopause is a physical process—much like adolescence—and may take several years to complete. This period is called perimenopause.
- Perimenopause: The period of time before menopause when many women experience emotional and physical changes related to decreased female hormones. This phase usually begins when women are in their forties.
- Premature menopause: When menopause happens before age 40.
- Surgical menopause: If a woman has surgery to have her ovaries removed, she will go through menopause, no matter what her age. Removal of the uterus but not the ovaries will not cause menopause, but will stop a woman's periods.

► **Signs and Symptoms of Menopause**

Some women have little or no symptoms of menopause; some women have many symptoms. An individual may have any, all, or (rarely) none of the following:
- Emotional changes: Depression, irritability, fits of anger, anxiety (low grade to panic attacks)
- Insomnia
- Hot flashes
- Night sweats
- Fatigue

- Vaginal dryness, painful intercourse
- Changed bleeding patterns < or >, irregular periods, shorter or longer cycles from her normal
- Short-term memory loss, forgetfulness
- Difficulty in concentrating
- Hair loss
- Decreased sexual desire

Emotional Changes

(See Emotional Problems 1 and 2. Rule out potential severe to moderate depression or suicidal tendencies.)

- Definition: Unusual, frequent, or sudden periods of depression, anxiety, irritability, anger, feeling "out of control" emotionally. Severe PMS symptoms. Sometimes lack of sleep can make you irritable or depressed.
- Cause: Hormone changes can cause depression, anxiety, irritability. Other major life changes can also lead to feelings of loss and depression, including "empty nest" syndrome and decreased self-esteem as a result of aging and body changes.
- Prevention/Tx:
  —Exercise
    ° One of the best ways to reduce negative emotional changes is exercise.
    ° Exercise increases energy, improves sleep patterns, and decreases depression.
    ° It also increases brain chemicals that give one a sense of well-being.
    ° Exercise gives a sense of accomplishment and decreases stress.
    o Exercise regularly (3-5 times per week or more): Swimming, tennis, hiking, yoga, biking, tai chi, running, walking, dancing.
  —Diet:
    ° Eat regular, well-balanced meals: Protein, vegetables, fruit, vitamin and mineral supplements.
  —Support:
    ° Support groups for women in midlife, meditation, counseling or psychotherapy.
  —Prescription meds:
    ° Hormone therapy *may* increase sense of well-being in perimenopausal and menopausal women,
    o Antidepressants may be needed for chronic depression.
  —Alternative medical approaches:
    o Some treatments such as biofeedback, acupuncture, acupressure, herbs, meditation, breathing, and homeopathy have been known to increase sense of well-being in perimenopausal and menopausal women. (See Best Books/Resources for additional information below.)

Hot Flashes/Night Sweats

(See Respiratory Problems I and 2 for night sweats. Rule out respiratory problems.)

- Definition:
  —Hot flashes: Sudden, intense feeling of being hot and sweating without external cause.
  —Night sweats: Hot flashes that come at night and awaken the woman from sleep.
- Cause: Hormone changes affect the body's temperature control.
- Prevention/Tx:
  —Hot spicy foods may trigger hot flashes or night sweats. Women may wish to avoid hot or spicy foods, hot or spicy drinks, alcohol.

—Emotions can trigger hot flashes.

—Dress in layers.

—Avoid using electric blankets, flannel sheets.

—Use cotton nightgown.

—HRT

—Alternative therapies (See Emotional Changes above)

Sleep Disorder

(See Emotional Problems 1 and 2. Rule out depression.)

- Definition: Difficulty falling asleep or staying asleep.
- Cause: Hormone changes, hot flashes, depression.
- Prevention/Tx:
- Rule: If not asleep within 15 min, get out of bed and do some other quiet activity (watch TV, read, sew, pay bills, or meditate).

   —Avoid all caffeine (coffee, cola) after 4-6 PM.

   —Exercise helps reduce sleep problems (see Emotional Changes above). In addition, yoga, stretching, and deep breathing are especially good.

   —Lavender oil under pillow

   —Warm milk, broth, herbal tea (nonstimulating, e.g., chamomile), soup

   —Warm bath

   —Melatonin (3 mg) 1-2 hrs before bed

   —HRT

   —Alternative therapies (See Emotional Changes above)

Sexual Difficulties

Painful intercourse/Vaginal Dryness

(See Urinary Problem; Vaginal Problem. Rule out vaginal infection, STI, urinary, or other problem.)

- Definition:

   —Painful intercourse with or without vaginal dryness. Sense of discomfort instead of pleasure.

   —Lack of moisture in vagina, causing discomfort, painful, or difficult intercourse.

- Cause: Decreased elasticity caused by decreased blood flow to vaginal tissue and thinning of vaginal wall.
- Prevention/Tx for painful intercourse and vaginal dryness:

   —Have sexual intercourse more often: it helps keep the vagina healthy and elastic.

   —HRT.

   —Use lubricants when having sexual intercourse (e.g., Astroglide, K-Y jelly). Do not use petroleum products as lubricants—they increase vaginal problems.

   —Use Replens 2-3 times each week to prevent vaginal dryness.

   —Avoid douching. (Overdouching can lead to vaginal dryness.)

   —Vitamin supplements: Vitamin E, Bioflavonoids

   —For vaginal dryness, wear cotton underwear and loose-fitting clothes.

Decreased Sex Drive

(See Emotional Problems 1 and 2. Rule out depression or other problem.)

- Replens 2-3 times each week to prevent vaginal dryness
- Definition: Lack of sexual desire or sex drive, disinterest in having sexual intercourse as often as in past.

- Cause: Possibly because of decreased testosterone levels, depression, or decreased self-esteem as a result of aging and body changes.
- Prevention/Tx for lack of sex drive:
  —Exercise (see Emotional Changes above)
  —HRT, progesterone cream
  —Testosterone cream/gel/capsule above
  —DHEA
  —Alternative therapies (see Emotional Changes above)
  —Sexual therapy

Urinary Problems

(See Urinary Problem; Vaginal Problem. Rule out potential infection.)

Caution: For UTI symptoms in perimenopausal and menopausal women: UTI symptoms (burning, frequency, urgency, cloudy urine, and pain) that follow sexual intercourse *may* be signs of decreased estrogen rather than an infection—more like "honeymoon cystitis." Never treat UTI symptoms over telephone without verified culture. Frequent inappropriate antibiotic therapy can lead to antibiotic resistance and/or increased allergic reactions.

- Definition:
  —Urinary incontinence (UI): Loss of control of bladder function. There are three types:
    o Stress: Loss of urine when coughing, sneezing, lifting, jogging
    ° Urge: Need to void immediately, overwhelming urge, unable to wait
    ° Mixed: Stress and urge combined
  —85% of affected people are women. People over age 60 are the largest group.
- Cause:
  —Relaxation of vaginal, rectal, urinary muscles, because of decreased estrogen.
  —Infection.
  —Stretching from childbirth, multiple pregnancies, and damage to muscles needed to control urination.
  —Trauma, surgery, bicycle accidents may damage muscles needed to control urination.
  —Overweight and gravity.
- Prevention/Tx:
  —Interim advice:
    ° Go to bathroom at regular times and often.
    ° Woman should keep a diary of how often she urinates, whether she has accidents, and the amount/kinds of fluids she drinks.
    o If she has symptoms of UI, she should have an appointment with MD/NP to evaluate and treat.
    ° This is a common problem and there are various treatments available. Behavior modification and biofeedback training may help up to 80% of people with this condition.
  —Kegel exercises:
    ° Kegel exercises help to strengthen the vaginal, rectal, and urinary muscles. This will help prevent UI from starting or getting worse.
    ° The sensation the woman is trying to achieve may be like: trying to stop from passing gas, or like "gripping" the penis with the muscles of the vagina (during intercourse). Another way to feel the sensation is to stop the stream of urine, when she goes to the bathroom.
    ° The basic exercise is to tighten, lift, and hold these muscles for 5 seconds, then relax for 5 seconds. Do 5 rounds, 1-2 times per day.

- ■ Relax and breathe during the exercise. Holding one's breath makes it harder to do the exercise correctly. Empty the bladder.
- ■ Start by doing Kegels when lying or sitting, for example, while riding in a car, watching TV, or lying in bed. After the woman can do the exercise easily, she can do it while standing, waiting in lines, etc. One can practice Kegels anywhere and any time—even during intercourse.
- ■ Use only the vaginal, urinary, and rectal muscles. Don't use stomach, leg, or buttock muscles.
- * One should see improvement (better control, fewer accidents, less urgency) after 4-6 weeks of practice.

► Best Books/Resources

One can find these and other informative books in a local bookstore or library:

Barbach, L., Ph.D. 1993. *The Pause: Positive Approaches to Menopause.* New York: Dutton Press.
Greenwood, S. 1996. *Menopause Naturally: The Second Half of Life.* Volcano, CA: Volcano Press.
Lark, S. M., M.D. 1992. *The Menopause Self-Help book.* Berkeley, CA: Celestial Arts.
Northrup, C., M.D. 1994. *Women's Bodies, Women's Wisdom.* New York: Bantam Books.

► Health Risks of Menopause

Cardiac Disease

(See Chest Pain Protocol. Rule out cardiac symptoms.)

What are risk factors for developing heart disease?

- • Diabetes: increases risk factor x 3—protection by estrogen is canceled out because of high sugar levels.
- • Family history of previous heart disease before age 60.
- • Age: Women are generally protected against heart disease by estrogen until menopause. Before age 60, they are 6 x less likely to have heart disease than men. After menopause, women begin to lose that edge. Heart disease is the leading cause of death in U.S. women after age 60+; 1 in 3 women after age 64 has heart disease.
- ® High BP: increases risk x 3.
- • Smoking: nicotine reduces estrogen levels; 4-5 x increase in risk factor.
- • Overweight.
- • Lack of exercise.

What Are Women's Risks for Heart Attack?

- • Women are diagnosed less quickly and referred for further testing less often than men. Women who have heart attacks are twice as likely as men to die.

Osteoporosis

- • Definition: Progressive loss of bone mass/strength associated with menopause
- • Contributing factors:
  —Family history
  —Smoking
  —Drinking
  —Lack of exercise
  —Steroid therapy
  —Unhealthy diet: e.g., high fat/high protein diet, overdieting
  —Decreased estrogen
  —Fair-skinned Caucasian and Asian women

- Prevention/Tx:

  —Exercise 20 min 5 days per week: Walking, running, tennis, Nordic track, dancing, weight lifting, hiking, aerobics, rowing, skiing.

  —Avoid caffeine, soft drinks, and processed foods—they decrease phosphates and rob the bones of calcium.

  —Take calcium/magnesium: 1000-1500 mg or three Turns daily.

  —Increase in daily diet: Lowfat dairy (milk/cheese/yogurt), dark green leafy vegetables (spinach, butter lettuce), fish, chicken; eat less animal fats.

  —Vitamin D: Milk fortified with vitamin D; 20 min per day of sunshine. However, avoid sun between the hours of 10 AM and 4 PM.

  —Hormone replacement therapy.

  —Mineral bone density (MBD) test: Get first test at age 50 to provide a "baseline" for later comparison.

  —Avoid smoking and drinking alcohol and caffeine.

  —Prescription medications for bone building or replacement may be needed.

▶ Treatments Associated with Menopause

Hormone Replacement Therapy Management FAQs

What Is Hormone Replacement Therapy (HRT)?

- Estrogen and/or progesterone replace the body's natural hormones lost at menopause. Currently, HRT comes in three forms: Pills, patches, and creams.

When Should Women Start Taking HRT?

- HRT may be started in the perimenopausal period. Discuss this issue with an MD/NP.

How Does a Woman Decide Whether She Needs to Take HRT?

- The need to take HRT should be based on careful consideration of the risks and benefits of this medication (See below).

What Are the Benefits of Taking HRT?

Estrogen is the most effective treatment available for menopausal symptoms, such as hot flashes, vaginal dryness, and sleep and mood disturbances. It can increase the quality of life after menopause. HRT is not prescribed to prevent cardiovascular disease at this time. It reduces the risk of colorectal cancer, hip fracture and osteoporosis. Most agree that it is an important option for the short-term treatment of menopausal symptoms.

What Are the Risks of HRT?

There is still much controversy and uncertainty regarding the risks of HRT. Consult an MD/NP to discuss risks/benefits. A careful review of your cardiovascular, colon cancer, breast cancer, and osteoporosis risks is important in determining the appropriateness of HRT therapy. HRT is not recommended for women with cardiovascular disease and may increase the risk of cardiac events in older women who use HRT for long periods of time. Breast cancer risk is important to discuss with your provider.

Who Should Not Be Taking HRT?

A woman should not take HRT if she has one or more of the following risk factors:

- Pregnancy: known or suspected
- Vaginal bleeding (undiagnosed)
- Cancer: Breast, endometrial
- Liver disease
- Thrombophlebitis history (discuss with an MD/NP)
- Known coronary artery disease

What Precautions Should Be Taken with HRT?

A woman should use caution and weigh the risks/benefits of taking HRT if she has one or more of the following conditions:

® Cancer: Family history of breast cancer, breast lumps, or abnormal mammogram. (She may need frequent breast exams.)

® Diabetes type I

® Fibroids

o Gallbladder disease

® Obesity

What Are Common Side Effects of HRT?

The following side effects can occur with hormone replacement therapy use:

° Headache

° Nausea and vomiting

® Breast tenderness or enlargement

e Enlargement of benign tumors ("fibroids") of the uterus

® Irregular bleeding

e Abdominal bloating/weight gain

® Painful periods

® Emotional changes: Depression, irritability

® Sex drive changes: > or <

® A spotty darkening of the skin, particularly on the face

What Are the Serious Complications of HRT?

Go to nearest ED if these symptoms occur:

® Pains in the calves or chest, sudden shortness of breath, or coughing blood (possible blood clot, MI)

® Severe headache, dizziness, faintness, or changes in vision (possible stroke)

Call for immediate appointment for following symptoms:

® Abnormal vaginal bleeding (possible uterine cancer) (See Treatments Associated with Menopause: Hormone Replacement Therapy Management FAQs above)

® Breast lumps (possible breast cancer)

® Yellowing of the skin or eyes

® Pain, swelling, or tenderness in the abdomen

How Can a Woman Reduce Risks of HRT?

Reduce the risks by doing the following:

® It is possible that a lower dose of HRT might have fewer risks.

® If she is taking hormones, she should see her MD/NP at least once a year for a checkup and re-evaluation of this therapy.

® If she develops unusual vaginal bleeding while taking hormones, she should call for advice and/or appointment.

® HRT is considered safe for short-term use.

What Can a Woman Expect Regarding Vaginal Bleeding While on HRT?

• The amount and length of time of vaginal bleeding can vary with each individual. While adjusting to hormones, bleeding may be irregular. Many women will not have periods at all (See Vaginal Bleeding Protocol to rule out unusual vaginal bleeding.)

Can a Woman Take HRT Forever?

® Asa result of one recent study (Women's Health Initiative 2002), this now is a controversial issue. Talk with your doctor or nurse practitioner.

Will Her Need for Hormones Change as She Ages?

- Maybe. She may need less as her body adjusts.

What Does HRT Cost?

- Depends on the type, insurance coverage and whether she uses generic prescriptions. The cost averages $30-50/mo.

► HRT Treatments

Creams (Estrogen, Vaginal Creams)

Why Use Creams?

- Estrogen and/or progesterone to replace body's declining hormones lost at menopause.

How Do Creams Work?

- Estrogen is absorbed directly through the mucous membranes of the vagina. This restores vaginal tone and moisture. It does not help with other symptoms of menopause, like hot flashes, insomnia. It does not reduce risk of heart attack, stroke, or osteoporosis. This method is useful for some people who cannot take HRT by patch or pill, because of other health problems.

How Effective Are Creams?

- This method helps reduce vaginal dryness making sexual intercourse more comfortable and pleasurable. It also helps reduce urinary tract symptoms.

Complications/Side Effects

- Sometimes creams can be irritating to the vagina because of chemicals in the cream. Sometimes the cream is not totally effective in relieving symptoms.

(For other FAQs regarding risks, contraindications, precautions, side effects, complications, and how to reduce risks of HRT, See Treatments Associated with Menopause above)

How Is the Cream Used?

- It is inserted into the vagina by applicator.

How Long Does the Cream Take to Work?

- Two to three weeks

Patch (Estrogen)

Why Is the Patch Used?

- The estrogen patch provides estrogen to the body through the skin. (Woman will need progestin if she still has her uterus.)

How Does the Patch Work?

- Estrogen is absorbed through the skin into the bloodstream.

What Are the Advantages of the Patch?

- Estrogen does not go through the liver, so it is less upsetting to the stomach. It is absorbed well in people who have difficulty absorbing oral medication. It is a better delivery method for patients with gallbladder or liver problems, and migraines. There is less breast tenderness with the patch.

How Effective Is the Patch?

- The patch is as effective as pills in reducing symptoms of menopause and reducing osteoporosis.

Complications/Side Effects

- Skin irritation and allergic reactions may be side effects.

(For other FAQs regarding risks, contraindications, precautions, side effects, complications, and how to reduce risks of HRT, see Treatments Associated with Menopause above.)

What To Do if the Patch Falls Off?

- If it falls off, try to apply the same patch to a new site, or use a new patch and follow the usual treatment schedule.

Can Women Swim/Shower/Bathe with the Patch?

- Yes. She may swim, bathe, or shower with the patch on.

Where Is the Patch Placed?

- On hip or abdomen, not breasts.

Pills (Estrogen, Progesterone, or Combination)

How Do the Pills Work?

- Pills work by being absorbed through stomach/intestines.

How Effective Are the Pitts?

- Pills are very effective, and work for most people.
- Reduce symptoms within 1 day to 1 mo (varies); most people notice improvement in first few weeks. Call if no relief in 2 weeks.

Side Effects (See information regarding risks, contraindications, precautions, side effects, complications, and how to reduce risks of HRT under Treatments Associated with Menopause above.)

What Are the Advantages of Taking the Pitts?

- Pills are convenient and less expensive than the patch. They are readily available. Pills offer more choices in managing menopausal symptoms. For example, all these types of pills can be taken daily or cyclically. Pills can be tailored to the individual to minimize bleeding and side effects.

Testosterone (Cream, Oral)

How Does Testosterone Work?

- Male synthetic or natural hormone—replaces testosterone normally produced by ovaries. Comes in oral or cream form. May enhance sexual pleasure and sex drive.

How Effective Is Testosterone?

- Effectiveness varies, depending on the individual.

Side Effects (Monitor carefully.)

- Acne
- Facial hair
- Enlarged clitoris
- Breast tenderness
- Lowered voice

Contraindications

- Liver disease
- Cancer

POSTPARTUM PROBLEM
Emotional Problems; Leg Pain; Painful Urination; Incisional Pain; Fever; Bleeding; Headache; SOB; Diarrhea; N/V; Abd. Pain

ASSESSMENT ACUTY LEVEL		DISPOSITION/ADVICE
Key Questions	**Emergent Symptom Patterns**	ED 0 min-1 hr
Vaginal Bleeding	+ Weak, dizzy, cold/mottled/pale skin, blue lips/nail beds, rapid/shallow breathing, unresponsive, loss of consciousness? (shock) (See Shock)	
SOB, Difficult Breathing	+ Chest pain/cough; anxious, restless, sweating, faintness, Hx BCP/phlebitis/immobilization/calf pain/surgery? (Pulmonary Embolus)	
Depression Symptoms	+ Suicidal/homicidal ideation, hallucinations? (Psychosis)	

Key Questions	**Urgent Symptom Patterns**	ED/UCC/Office 1-8 hr
Vaginal Bleeding	+ 1 pad/hr after rest, passing clots? (> Risk Hemorrhage)	
Fever ± Chills	+ Abd. pain (lower)? (Endometritis, Septic Pelvic Thrombosis)--	*-Rule of Thumb: > 38°C or 100.4°F on any 2 of first 10 days after delivery = postpartum infection
	+ Foul-smelling lochia? (Infection)	
	+ Perineal pain? (Infection of Episiotomy/Tear)	
	+ Incision discharge: puslike, foul-smelling, incision edges separated ± pain? (Wound Seroma/Separation)	
Depression Symptoms	+ Problems w eating, sleeping, feeling isolated/hopeless, anxiety, crying, frightening thoughts/fantasies? (Depression)	
Painful Urination	+ Pain (sev.-mod.), radiating from abd./flank/back to groin, colicky then constant & severe, fever/chills, N/V, ± hematuria, ffequency/urgency? (pyelonephritis) (See Urinary Problem)	
	+ Frequency, urgency, ± blood-tinged urine, ± nocturia, ± cloudy, foul or strong-smelling urine, ± fever? (UTI) (See Urinary Problem)	

(continued)

Key Questions	Urgent Symptom Patterns	ED/UCC/Office 1-8 hr
Painful Urination (continued)	+ Inability to empty bladder completely,	
	± Hx anesthesia? (Urinary Retention)	
Headache (severe)?	+ Hx of spinal, epidural anesthesia, unrelieved by home Tx? (Spinal Headache) - - - - - - - - - - - - - - - - - - ➤	SA: Have pt. sit upright; > pain = +
Leg Pain	+ Gradual onset, numbness, swelling, unilateral calf tenderness/warmth, Hx of BCP, recent surgery/Fx, recent prolonged immobilization? (Deep Vein Thrombosis)	
Unusual Pain/Symptoms	+ Postop or postprocedure? (Poss. Complications/Infection)	
Symptoms of Infection	+ Failure to improve on antibiotics x 48 hr? (Ineffective Rx)	

Key Questions	Acute/Nonacute Symptom Patterns	FA 8+ hr
Heaviness, Bearing Down Sensation	+ Incontinence, discomfort w walking/sitting, backache, painful intercourse, cervix protrudes from vagina? (Uterine Prolapse)	
Loss of Bowel/Bladder Control	+ Hx of big baby, forceps, large episiotomy, difficult delivery? (Rectocele, Cystocele, Recto-Vaginal Fistula)	

Cross-References

Breastfeeding Problem	Postpartum Emotional Problem SI	Postpartum Problem SI	Urinary Problem

POSTPARTUM PROBLEM
Supplemental Information

Quick Reference:
- ▶ Rules of Thumb
- ▶ Activity
- ▶ Constipation
- ▶ Cramps
- ▶ Diet
- ▶ Family Adjustment Problems
- ▶ Hemorrhoids Tx
- ▶ Incisional Pain Care

- ▶ Night Sweats
- ▶ Perineal Pain/Swelling
- ▶ Rectal Bleeding
- ▶ Sexual Activity and Birth Control
- ▶ Vaginal Bleeding
- ▶ Varicose Veins/Leg Edema
- ▶ Tutorial

See also: Directory of Hotlines/Web Sites for Support Groups, Appendix E

▶ Rules of Thumb

All postpartum problems < 6 wk that need appointments go to ED or delivery.

▶ Acitivity
- You may feel tired for 2 wk or longer (6 wk for C-section).
- Rest when baby sleeps if possible. Balance rest and activity; don't stay in bed all day. Interrupted sleep at night can lead to crying, anxiety, poor concentration, depression, fatigue—not uncommon Sx in parents of a newborn.
- Don't lift anything heavier than baby.
- Don't climb stairs more than necessary (C-section).
- Sit up. Walk in home, walk outside as able (progressive ambulation).
- Get help with shopping, cleaning, laundry.
- Make list of chores for family to help.
- Do not return to work before 6 wk if possible.
- Try to walk outside w baby for fresh air and sunshine at least 1 x day

▶ Constipation
- Bowels may move more slowly after delivery because of hormonal effect.
    - —Drink 3-4 quarts fluid/day.
    - —Eat fresh fruits and vegetables, bran, and drink prune juice.
    - —Try bulk-forming laxatives [Metamucil (psyllium seed) 1 tbsp. 2-3 x a day] and/or stool softener [Colace (docusate sodium) 100-200 mg/day].
    - —Passing more gas is also common when your bowels start working again.
- • To avoid gas: Avoid carbonated beverages or gassy foods like beans, cabbage, broccoli, and fried foods.

► Cramps

Painful contractions of uterus during first 48-72 hr. More common and stronger in women who have had more than one baby. For comfort:

- Go to the bathroom/urinate every 1-2 hr.
- Put hot water bottle/compress to lower abdomen.
- Lie on stomach.
- Apply pressure to lower abdomen with pillow.
- Massage lower abdomen.
- While lying flat on back or on side, bend knees into the chest.
- Take Tylenol as appropriate or ibuprofen every 4 hr.
- You may need to take med around the clock. Call Advice RN if no relief.

► Diet

- General:
  —Eat small, frequent meals.
  —Drink 3-4 quarts of juice, milk, water, or decaffeinated herbal tea per day.
  —Eat 5 servings per day of fresh fruits and vegetables.
  —Eat 4 servings of protein foods (e.g., dairy products, meat, fish, eggs, beans, legumes) per day.
  —Eat 5 servings of grains and breads (e.g., pasta, bread, rice, crackers, tortillas) per day.
  —Eat 4 servings of dairy products (e.g., cheese, milk, yogurt, ice cream) per day.
- To prevent anemia:
  —Continue taking prenatal vitamins.
  —Eat more eggs, fish, meat, dark green leafy vegetables, raisins, prunes, oysters, clams, beans, cheese. Use iron skillet or pot. More iron will build up your blood.

► Family Adjustment Problems

- Risk factors (See also Postpartum Emotional Problem SI):
  —Domestic violence
  —Father of baby not involved; partner conflicts
  —Inadequate social/financial support
  —Pressure to return to work very early
  —Sibling issues
  —Fussy baby, difficult to console
  —Feeling inadequate, unrealistic expectations, especially first-time mom
  —Homeless, shelter-based
  —Baby sick/hospitalized
  —Difficult birthing experience
- Family adjustment Tx:
  —Take care of yourself. Your health and well-being are important to your family. A new baby means many changes for you and your family. At times you may feel overwhelmed. All new moms/families need to ask for help [See Abuse 2 (Physical) SI; Postpartum Emotional Problem].

► Hemorroids Tx

    (See Rectal Problem)

    ® Use soft pillow for sitting.

    ® No laxatives

► Incisional Pain Care

    (Rule out infection/complications)

    It is normal to have some pain after a C-section or postpartum tubal ligation. It can be worse especially when changing position. For comfort:

- Splint incision. Press a pillow into your abdomen when you cough or move.
- If breastfeeding, use football hold or side-lying position to nurse, or place pillow on abdomen under baby to cushion incision.
- Take prescribed pain meds. If pain unrelieved, call back.
- The incision will heal in 10-14 days. It is normal for Steri strips to come off before that time.
- Shower daily; pat wound dry.
- Wear loose clothing (cotton is best).

    « Call if signs of infection: red, hot, fever, > pain, swelling, pus, foul odor, opening of wound edge.

► Night Sweats

    (Rule out fever, engorged breasts.)

    You may wake up at night soaked with sweat. This is caused by hormonal changes after birth. It is normal and will pass within about a week.

► Perineal Pain/Swelling

    Discomfort from episiotomy, hemorrhoids, or trauma to tissues during birth

- Home Tx goal: Comfort, prevent infection.
- Sitz bath: As often as you like, at least 2 x day. Shower first if possible (see Home Tx SI, Appendix A: Sitz Bath).
- Witch hazel: Wet a very clean washcloth w witch hazel. Place on stitch, cover w pad.
- Peri bottle: Use any clean liquid soap bottle or ketchup squeeze bottle. Fill w warm water. Spray entire area between your legs from front to back (private parts) every time you go to bathroom.
- Ice packs: 20 min q hr. (see Home Tx SI, Appendix A: Ice Pack)

    ® Pain: Tylenol as appropriate

- For stinging/burning when you urinate, spray water over your vaginal area to dilute the urine. Drink 8 glasses of fluids (water, juice) per day.

► Rectal Bleeding

- Home Tx:
  —Apply small plastic bag filled w 3 ice cubes and wrapped in light cloth to hemorrhoids w mod. pressure for 15 min of each hr.
  —Avoid sitting up for long periods.
  —Witch hazel compresses to hemorrhoids between ice packs
  —If bleeding gets worse or won't stop, call back.

► Sexual Activity and Birth Control

- You may have vaginal intercourse after vaginal discharge has stopped completely, the stitches are healed, and you are ready.
- Vaginal dryness (especially w breastfeeding) is not unusual and water-based lubricants like Astroglide can be used.
- Changes in sexual desire are common (may be caused by hormones, fatigue, feeling overwhelmed, family adjustment).
- Milk may drip during sexual intercourse because of sexual excitement or orgasm.
- You can still get pregnant even though your period has not yet returned.
- The first 6 wk: No diaphragm, sponges, cervical caps, or tampons!

► Vaginal Bleeding

- Definition: > 1 pad/hr while up; or gushes or does not slow down after rest.
  —Change pad. Go to bed x 1 hr, then check pad. If bleeding does not slow down, call RN.
  —Do not take ASA, Motrin, NSAIDs.
  —Rest as much as you can.

► Varicose Veins/Leg Edema

Because of the pressure of the pregnancy on blood vessels, postpartum women often have varicose veins in their leg(s) and genitals and/or swelling of the feet/legs. For comfort:

- Elevate legs whenever possible, but at least 20 min 4 x day.
- Avoid sitting or standing for long periods of time.
- Varicosity position 2-5 min 3-4 x a day: Lie on floor w legs extended straight into air at right angle from body w buttocks, heels, and legs pressed against the wall.
- Wear loose, nonrestrictive clothing.
- Wear full-length supportive stockings.
- Avoid crossing legs at knee.
- Avoid high-heeled shoes, knee-high socks.
- If your veins start to ache, you have been in one position too long and need to change position.
- Do not massage varicose veins.
- Call the RN if you notice painful hot spots, or calf pain when you walk on your heels.

► Tutorial

Red Flags

- Age: The childbearing years are a time of high risk because of the risks related to birth, birth control, and sexual activity.
- Emotional Distress: Pregnancy and the postpartum period are risk factors for depression and domestic violence.
- Debilitation. Alcohol and drug abuse can lead to higher-risk pregnancies.

Rules of Thumb

If a patient is very worried or calls frequently within short time periods, give her an SDA or tell her to come in now.

Red Herrings

Multiple somatic complaints may be a hidden agenda for depression, domestic violence, or drug seeking. Failure to follow up or sporadic postnatal care may be the result of drug abuse, domestic violence, or emotional or financial instability. Therefore, when these callers do contact healthcare providers—"seize the opportunity" to see them or to counsel them.

Hotlines and Web Sites

Web site and hotline information is provided for professionals, patients, and their families. The listings below were current as of April 13, 2008.

Organization	Type	Contact Info
Breastfeeding.com	Info	http://www.breastfeeding.com
Domestic Violence Hotline	Info/Referral	http://www.ndvh.org/(800) 799-7233
Mothers of Twins Clubs	Info/Support	http://www.nomotc.org/
Pacific Postpartum Support Society	Support/Info	http://www.womenshealth.gov
Postpartum Depression	Support/Info	http://www.postpartum.net
PSI: Postpartum Support International	Support/Info	www.postpartum.org

POSTPARTUM EMOTIONAL PROBLEM
Supplemental Information

Quick Reference:
- ▶ Postpartum Blues
- ▶ Postpartum Depression
- ▶ Postpartum Blues/Depression Risk Factors
- ▶ Referrals

▶ Postpartum Blues

- Postpartum blues usually happen during the first 10 days after birth. Sometimes it still happens up to 8 wk after birth. It is common to feel teary, anxious, and to have mood swings, fatigue, or poor concentration. These feelings are caused by hormonal changes, the demands of the new baby, and getting used to being a new parent.
- If this depression lasts longer than 10 days or you feel worse, call for an appt.
- Postpartum blues prevention/Tx
  - —Go where other people are: Park, restaurant, shopping, walk w friends.
  - —Join a New Mom Group or get together w other new moms on a regular basis. (It helps to talk to other new moms about this experience.)
  - —Attitude: Take it slow and easy at first. Try to have a "honeymoon" period w baby: relax in bed, quiet walks, eat well. Keep it simple.
  - —Get help when possible. Get help with cooking, housecleaning, limit visitors, etc. Turn off the telephone. Send laundry out. Use paper plates.
  - —Sleep when baby sleeps. Rest as often as you can.

▶ Postpartum Depression (Postpartum psychosis, major affective disorder)

- Definition: In first 2 wk, confusion, extreme fatigue with insomnia, agitation, feelings of hopelessness, shame, delusion, auditory hallucinations, hyperactivity, rapid speech, or mania
- Complications:
  - —Impaired bonding
  - —> Risk child abuse
  - —Suicide

▶ Postpartum Blues/Depression Risk Factors

- Abusive and/or substance-abusing partner
- Difficult, lengthy labor and delivery, C-section
- Hxof PMS (severe)
- Fetal loss/death
- First pregnancy
- Lack of social supports/social isolation; uninvolved father of baby/partner
- Overly high expectations in any low-risk mother, whether in stable social relationships, or with a positive pregnancy experience
- Multiple life stresses

- Psych. Hx of patient or family: manic depression, psychotic disorders, major depression
- Posttraumatic stress disorder
- Stress Hx
- Unwanted pregnancy

▶ Referrals

- Make friends w other moms in clinic lobby
- Economic concerns—General assistance
- Home visit—PHN
- Warm line—Parent support
- New Mother Support Groups
- Teen mom, single mom
- Domestic violence—shelter
- La Leche League
- Nutrition

PREGNANCY PROBLEM 1
Labor; Abdominal Pain; Vaginal Discharge/Bleeding

ASSESSMENT ACUITY LEVEL		DISPOSITION/ADVICE
Key Questions	Emergent Symptom Patterns	ED 0 min-1 hr
Advanced Labor	+ Contractions q 5 min, wants to push, ± body part/head seen in vagina? (Call 911)	
Vaginal Discharge (sudden)	+ Watery, gush brown/green, frequent, reg. UCs q 5 min, vaginal bleeding (into shoes), during contraction needs to "hold on to something," can't speak?----------------------- ------ -----------------------	SA: Place white towel or Peri pad between legs + Clear to cloudy pea soup, green specks/yellow (meconium) fluid w/o odor = + amniotic fluid
Abdominal Pain	+ W or w/o bleeding, sudden onset, hard/balled up uterus, 2nd/3rd trimester? (Abruptio Placenta, Uterine Rupture, Appendicitis, Cholecystitis)--------- ▶	Refer to L&D
Cord	+ Shiny, twisted like phone cord is coming out of vagina? (Prolapsed Cord)-------------------------- - - -➤	First Aid: + Tell mother to lie on left side w knees flexed or on hands & knees + Stay on telephone until ambulance comes
Depression Sx	+ Suicidal/homicidal ideation, hallucinations? (Psychosis)	
Vaginal Bleeding	+ Sudden onset (dripping down leg), w or w/o pain, bright red or clots, Hx of cerclage, 2nd or 3rd trimester? (Placenta Previa) + Sharp, progressive, unilateral pelvic pain, ± radiates to shoulder, pale, lightheaded, fainting, ± Hx: STI, PID, any abd./tubal surgery, prior IUD use, missed period x 3-6 wk; spotting, painful intercourse? (Ectopic Pregnancy) + Weak, dizzy, cold/mottled/or pale skin, blue lips/nail beds, rapid/shallow breathing, unresponsive, loss of consciousness? (Shock) (See Shock)	•*- Lie on one side or on back w one hip supported w pillow, legs elevated if possible, until help arrives

Key Questions	Urgent Symptom Patterns	ED/UCC/Office 1 -8 hr
Trauma	+ Suspicious history/potential risk of assault? (Abuse, ~~Possible Intimacy~~ - v_emerit- - → ᴉɴᴜᴡ: ED	
Depression Symptoms	+ Problems w eating, sleeping; feeling isolated/hopeless, anxious; crying, frightening thoughts/fantasies? (Depression)	
Labor Symptoms	+ High-risk pregnancy? (Preterm Labor) (See High-Risk Pregnancy IAQ)	
	+ Regular UCs 6/hr, ± membrane rupture, clear, watery discharge, blood tinged, < 1 pad/hr (Labor Onset)	
	+ High-risk pregnancy? (Poss. Upgrade) (See High-Risk Pregnancy IAQ)	
Vaginal Bleeding/Cramps (> 1 pad/hr)	+ > 19 wk? (Previa, Abruption, SAB)---------------------	Refer to L&D if > 20 wk gestation
	+ < 19 wk? (Ectopic, Missed AB, SAB)	
Pressure/Cramping	+ Recent onset, lower backache, upper thigh or uterine pain/discomfort/cramping, burning on urination, pelvic pressure, hard/balled-up uterus, diarrhea? (Preterm Labor)	Refer to L&D if > 20 wk gestation

Key Questions	Acute/Nonacute Symptom Patterns	FA 8+ hr ± Home Tx
Contractions	+ W/o emergent symptoms, decreased fetal movement/ ruptured membranes, heavy bleeding ruled out? ——	Refer to L&D if > 20 wk gestation
Vaginal Discharge (All)	+ Exposure to STI? (STI)	

Cross-References Postpartum Emotional Problem	Pregnancy Problem 2	Pregnancy Problem SI

PREGNANCY PROBLEM 2
Trauma; Headache; Chest Pain; < Fetal Movement; N/V; Swelling; Burning on Urination; Itching

ASSESSMENT	ACUITY LEVEL	DISPOSITION/ADVICE
Key Questions	Emergent Symptom Patterns	ED 0 min-1 hr
Chest Pain (Sev.-Mod.)	+ SOB, cyanosis? (Pulmonary Edema, Amniotic Fluid Embolism)	
Severe Headache	+ ± Trauma (sudden/sharp or gradual/dull/throbbing), neck pain/stiffness, resp. changes, progressing: irritable/lethargic/± loss of consciousness; visual changes, weakness, N/V, staggering, slurred speech? (Intracranial Hemorrhage, Traumatic/Spontaneous)-->-	First Aid: If Hx of HTN or tox-emia, have pt. lie on left side
	+ 2nd/3rd trimester: blurred vision, Hx rapid wt gain, swelling (hands/feet/face), N/V, epigastric pain, fatigue, Hx of hypertension ± seizure? (Severe, Preeclampsia)	
Decreased Fetal Movement	± Risk factors for fetal demise? (See High-Risk----------► Pregnancy IAQ)	SA: Do kick count assessment
Depression Symptoms	+ Suicidal/homicidal ideation, hallucinations? (Psychosis)	
Key Questions	Urgent Symptom Patterns	ED/UCC/Office 1 -8 hr
Trauma	+ Suspicious history/potential risk of domestic abuse? (Possible Abuse)	
All Symptoms	+ High-risk pregnancy? (See High-Risk Pregnancy IAQ)	
Depression Symptoms	+ Problems w eating, sleeping; feeling isolated/hopeless, anxious; crying, frightening thoughts/fantasies? (Depression)	
Swelling (Hands/Feet/Face)	+ 2nd/3rd trimester: headache/blurred vision, Hx rapid wt gain, N/V, epigastric pain, fatigue, Hx of hypertension? (Mild Preeclampsia)	
Pain/Burning w Urination	+ Pain (sev.-mod.), radiating from abd./flank/back to groin, colicky then constant & severe, fever/chills, N/V, dysuria, ± hematuria, frequency/urgency? (Pyelonephritis) (See Urinary Problem)	

(continued

Key Questions	Urgent Symptom Patterns	ED/UCC/Office 1-8 hr
Nausea & Vomiting (Sev.) (> 1/Hr)	+ Voids < 1 in 8 hr, unable to hold down fluids x 12 hr, muscle weakness, dry mouth? (Dehydration, Hyperemesis Gravidarum)................ ....▶	SA: Urine output < 1 x 8 hr or dark yellow = poss. dehydration: Refer to L&D
Pain (Calf, Groin, Thigh)	+ Leg pain, edema, Hx varicosities, hot, red, swollen? (Thrombophlebitis) -........... -.....................................•*-	Rest, elevate leg that is swollen
Fever	+ > 38°C or 100.4°F? (Amnionitis, Listeriosis)	
Painful Urination	+ Frequency, urgency, ± blood-tinged urine, ± nocturia, ± cloudy, foul or strong-smelling urine, ± fever? (UTI)	
Painful Lesion(s) (Vaginal, Labial)	+ Cluster of tiny clear blisters, begins w tingling, itching, pain, followed by yellow, crusty crater after 1 -2 days; first time; w severe throat pain, ± sev./mod. dehydration; w sev. vaginal pain, difficulty urinating, close to delivery date? (Herpes)	

Key Questions	Acute/Nonacute Symptom Patterns	FA 8+ hr ± Home Tx
Itching (Generalized)	+ > 20 wk "nothing works"? (Cholestasis of Pregnancy, Pruritus Gravidarum, > Risk Stillborn, Possible Induction)---▶	Do frequent kick counts
All Other Concerns	(See Pregnancy Problem SI)	

Cross-References Pregnancy Problem SI	Pregnancy Problem 1	Urinary Problem

HIGH-RISK PREGNANCY INITIAL ASSESSMENT QUESTIONS (IAQ)

► **Key Risk Factors for Preterm Labor**
- Cervical length less than 3 cm by sonogram
- ® Fetal fibroplastin
- History of preterm delivery

► **Other Risk Factors**
- ® Age < 18
- ® History of LEEP/cone biopsy/incompetent cervix
- Multiple gestation (> stress on uterine muscle—overstretched)
- Polyhydramnios (> stress on uterine muscle—overstretched)
- Prenatal care—little or none
- Previous preterm delivery (history > risk)
- Pyelonephritis (systemic infection > uterine irritability)
- More than two 2nd trimester TABs

► **Soft Indicators**
- Physical or mental stress (extreme)
- Uterine anomalies
- Vaginal bleeding/placenta previa

► **Fetal High-Risk Surveillance**
- ® Decreased amniotic fluid
- ® Diabetes
- ® Domestic violence
- Emotional problems (severe)
- History of fetal demise
- Hypertension [chronic or pregnancy-induced hypertension (PIH)]
- Intrauterine growth retardation
- Multiple gestation (twins, triplets, etc.)
- ® Postdates (> 41 wk)
- ® Prenatal care—little or none
- Preterm labor
- Rh sensitized
- Substance abuse
- Vaginal bleeding
- PROM

► **Difficult Pregnancy Risk Factors**
- Age < 18 or > 35 (development < 18, > 35, DM, HTN, genetic defects)
- Asthma (> risk emotional trigger)

   ° Cardiac disease (> risk fluid retention, hypertension)

   ° C-section/uterine surgery history (> risk uterine rupture with labor)

   ® Diabetes (> risk: stillbirth, cephalopelvic disproportion (CPD), shoulder dystocia, fragile infant, C-section)

   ® Domestic violence

   o Ectopic history (> risk ectopic)

- Grand multipara (> 5 births) (> risk uterine rupture, hemorrhage)

- Homeless (no support, stability, overall health risk)

- Hypertension (chronic/recent: > risk placental insufficiency, intrauterine growth retardation (IUGR), stroke, convulsions, and abruption)

8 Incompetent cervix or cerclage (> risk infection, bleeding, premature delivery) (cerclage: ribbon to hold cervix closed; premature labor, delivery)

o IUD in place in second trimester (> risk infection, preterm labor, uterine rupture, SAB after removal within 14 days)

- Multiple gestation (twins, triplets, etc.) (> risk: preterm labor, hemorrhage, atony, DM, HTN, possible exposure to infections, parasites)

- Prenatal care—little or none (> overall risk)

- Preterm delivery history (> risk preterm labor)

- Recent arrival/travel outside U.S. (parasites, inadequate prenatal care)

- STI in pregnancy history (> risk infection, SAB, > fetal risk)

- Substance abuse history (> risk fetal alcohol syndrome, prematurity, addicted or withdrawing babies)

- Uterine anomalies (> risk preterm labor, hemorrhage, C-section, painful fibroids)

PREGNANCY PROBLEM
Supplemental Information

Quick Reference:
- ▶ Rules of Thumb
- ▶ Backache
- ▶ Breast Tenderness
- ▶ Constipation
- ▶ Contraction Timing
- ▶ Dizziness, Fainting, Lightheadedness
- ▶ Fatigue
- ▶ Foot Pain
- ▶ Headache
- ▶ Heartburn
- ▶ Hemorrhoids
- ▶ Insomnia

- ▶ Kick Count Assessment
- ▶ Leg Cramps
- ▶ Nausea (Morning Sickness)
- ▶ Nosebleed
- ▶ Sexual intercourse
- ▶ Shortness of Breath
- ▶ Stuffy Nose
- ▶ Swelling (Face; Feet/Legs; Hands/Fingers)
- ▶ Urinary Frequency
- ▶ Varicose Veins (Legs, Vulva)
- ▶ Tutorial

See also: Directory of Hotlincs/Web Sites for Support Groups, Appendix E

▶ **Rules of Thumb**

® Multiple somatic complaints may be a red flag for domestic violence.

® Pregnancy may be a high-risk period for domestic abuse.

- Determine all gestation by using dating guide wheel (guide for estimating due date).
- When pregnant or breastfeeding, never take any medication, OTC or Rx, without MD advice.

▶ **Backache**

(Preterm, Labor UT1 Ruled Out)

° Prevention/Tx:

—Always stand straight and tall.

—Keep knees bent, feet wide apart. Roll shoulders back.

—Wear shoes w low heel and good support.

—Walk 4-5 x wk. Try to go farther each time. Go w a friend, partner.

—Apply hot water bottle or heating pad on low setting to back.

—Apply ice pack to back 15 min of each hr (See Home Tx SI, Appendix A: Ice Pack).

—Backrub by partner.

—Rest: Sideways on couch w knees and arms bent, pillow between knees and arms. Rest on floor w legs bent, feet and leg on chair: Pelvic tilt. Arm to side. Tylenol: q 4-6 hr prn.

► **Breast Tenderness**

- Prevention/Tx:

  —Wear support bra.

  —Use cool compresses or ice packs to provide temporary relief (See Home Tx SI, Appendix A: Cold/Cool Compress, Ice Pack).

  —Don't stimulate nipples by touching, rubbing, or sucking. It may cause little contractions of uterus.

► **Constipation**

See Bowel Problem 2.

► **Contraction Timing**

- Use a watch w second hand ("sweep").
- Write the time each contraction starts and length of contraction in seconds = Duration.
- Time number of minutes from beginning of one contraction to beginning of next contraction = interval.
- False labor = Irregular contractions (intervals), e.g., 5-3-10-15-2-6 min apart.
- True labor = Regular contractions of consistent duration that occur at regular intervals, e.g., 45 sec long and every 5 min.

► **Dizziness, Fainting, Lightheadedness**

(Preeclampsia Ruled Out)

- Causes:

  —Adjustment to increased blood volume in pregnancy

  —Decreased blood sugar.

  —Hyperventilation.

  —Pregnancy-induced hypertension: Check for > BP, edema, visual changes, complications (e.g., injury from fall).

  —Dehydration.

- Prevention/Tx:

  —Avoid sudden changes in position. Get up slowly from lying position. Roll to side and push up to sitting position.

  —Do not stand or lie flat on back for prolonged periods of time.

  —Remember to take iron supplements and eat iron-rich foods as advised for anemia.

  —Do not skip meals. Eat small, frequent meals to help keep constant blood sugar level, e.g., crackers w cheese, apple, yogurt, soup, tortillas, etc.

  —Avoid hot, stuffy rooms—open windows.

► **Fatigue**

(Depression, Abuse Ruled Out)

- Weariness and fatigue are common in pregnancy. You will need more sleep.
- Causes:

  —Early pregnancy: Hormone changes.

  —Later in pregnancy: Discomforts of the growing baby, waking in night to urinate frequently, heartburn, shortness of breath, worries or thoughts that may keep you awake. Stress on your body caused by carrying extra weight.

  —Domestic violence, depression.

- Complications:
  —You may need counseling for worries, concerns, anxiety.
- Prevention/Tx:
  —You may need rest/sleep up to 8-12 hr per day.
  —Nap/rest during the day as work/school/child permit.
  —Try sleep aids: Warm milk, herbal tea, music. Before sleep, shower, make love.
  —Urinate before sleep.
  —Use pillow for comfort.
  —Take deep breaths.
  —No coffee, coke, or regular tea (avoid caffeine).
  —General good health will help: Eat well-balanced diet; take moderate and regular exercise. Take after-dinner walk.
  —Think realistically: You may need to change your schedule, reduce activities.
  —Get as much help from family and friends as you can so you can get more rest.
  —Don't take on more responsibilities.
  —Avoid sleep meds.
  —Mint tea, cinnamon tea
  —Sleep w pillow behind back, between arms and knees.

► Foot Pain

- Causes:
  —Excessive weight gain (40-60 lb) and lower back curvature of the spine may affect stability of the feet, causing arch breakdown.
  —Edema from decreased circulation, excess salt intake, weight gain.
- Prevention/Tx:
  —Invert feet—e.g., turn feet in, when walking barefoot to hold arch up.
  —Wear shoes w arch supports.
  —Elevate feet above level of heart—higher than chair level if sitting.
  —Try support pantyhose, soaking, and massage.

► Headache

(Preeclampsia ruled out)

- Causes: Physical, hormonal, emotional changes of pregnancy
- Prevention/Tx:
  —Increase rest periods.
  —Eat small, frequent meals.
  —Increase clear liquids to 3 qts/day.
  —Apply cold washcloth or ice pack to forehead and/or back of neck (See Home Tx SI, Appendix A: Ice Pack).
  —Lie down in quiet, dark room.
  —Tylenol as appropriate (no ASA or ibuprofen unless ordered by MD or NP).

► **Heartburn**

- Causes: During pregnancy, stomach muscles relax, the growing womb presses against stomach, and stomach acids back up, causing pain.
- Prevention/Tx:
  —Avoid tight fitting clothes that cinch the waist.
  —Avoid greasy, spicy foods.
  —Avoid coffee, coke.
  —Avoid cigarettes.
  —Eat small, frequent meals, 5 x day instead of 3.
  —Rest w head slightly elevated or sitting up. Lying down may make it worse.
  —Sip liquids, water, milk, soda water, or yogurt.
  —Try walking or resting—whichever works.
  —Try sitting cross-legged and raise and lower arms quickly, bringing the backs of your hands together over your head.
  —Maximum 1-2 Turns (non- or low-sodium Turns) as appropriate daily (check w MD first).

► **Hemorrhoids**

- Hemorrhoids are more common in pregnancy because of pressure of baby (See also Rectal Problem).
- Prevention/Tx:
  —Knee chest position as needed.
  —Wear loose clothing.
  —Exercise daily.
  —Avoid knee-high stockings.
  —Wear maternity support pantyhose ("Loving Lift" by MediCal).
  —Avoid standing for extended periods of time.
  —Lie down w legs elevated for 20 min, 4 x day.
  —Try refrigerated witch hazel pads (e.g., Tucks) or make your own compresses.
  —Cool sitz bath (see Home Tx SI, Appendix A: Sitz Bath)

► **Insomnia**

(See also Fatigue above).

- Causes: In later months, it is normal to have insomnia. It is usually caused by difficulty in finding a comfortable position or baby kicking at night.
- Prevention/Tx:
  —Exercise daily.
  —Take bath before going to bed.
  —No coffee or cokes.
  —Drink warm milk, eat cracker, toast.
  —Relaxation exercises
  —No sleep meds—they could hurt the baby.

► **Kick Count Assessment**

- Do kick counts daily. Eat a snack and drink 1-2 large glasses of fluids.
- After eating and drinking, lie down on either side, or sit slumped in a chair. Put your hands on your belly, over your baby.

® Count the number of times the baby moves. If the baby moves 10 x or more in 2 hr, that is fine.

® If baby moves < 10 x in 2 hr, call Labor and Delivery.

® Once 10 kicks are counted (within 1-2 hr), you may stop.

► Leg Cramps

® Causes: Not enough calcium in diet, new exercise, or no known reason

® Prevention/Tx:

—Drink more milk, eat cheese, yogurt, tofu, broccoli, bok choy, okra. Make soups w bones and add 1 tablespoon cider vinegar.

—Exercise daily (walk).

—Take warm baths at bedtime.

—Avoid pointing toes.

—Try flexing feet at ankles while sitting on floor.

—Massage cramped muscles.

—Avoid prolonged standing or sitting (e.g., at work).

► Nausea (Morning Sickness)

(Hyperemesis ruled out)

® Cause: Hormonal. May happen any time, day or night. Usually goes away after 3rd mo.

® Prevention/Tx:

—Before getting out of bed: Eat dry crackers (e.g., saltines). Get out of bed slowly.

—Between meals: Eat dry crackers (e.g., saltines), tortillas, rice, plain pasta, or bread.

—Eat small, frequent meals.

—Avoid sudden movement.

—Don't eat greasy or spicy foods.

—Sip carbonated water, spearmint, chamomile, peppermint, or ginger tea.

—Avoid strong odors.

—Eat meat, eggs, fish, which may prevent low blood sugar.

—Appt. for evaluation if unable to eat in 24 hr.

► Nosebleed

® Causes: Mucous membranes of nose and gums are filled with tiny, fragile capillaries that have become more fragile or breakable.

® Prevention/Tx:

—Loosen clothing around neck.

—Ice pack across nose.

—Pinch nostrils for 10-15 min.

—If no relief in 10-15 min, call back.

—Sit w head tilted forward or lie back w head and shoulders elevated.

—Don't swallow blood—spit it out.

—Use mouth breathing.

—Don't blow nose—it may start bleeding again.

- Women's Health Protocols

► **Sexual Intercourse**
- Avoid sexual intercourse in the 1st or 3rd trimester in the following situations:
  —1st trimester (psychological help mainly)
    ° Previous Hx of > two SABs
    o Vaginal bleeding or spotting in current pregnancy
  —3rd trimester
    o Hx preterm delivery or PROM, check with MD for individual recommendations.
    ° Vaginal bleeding or spotting in current pregnancy (until Previa ruled out).
- If none of the above are present, you may have sex any time during your pregnancy.
- Consider alternate positions for comfort as pregnancy progresses.

► **Shortness of Breath**
(Respiration/Cardiac Problem Ruled Out)
- Cause: The baby gets bigger and presses on the lungs so they can't expand enough. You will feel better when the baby drops down (2 wk to right before delivery).
- Prevention:
  —Regular moderate activity.
  —Avoid overexertion.
  —Sit and stand up straight.
- Home Tx:
  —Reassurance.
  —Sleep propped up w pillows.
  —Stretch arms overhead to expand lungs. (Hispanic clients may resist this because of belief it results in breech birth.)
  —Slow, deep relaxation, breathing.
  —Lie on side if SOB occurs when on back.

► **Stuffy Nose**
- Sometimes pregnancy causes stuffy nose or allergies.
- Prevention/Tx:
  —Avoid cigarette smoke.
  —Use a humidifier.
  —Boil water. Place in bowl w towel over head, breathe steam.
  —Place bowls of cold water in each room.
  —Place warm, moist towels on face.
  —Increase clear liquids intake.
  —Try Saline Nose Drops (See Home Tx SI, Appendix A: Saline Nose Drops) x 3 days only. More will cause rebound stuffiness.

► **Swelling of Face**
(Preeclampsia ruled out)
- Causes:
  —Fluid retention related to increasing blood pressure from pregnancy-induced hypertension
  —Fluid retention as a result of hormones of pregnancy

- Prevention/Tx:
  - —If patient is experiencing headache and spots in front of eyes or has elevated BP Hx, needs BP checked.

► Swelling of Feet and Legs (Edema)

(Preeclampsia Sx ruled out)

- Causes:
  - —Pressure of baby decreases fluid return in legs, esp. in the last 3 mo of pregnancy.
  - —Feet and legs may become swollen, painful, and sore.
  - —Excess salt in diet,
- e Prevention/Tx:
  - —Elevate legs above level of heart (displace uterus left or right). Roll hand towel w rubber band around it. Stick under left or right hip.
  - —Gently massage feet.
  - —Wear maternity support pantyhose; put them on before getting out of bed—it will work better to prevent swelling.
  - —Avoid bands around abdomen and legs. Wear *maternity* support pantyhose.
  - —Eat more protein: Meat, fish, eggs, nuts, cheese. Protein is important for growing baby.
  - —Don't eat a lot of salty foods or drink sodas. No diet sodas.
  - —Rest or sleep positioned on left side as much as possible.

► Swelling of Hands and Fingers

(Feeling of tingling, numbness)

- Causes:
  - —Enlargement of breast tissue high in armpit, resulting in pressure on nerves and blood vessels. This is a normal occurrence from increase in hormones.
  - —Jewelry that constricts circulation.
  - —Increase in salt in diet.
  - —Excess fluid in arms increases pressure on nerves (carpal tunnel syndrome).
- Prevention/Tx:
  - —Place hands on shoulders and rotate elbows in a circle.
  - —Do arm circles and "walk up walls" w fingers.
  - —Wear a well-fitting bra (not too constrictive).
  - —Decrease Salt in diet.
  - —Avoid tight jewelry.

► Urinary Frequency

(Vaginal infection, UTI ruled out)

- Cause: Pressure of growing baby on bladder normal in 1st and 3rd trimesters.
- Complication: Possible bladder infection.
- Prevention/Tx:
  - —Drink most of fluids during day.
  - —Do not let bladder get too full—to avoid losing muscle tone and increasing risk of infection.
  - —Burning, urgency, foul-smelling or cloudy urine are signs of infection and need to be seen in 8 hr.

- Women's Health Protocols

► **Varicose Veins of Legs**
- Cause: Weak areas in walls of veins; more common in pregnancy caused by pressure of baby.
- Prevention/Tx:
  —Wear loose clothing.
  —Exercise daily.
  —Avoid knee-high stockings or high-heeled shoes.
  —Wear maternity support pantyhose ("Loving Lift" by MediCal).
  —Avoid standing or sitting for long periods of time.
  —Lie down w legs elevated for 20 min, 4 x daily.

► **Varicose Veins of Vulva**
- Cause: Weak areas in walls of veins; more common in pregnancy caused by pressure of baby
- Prevention/Tx:
  —Lie w hips and legs elevated several times a day, either on back or on side.
  —Ice packs 15 min each hr, 4 x day may help (See Home Tx SI, Appendix A: Ice Pack).
  —Sexual intercourse may help to decrease pelvic congestion if not contraindicated.
  —Wear firmly applied perineal pad for support. Special pads are available from surgical supply companies.
  —Knee chest position prn.
  —Cool Sitz baths (See Home Tx SI, Appendix A: Sitz Bath).

► Tutorial

Red Flags
- Age. The childbearing years are a time of high risk because of the risks related to birth, birth control, and sexual activity.
- Emotional Distress. Pregnancy and the postpartum period are risk factors for depression and domestic violence.
- Debilitation. Alcohol and drug abuse can lead to higher-risk pregnancies.

Rules of Thumb
- All amenorrhea is a possible pregnancy until proven differently.
- Once an ectopic, always an ectopic.
- If a patient is very worried or calls frequently within short time periods, give her an SDA or tell her to come in now.

Red Herrings
- Multiple somatic complaints may be a hidden agenda for depression, domestic violence, or drug seeking.
- Failure to follow up or sporadic prenatal care may be the results of drug abuse, domestic violence, or emotional or financial instability. Therefore, when these callers do contact health care providers—"seize the opportunity" to see them or to counsel them.

Web Sites and Hotlines

Web site and hotline information is provided for professionals, patients, and their families. The listings below are current as of April 13, 2008:

Organization	Type	Contact Information
Breastfeeding.com	Info	http://www.breastfeeding.com
Domestic Violence Hotline	Info/Referral	http://www.ndvh.org/ (800) 799-7233
Mothers of Twins Clubs	Info/Support	http://www.nomotc.org/
Pacific Postpartum Support Society	Support/Info	www.womenshealth.gov
Postpartum Depression	Support/Info	http://www.postpartum.net
PSI: Postpartum Support International	Support/Info	www.postpartum.org

VAGINAL BLEEDING (NONPREGNANT)
Abnormal Bleeding: Painful, Irregular, Excessive; Absence of Menses

ASSESSMENT	ACUITY LEVEL	DISPOSITION/ADVICE
Key Questions	Emergent Symptom Patterns	ED 0 min-1 hr
Bleeding (Severe)	+ Postpartum? (See Postpartum Problem)	
	+ Weak, dizzy, cold/mottled/or pale skin, blue lips/nail beds, rapid/shallow breathing, unresponsive, loss of consciousness? (Shock: Hemorrhage/Fibroids, Ectopic Pregnancy) (See Shock)	
Bleeding (Any Abnormal)	+ Sharp, progressive, unilateral pelvic pain, ± radiates to shoulder, pale, lightheaded, fainting, ± history: STI, PID, any abd./tubal surgery, prior IUD use, missed period x 36 wk, spotting, painful intercourse? (Ectopic Pregnancy, Ovarian Torsion, Ruptured Ovarian Cyst, or Endometrioma)	
	+ Fever, N/V, sev. intractable diarrhea, sunburn-like rash, muscle aches, headache, confusion, dizziness, fainting; history of menses, postpartum, post-GYN surgery, history of tampon, sponge, cap use? (TSS)	

Key Questions	Urgent Symptom Patterns	ED/UCC/Office 1-8 hr
Bleeding w/o Trauma (Mod. to Sev.)	+ > 1 pad/hr x 3 hr, clots > 5 or walnut-sized or larger, "running down leg"? (DUB, SAB, Fibroids)	
	+ Unusually heavy, history of TAB, GYN surgical procedure? (Postop Complications)	
	+ History of bleeding problems, anticoagulant therapy? (Coagulopathies, von Willebrand Disease, > Risk Hemorrhage)	
	+ IUD usage? (Possible Anemia Risk)	
	+ Pelvic pain, vaginal discharge: foul smelling, bloody/any color; fever (> 38°C or 100.4°F)/chills, walks bent over, ± history of STI exp., ± IUD user? (PID)	

Key Questions	Acute/Nonacute Symptom Patterns	FA8 + hr ±Home Tx
Bleeding (Light)	+ Prolonged period > 10 days? (DUB, Anemia, Threatened Abortion)	
	+ Short cycle <21 days x 3 cycles? (DUB, pregnancy)	
	+ Age > 45, after 1 yr w/o bleeding (postmenopause)? (DUB, Endometrial Cancer)	
	+ After new Rx HRT x 6 mo? (Endometrial Cancer)	
	+ Breakthrough on BCP > 3 mo? (Breakthrough Bleeding)	
	+ Midcycle spotting, assoc, w abd. pain, dull low backache, regular period? (Mittelschmerz)	
	+ Painful periods, painful intercourse, dull backache? (Endometriosis, Fibroids)	
	+ > Vaginal bleeding + history of OTC meds? (Drug Side Effect)	
	+ Sporadic, postcoital? (Cervical/Vaginal Bleeding)	
Absence of period	+ x 3 consecutive mo + negative pregnancy test? (Pregnancy, TB, Post-TAB, Endocrine Disorders, Emotional Stress, Nutritional Disorders)	
	+ Fear of obesity, preoccupation w dieting/food, excessive exercising, wt. loss > 15% body mass, fine hair on body, cold intolerance, constipation, social isolation, depression, poor concentration? (Eating Disorder)	

Cross-References

Birth Control Options	Menopause Options	OB/GYN SI	Vaginal Problem: STI SI

VAGINAL BLEEDING (NONPREGNANT)
Supplemental Information

Quick Reference: ► Increased Vaginal Bleeding (All Salicylates)

► Menstrual Cramps

► Toxic Shock Syndrome

► Tutorial

See also: Directory of Hotlines/Web Sites for Support Groups, Appendix E

►   Increased Vaginal Bleeding (All Salicylates)

o Pepto Bismol

s ASA

® Motrin

►   Menstrual Cramps

® Signs and symptoms: Pain before and during period, low abdominal pain, dull/constant ache, may travel to back or legs.

® Cause: Contraction of uterine lining caused by chemical release in body; stress thought to make it worse.

® Complication: None.

• Tx:

—Motrin, Tylenol, Aleve

—Heating pad to abdomen 20-30 min prn

—Exercise: Stretching, walking, climbing stairs, and dancing

►   Toxic Shock Syndrome

e Toxic Shock Syndrome: Exact cause unknown. Rare but serious disease caused by *Staph* bacteria.

® Signs and symptoms:

—Nausea, vomiting, diarrhea (severe, intractable)

—Fever (38.9°C-40.5°C or 102°F -105°F)

—Sunburnlike rash

—Flu, muscle aches, weakness

—Headache, confusion, and disorientation

—Dizziness, fainting

—History of recent menses, postpartum, post-GYN surgery, barrier methods of birth control (diaphragm, cervical cap, and sponge)

® Complications: Shock, death

® Prevention:

—Wash hands before putting anything in vagina.

—Use sanitary pads instead of tampons.

—If you use tampons, never leave the tampon in for more than 8 hr or overnight.

—Use diaphragms, cervical caps, or sponges during menses with caution.

—Toxic shock syndrome may return with future periods.

▶ Tutorial

Red Flags

- Any abnormal bleeding, with or without sharp, progressive, unilateral pelvic pain, that radiates to shoulder, symptoms of lightheadedness or fainting and/or pallor.
- History of STIs (sexually transmitted infections), PID, any abdominal/tubal surgery, prior IUD use, spotting, or have missed a period for 3-6 wk, or painful intercourse.
- All women of childbearing years.
- History of ectopic pregnancy.
- Vaginal bleeding with associated abdominal pain needs to be evaluated carefully. The combination of symptoms is often an indicator of possible SAB or ectopic pregnancy.

Rules of Thumb

- Once an ectopic, always an ectopic.
- Any woman of childbearing age with abdominal pain and/or unusual bleeding is treated as an ectopic until proven otherwise.

Red Herrings

- Menopausal callers: Don't assume a female is in her postchildbearing years.
- No matter how reliable the form of contraception, always consider pregnancy (ectopic, early miscarriage).
- Postoperative pain unrelieved by prescribed medications should be evaluated further.
- Patients who have been "seen recently" may still need to be seen today.

Assessment Tips

Number of pads per hour:

- Severe = one large pad (saturated) per hour x 3 hr.
- Moderate = one pad every 2 hr.
- Light = one pad every 3-4 hr.
- Weight gain or loss affects period. Extreme weight loss can lead to < vaginal bleeding or complete absence of period.

VAGINAL PROBLEM (NONPREGNANT)
FB; Trauma; Discharge; Pain; Lesion; Itching; STI Exposure

ASSESSMENT	ACUITY LEVEL	DISPOSITION/ADVICE
Key Questions	**Emergent Symptom Patterns**	**ED 0 min-1 hr**
Laceration/Bleeding	Weak, dizzy, cold/mottled/or pale skin, blue lips/nail beds, rapid/shallow breathing, unresponsive, loss of consciousness? (Shock) (See Shock)	
Key Questions	**Urgent Symptom Patterns**	**ED/UCC/Office 1-8 hr**
Discharge (in School Age)	+ Foul-smelling, bloody/any color; pelvic pain, fever (> 38°C or 100.4°F)/chills, walks bent over, +/- Hx of STI exp., +/- 1UD User? (PID) (See Abdomen Problem 2; SI)	
	+ Any unusual? (*Trichomonas, Candida,* bacterial vaginosis, chlamydia, FB, atrophic vaginitis, carcinoma, gonorrhea, allergic vaginitis)	
Pain/Burning	+ Frequency, urgency ± blood-tinged urine, + nocturia, ± cloudy, foul or strong-smelling urine, ± fever? (UTI) (See Urinary Problem)	
Unsuccessful removal of FB?	+ tLost tampon, sponge, sexual ioysy ------ ----➤	Squat down; tilt hips forward; use longest finger to remove item
Key Questions	**Acute/Nonacute Symptom Patterns**	**FA8+ hr ± Home Tx**
Known STI Exposure	+ W or w/o symptoms? (± Sx)? (STI)	
"Lump" or "Ball"	+ ± Pain, on labia or vaginal opening? (Bartholin cyst)	
Itching	+ ± Lesions? (Condylomata, Flerpes, Yeast Infection, Atrophic Vaginitis, *Trichomonas,* Cancer)	
	+ W/o lesions? (Pruritus, Atrophic/Contact Dermatitis)	
	+ Hx poss. lice exposure? (Pubic Lice)	

(continued)

Key Questions	Acute/Nonacute Symptom Patterns		FA8+ hr ± Home Tx
Lesion (Any)	+ Asymptomatic? (Granuloma, Condylomata, Syphilis)		
	+ Hx of AIDS, chemo? (Immunosuppressed)		
	+ Cluster of tiny clear blisters, begins w tingling, itching, pain, followed by yellow, crusty crater after 1-2 days; w severe vaginal pain, difficulty urinating? (Herpes)		
Vaginal Pain	+ W intercourse? (Dyspareunia)		
Discharge	+ Hx of recent (2-3 wk) cryo or LEEP, profuse watery, foul-smelling (normal healing process from cryo or LEEP)? (See OB/GYN SI)		
	+ ± Slight odor, clear, profuse, assoc, w menstrual cycle changes; color + consistency changes w menstrual cycle? (Normal Vaginal Discharge)		

Cross-References			
Abdomen Problem	OB/GYN SI	Urinary Problem	Vaginal Problem: STI SI
	Penile/Scrotal/Testicle Problem	Vaginal Bleeding	

VAGINAL PROBLEM: SEXUALLY TRANSMITTED INFECTIONS
Supplemental Information

Quick Reference:
- ► AIDS/HIV
- ► *Chlamydia*
- ► Contact Dermatitis
- ► Genital Warts/Condyloma
- ► Gonorrhea
- ► Hepatitis
- ► Herpes

- ► PID
- ► Pubic Lice
- ► STIs
- ► Syphilis
- ► Urethritis
- ► Vaginitis

See also Directory of Hotlines/Web Sites for Support Groups, Appendix E.

► AIDS (Acquired Immune Deficiency Syndrome); HIV

    ® Definition: An infection by a virus that damages the body's ability to fight infections. Most at risk:

        —Gay, bisexual males, African-American females

        —IV drug users

        —People who have had blood transfusions

        —Sexual partners of above groups

        —Infant born to infected mother

    ° Signs and symptoms: Chronic fatigue, fever, chills, night sweats, sudden weight loss > 10 lb, unexplained swollen glands, pink/purple flat or raised blotches on or under skin, chronic diarrhea, persistent white spots in mouth, dry cough, shortness of breath. Incubation period: 2 wk-6 mo after contact: symptoms may not develop for 2-6 yr.

    ® Complications:

        —Persons w AIDS can become extremely ill because their immune system is damaged and cannot fight infections.

    ® Tx: There is no known cure for AIDS. There are some treatments that help.

    ® Prevention (See also STIs: Prevention below)

        —Avoid contact w all body fluids of anyone w AIDS or symptoms of AIDS.

        —Never share IV needles.

► *Chlamydia*

    • Definition: A bacterial infection in women that can cause cervicitis, urethritis, and PID. In men, may cause nongonococcal urethritis (NGU) or infection of the prostate and epididymis.

    • Signs and symptoms: Incubation period is 1-3 wk.

        —Women: Pelvic pain, painful or frequent urination, vaginal discharge, vaginal or vulvar pain, and/or bleeding after intercourse. Many women have no symptoms.

        —Men: Discharge from penis, painful urination. May have no symptoms.

    ® Complications:

        —Severe infection of the reproductive organs

        —Infertility (inability to have children)

—*Chlamydia* can be passed by mother to baby during childbirth.

—Can spread infection to sexual partner(s)

—Do not have sex w anyone w symptoms.

- Tx: antibiotics
- Prevention: (See STIs: Prevention below)

► **Contact Dermatitis**

- Tx Goal: Comfort. Prevention.
- Check for use of new products (e.g., soap, detergent).
- Use unscented pads, tampons, soaps.
- Do not douche or take bubble baths.

► **Genital Warts/Condyloma**

- Definition: Warts caused by a virus (human papillomavirus, HPV).
- Signs and symptoms: Small, painless, cauliflower-like bumps; may also be flat, skin-colored. May occur w itching, burning, or irritation. Incubation period is 1-6 months.

  —Female: Internal (vaginal) or external (vulvar). Inside the vagina where the woman might not notice them.

  —Male: External (penis, scrotum); internal (lining of the urethra).

- Complications:

  —Some types of HPV may lead to cervical cancer.

  —Warts may grow larger or spread to new areas and become harder to remove.

  —Cervical warts can lead to more serious problems.

  —Cervical or vaginal warts can be passed by mother to baby during childbirth.

- Tx: Warts can be removed by burning w chemicals/electric current/laser, freezing, or minor surgery.
- Prevention: Avoid skin-to-skin contact w genital warts (See also STIs: Prevention below).

► **Gonorrhea**

- Definition: Bacteria. In women, can infect cervix, urethra, uterus, and tubes. In men, can infect urethra, prostate, and epididymis.
- Signs and symptoms: Incubation period is 3-21 days.

  —Women: Pelvic pain, painful urination, vaginal discharge, or fever. Eight out of ten women w gonorrhea have no symptoms.

  —Men: Painful urination, drip, or discharge from penis. May have no symptoms.

- Complications:

  —Serious infection of reproductive organs.

  —Infertility (inability to have children).

  —Heart problems.

  —Skin disease.

  —Arthritis (joint problems).

  —Gonorrhea infection can be passed from mother to newborn during childbirth.

  —Can spread infection to sexual partner(s).

- Tx: Penicillin or stronger antibiotic.
- Prevention: See STIs: Prevention below.

► Hepatitis

(See Hepatitis SI, Appendix C.)

► Herpes

- Definition: An infection by a virus.
- Signs and symptoms: Painful blister(s) that break into open sore(s), usually on or near the mouth, sex organs, or rectum. May be found on woman's cervix (inside vagina) where she may not notice them. Incubation period is 2-20 days. Sores will dry up and disappear in 5-21 days.
- Complications:

  —The sores will heal on their own, but may return w illness or stress.

  —Herpes can be passed by mother to newborn during childbirth, causing serious illness or death.
- Tx: The virus stays in the body and can never be cured. Treatment w acyclovir (oral or topical) may help some symptoms. Comfort: (1) cold milk compress, (2) blow dry at cool setting, (3) zinc oxide.
- Prevention (See also STIs: Prevention below).

  —Do not have sex w anyone w symptoms.

  —Avoid direct contact w a herpes sore, or discharge from a sore.

  —Herpes is contagious a few days before a sore appears and for a week after the skin has healed.

  —Avoid foods w chemicals that sometimes cause outbreak: Nuts, coffee, caffeine, chocolate.

► PID (Pelvic Inflammatory Disease)

- Definition: An infection of the uterus, tubes, and pelvic organs. May be caused by gonorrhea, *Chlamydia*, or other STI.
- Signs and symptoms: Some women have mild or no symptoms. Pelvic pain, vaginal discharge: foul-smelling, bloody/any color; fever (> 38°C or 100.4°F)/chills, Hx of STI exp., IUD user w fever, joint pain, swelling, walks bent over. Sometimes months go by before PID develops.
- Complications:

  —Pelvic abscess (may require surgery)

  —Infertility (inability to have children)

  —Repeat episodes of PID

  —Chronic pelvic pain

  —Increased risk of tubal pregnancy
- Tx:

  —Pain: Tylenol, Motrin, Aleve

  —Antibiotics

  —Bedrest and "pelvic rest" (no sexual intercourse for a few weeks)
- Prevention:

  —Do not have sex w anyone w symptoms (See STIs: Prevention below).

  —For recurrent outbreaks take daily: Lysine, 1000 mg; zinc, 25 mg; Vitamin C, 2000 mg. Double dose during an outbreak.

► Pubic Lice

- Tx:

  —Use RID or R&C if not pregnant. Use per package instructions.

  —Wash all linen, clothes in hot water. Vacuum furniture, carpets. Put pillows in dryer x 20 min.

► **STIs (Sexually Transmitted Infections)**

- Definition: A group of infections that spread from one person to another through sexual contact. This includes any sexual contact that involves your mouth, sex organs, or anus.
- You can have an STI and not have any signs or symptoms. The only way to know is to have a test. The only way to be cured is to get antibiotics. Get tested regularly.
- Simple blood tests can diagnose it.
- STIs are related to having sex. The earlier STIs are found, the easier they are to cure.
- Most STIs can be cured completely if treated right away.
- If you have symptoms, get antibiotics as soon as possible. Otherwise, it could get worse.
- Tx is confidential.
- All people w whom you had sex recently must be tested and treated too.
- Signs and symptoms: If you are having sex, watch for these possible warning signs:

  —unusual discharge from vagina, penis, rectum

  —sores, bumps, swelling, or blisters near mouth, anus, vagina, or penis

  —painful urination

  —pain in abdomen

  —fever

- Prevention

  —Use condoms. When a man wears a condom during sex, it prevents the passing of infection from one person to another. It is about 90% effective.

  —Know your partner. If you notice that your partner has unusual symptoms (see Signs and symptoms above), *Don't have sex.* The more sexual partners you have, the greater your chances are of getting an infection.

  —Washing: Wash your vagina or penis and urinate right after having sex. It *may* help prevent infection.

► **Syphilis**

- Definition: An infection from a bacteria
- Signs and symptoms: Early stage: A painless sore on the mouth, sex organs, or anywhere on the body. Without Tx, the sore will go away by itself in a couple of weeks, but syphilis is still present. Many infected people do not notice the sores. Incubation period is 10-90 days.
- Complications

  —Second stage (6 wk-4 mo after contact): Sores, rash, fever, hair loss, body aches, sore throat, enlarged lymph nodes

  —Third stage (years later): Damage to heart, blood vessels, brain, eyes

  —Syphilis can be passed by mother to baby during childbirth. It may cause severe damage or death.

- Tx: Penicillin or stronger antibiotics
- Prevention (See also STIs: Prevention above)

  —Avoid sexual contact w someone who carries the organisms.

  —Avoid any contact w syphilis sore.

  —Monthly testing after Tx

► **Urethritis**

- Definition: An infection of the urethra due to gonorrhea, chlamydia, trichomonas, or other organisms. In men, urethritis w/o gonorrhea is called NGU (nongonococcal urethritis).
- Signs and symptoms: Gonorrhea incubation period is 3-21 days; NGU 1-4 wk.

—Women: Painful or frequent urination

—Men: Painful or frequent urination, drip or discharge from penis

® Complications

    —In men, infection of the reproductive organs

    —Infertility (inability to have children)

    ■—Can spread to sexual partner(s)

0 Tx: Usually two drugs are given to treat both organisms.

    —Ampicillin or similar antibiotic

    —Tetracycline or similar antibiotic

    —Antispasmodic: Pyridium

• Prevention: Do not have sex w anyone w symptoms (see STIs: Prevention above).

► Vaginitis

® Definition: Most common infections are yeast, trichomonas, and gardnerella.

0 Signs and symptoms: Change in vaginal discharge (more than usual, different color, bad or fishy odor), itching or burning in or near vagina, painful urination

• Complication: Extreme discomfort that will get worse. Can spread to sexual partner(s).

0 Tx: Depending on type of infection: Vaginal creams, tablets, douches, or oral antibiotic med (Rx or OTC)

® Prevention (See also STIs: Prevention above)

    —Do not have sex w anyone w symptoms.

    —Yeast infections can also occur in women who have not had sexual contact.

APPENDIX A
Home Treatment Supplemental Information

Listed below are common home remedies that must be approved in-house by medical staff.

Standards for home treatments: All home treatments must be approved foods, drinks, activities done at home by patient or caretaker.

1. Effective: Provide some relief from symptoms.
2. Harmless: No ill effect can come from using it as directed.
3. Accessible: Low cost, easily available to most clients.

Directory

Baking Soda Bath	Hot Pack	Rehydration Guidelines
Baking Soda Paste	Hot Soapy Soak	"RICE"
"BRAT" Diet	Ice Collar	Rice Water
Breast Cold Pack	Ice Massage	Saline Gargle/Mouthwash
Clear Liquids	Ice Pack	Saline Nose Drops
Clove Remedy	Increase Fluids	Sitz Bath
Cold/Cool Compress	Jell-O Water	Soft Diet
Cold Pack	Mint Tea	Steam Treatment
Cornstarch Bath	Motion Sickness Remedies	Tooth Transport
Cornstarch Paste	Nausea Remedies	Vinegar Douche
Elevate	Night Air	Warm Compress
Eyewash	Nose Pinch	Warm Soapy Soak
Gatorade	Oatmeal Bath	Warm (Tepid) Bath
Ginger Tea	Popsicle	
Honey-Lemon Mix	Pressure Points	

Home Treatment	Formula	Purpose
Baking Soda Bath	Add 7, cup baking soda to tub of warm water	Itching; skin irritation
Baking Soda Paste	A smooth paste of baking soda and water	Pain/itching; bee sting; insect bites; chickenpox lesions
"BRAT" Diet	Bananas (ripe), rice (white), applesauce, toast (white), and other foods easily digested	GI upset; diarrhea
Breast Cold Pack	Baggie of frozen vegetables, wrapped in thin dry cloth or pillowcase, placed on breasts after feedings for 10 minutes or less; cool cabbage leaves are effective as well	Breast engorgement
Clear Liquids	Drinks you can see through: water, soda, clear fruit juice, Gatorade, herb tea, chicken broth, boullion,)ell-0	GI upset; diarrhea
Clove Remedy	Place whole clove between gum and painful tooth	Toothache
Cold/Cool Compress	Cold, damp cloths, wrung out; change every 10 min	Swelling; discomfort
Cold Pack	Bags of frozen peas, corn, lima beans, wrapped in pillowcase, dish towel or soft cloth use cold pack for 10-20 minutes every 2-4 hr for 24 hr	Reduce swelling, muscle spasms and pain

(continued)

Home Treatment	Formula	Purpose
Cornstarch Bath	One handful of cornstarch added to tub of tepid water soak for about 15 min	Itching
Cornstarch Paste	A smooth paste made from cornstarch and water	Itching
Elevate	Raise above the level of the heart	Swelling/bleeding
Eyewash	Hold eye open put head under gentle lukewarm kitchen tap; or have someone pour lukewarm water gently in steady stream into eye X 20-30 min. Fill bowl w water, open eyes and put face into bowl x 5 min or gently flood eye w water for 15 min by the clock. Bring chemical to hospital for MD to see	Eye irritation; chemical/toxic burn
Gatorade	Drink Gatorade or similar drink drink slowly but frequently until urine becomes light, clear yellow	Dehydration, electrolyte replacement
Ginger Tea	Make a tea with ginger drink small amounts slowly until upset disappears	Nausea
Honey-Lemon Mix	Two parts honey to one part lemon juice; one part alcohol (brandy, rum, vodka, etc.) may be added if desired (check for Hx alcohol abuse). The honey soothes the throat and helps to bring up mucus; lemon juice helps to make mucus more watery and easier to cough up; alcohol reduces cough. This Rx may be taken by teaspoon as needed for cough	Cough
Hot Pack	Put cloths soaked in hot water and wrung out in plastic bag; place on swelling for 20 min on and off. Don't place directly on skin (use with caution for children under 18 yr or elderly, or use warm compress)	Swelling; muscle spasm
Hot Soapy Soak	Fill tub or bucket w hot water and enough liquid hand soap or liquid dish soap to make bubbles. Soak for 10-15 min 3 x per day in the morning, afternoon, and before you go to bed at night. For hands/fingers, wash dishes in hot soapy water 3 x a day the infection should get better after three soaks. (Use with caution for children under 18 yr or elderly, or use warm soapy soak)	Minor infections
Ice Collar	Put crushed ice in plastic bag, cover w towel, and drape across patient's neck. Wet dishtowel frozen around a large cylinder (e.g., can) also good. Reduces discomfort	Sore throat; swollen glands
Ice Massage	Wrap a cloth around a frozen juice can or put frozen juice can in a sock and roll the can over the muscle in spasm. Cold and massage help relieve muscle spasm	Muscle spasm
Ice Pack	Fill a Ziploc bag w crushed ice; wrap the bag in pillowcase, dishtowel, or soft cloth. Use the ice pack for 10-20 minutes every 2-4 hr for 24 hr	Swelling; muscle spasm, and pain (See also Cold Pack)

(continued)

Home Treatment	Formula	Purpose
Increase Fluids	Drink one glass of water each hr while awake, up to 6-8 glasses. Elderly patients or those w heart disease should drink one glass every 2 hr while awake	Dehydration/constipation
Jell-O Water	Mix hot water w Jell-0 to taste	Sore throat, cough
Mint Tea	Mint herbal tea; drink small amounts slowly until upset disappears	Nausea
Motion Sickness Remedies	Keep your head still. Avoid bad odors—engine fumes, cigarette smoke, and strong smelling foods. Avoid smoking. Avoid others who are getting sick. Travel at night. Sit in the front seat of the car or drive the car. Get fresh air—in car, open the window; on a plane, turn on overhead vent. Avoid alcohol. Avoid fatigue—it increases the chance of motion sickness. Always get enough sleep. Try acupressure wristbands (See also Nausea and Rehydration Guidelines)	Relieve nausea, prevent vomiting
Nausea Remedies	Rest in a quiet, cool room. Take ice chips or drink in small amounts: room temperature Jell-O or clear juice; e.g., soft drinks, 7-Up, ginger ale—fizzy or flat, whichever works best. Try warm, clear liquids like ginger, peppermint, or chamomile tea Try small amounts of soda crackers, white toast, plain pasta, or rice avoid spicy, greasy foods, caffeine (cola and coffee) (See also Rehydration Guidelines)	Relieve nausea
Night Air	Damp, cool night air	Croup cough, wheezing
Nose Pinch	Pinch soft part of nose x 5 min by the clock	Nosebleed
Oatmeal Bath	Fill thin cloth or toe of old nylon stocking w uncooked oatmeal (about 1 cup); tie it closed; allow it to float in bathtub of warm water. Bag of oatmeal can be cooked for ¹/₂ hr, then squeeze the bag in warm bath water to extract the gelatinous starch. Be careful, the tub may be slippery. Place bath towel in bottom of tub	Skin irritation, itching
Popsicle	Give popsicle to cut down on bleeding, pain, and act as a distraction	Cut lip
Pressure Points	Raise extremity above heart to < bleeding; Arm Wound: Apply pressure (firm and continuous) to pulse point inside the upper arm; use four fingers; Apply pressure firmly against bone until you can no longer feel pulse Leg Wound: Place victim on back and feel for pulse in groin area—at top of leg or where leg bends. Use the heel/palm of hand, keep arm straight, press artery against bone. If you need to, use both hands	To decrease bleeding

(continued)

Home Treatment	Formula	Purpose
Rehydration Guidelines	First 24 hr: Slowly give small amounts of the following: + Water, ice chips, popsicles, Gatorade, soda, diluted clear fruit juice + */2 to 1 cup every 30-60 min + Give more if person is able to hold it down. Slowly give larger amounts and more often as long as the person does not throw up. If the person vomits, allow to rest for 30 min and try again. When the person has not vomited x 8 hr, start "BRAT" and soft diet (See "BRAT" Diet; Soft Diet) After 24 hr w/o vomiting, begin solids. Do not take any dairy products (milk, cheese, ice cream, yogurt) for 24 hr. Use the "BRAT" diet x 24 hr (See "BRAT" diet) After 24 hours on above diet: After 2 days, begin slowly giving solids. If not tolerated, person needs to be evaluated	To prevent dehydration
"RICE" (Rest, Ice, Compression, Elevation)	Using several pillows, large blankets, or bolsters, raise arm or leg above the level of the heart. Remove any jewelry. Using RICE x 24 hr will reduce swelling and avoid further injury. Do not use the injured part or walk on it (See also Cold Pack; Ice Pack)	Reduce swelling/pain/injury of extremities
Rice Water	Boil white rice in water, drain off before absorbed	Diarrhea
Saline Gargle/ Mouthwash	Use '/4 teaspoon salt to one cup of water, warm or cool, whichever feels better	Sore throat
Saline Nose Drops	Use '/, teaspoon salt to one cup of warm water; use w a dropper prn nasal congestion; put in 3 gtts w nose dropper; wait 3 min and blow nose	Nasal congestion
Sitz Bath	A shallow, warm tub bath, 3 x or more per day x 20 min	Rectal irrigation; hemorrhoid, vaginal irrigation; vaginal lesion or boil
Soft Diet	Don't eat or drink anything that is very hot or very cold. First 12-24 hr: clear liquids (See Clear Liquids). After diarrhea stops x 2 days: white toast, crackers, nonsweetened cereals of rice or corn, bread (not whole grain), white rice, macaroni, potatoes, cooked yellow vegetables (squash or carrots), light-colored fruits (applesauce or bananas), and meats; soft-boiled/poached eggs, boiled chicken. For 3-4 days, avoid the following: milk, cheese, ice cream, yogurt, alcohol, coffee, caffeine drinks, diet soda, raw fruits and vegetables, fatty/very sweet/spicy foods	Diarrhea
Steam Treatment	Run hot shower w doors and windows closed; breathe steam for 20 min 3 x a day	Respiratory congestion or croup, cough, wheezing

(*continued*)

Home Treatment	Formula	Purpose
Tooth Transport	Hold tooth in mouth between gum and cheek during transport to MD, or place in glass of milk	Avulsed tooth
Vinegar Douche	Use 1 tbsp. of white vinegar to 1 qt. of tepid water in a douche bag	Yeast infection
Warm Compress	Soak cloths in warm water, wring out, and place on skin for 20 min on and off	Swelling; muscle spasm
Warm Soapy Soak	Fill tub or bucket w warm water and enough liquid hand soap or liquid dish soap to make bubbles. Soak for 10-15 min 3 x per day: in the morning, afternoon, and before you go to bed at night. For hands/fingers, wash dishes in warm soapy water 3 x a day; the infection should get better after three soaks	Minor infections
Warm (Tepid) Bath	Warm (not hot) water deep enough to cover patient's legs. Splash water on trunk. Get head wet. Do not submerge in water. Keep pt. in tub 20-30 min. The water will draw heat from body as it cools. Try not to make water so cool as to start pt. shivering. Make it comfortably warm	Fever

Position Statement of the Emergency Nurses Association

Access to Quality Healthcare

Description

The Affordable Care Act (ACA) constitutes the broadest change to American healthcare since the institution of Medicare in 1965.[1] The ACA has had the greatest impact on families and adults aged 18-64, while Medicare primarily (although not exclusively) affects adults 65 years old and older. As a result of the ACA, between January 2012 and March 2016, the number of uninsured American adults is estimated to have declined by between 43% and 48%.[2] As of February 2016, however, there were still between 20.8 and 26.5 million non-elderly uninsured adults, and 19 states had chosen not to expand Medicaid, the vehicle by which the ACA offers health insurance to the poor.[2,3,4]

Although the ACA has increased the number of individuals who have insurance, increased access to insurance does not necessarily correlate with increased access to quality healthcare. Many people continue to have high-deductible health plans (HDHPs) and limited networks from which to choose a primary care provider (PCP).[5] By April 2014, 85% of patients who had obtained private health insurance through the ACA marketplace had HDHPs, defined in 2015 as a minimum annual deductible of $1,300 for individuals and $2,600 for families (in 2016, out of pocket expenses were capped at $6,850 per person and $13,700 per family, per year).[6–8] Deductibles for employer-sponsored insurance rose three times faster than premiums, and seven times faster than wages and inflation combined, between 2010 and 2015,[10] and a 2015 survey found that 75% of insured patients who had problems paying their medical bills stated that it was because they could not afford copays, deductibles, or coinsurance.[11] Others have plans that include up to 50% coinsurance.[9] Medicare-insured patients also face difficulties paying for needed services and medications, whether because of fixed incomes (half of which were less than $23,500 in 2013), annual increases in premiums and deductibles, or difficulty affording medications.[59]

The consolidation of health insurance companies has contributed to this problem. Often touted as good for the consumer because increased market share means increased buying power and lower healthcare costs, consolidation has instead resulted in increased premiums and deductibles.[60] Furthermore, increased competition within the healthcare insurance industry has been associated with decreased costs for patients, but consolidation has resulted in exclusive, non-overlapping market territories and increased barriers to entry for smaller companies.[60] In 2014, private insurance premiums averaged $16,834 per family, and out of pocket spending averaged $800 per individual; the four largest insurance companies commanded approximately 83% of the market share (up from 74% in 2006), and the largest of them recorded $5.6 billion in profits.[60,61]

This problem of unaffordable healthcare is especially prevalent among those with chronic health conditions[12] and is often compounded by a lack of patient knowledge of helpful resources: 47% of those patients who had problems paying their medical bills were unaware of hospital-fee-reduction programs[13] and 37% of patients in another survey did not know that their insurance plan fully covered preventive care services.[14]

Access to quality hospital-based healthcare is impeded by emergency department (ED) overcrowding, which is associated with increased patient mortality, length of stay, cost, and an overall decreased access to timely treatment, regardless of insurance type.[15–17] EDs are a major gateway for hospital admissions and by law must provide care to all patients regardless of citizenship, legal status, or ability to pay.[2,18,19] As a result, EDs have become the healthcare system's safety net, treating the non-emergent and primary care needs of those who cannot access a PCP, while also being reimbursed poorly or not at all by Medicaid-insured and uninsured patients. The problem of overcrowded EDs is exacerbated by a shortage of PCPs[20,21] and a dearth of healthcare workers specifically trained to treat those patients with behavioral health problems who comprise 12.5% of ED visits, spend almost 3 times longer in the ED, and are 2.5 times more likely to be admitted than other patients.[22]

The greater the number of barriers to primary care access, the greater the ED utilization,[23] and Medicaid-insured patients continue to have more barriers and receive lower quality healthcare than privately insured patients. Contributing factors include:

1 Limited physician willingness to accept Medicaid insurance[23–25]
2 Discrimination against and stigmatization of Medicaid-insured patients by healthcare providers[26]
3 Medical and non-medical hurdles associated with lower socio-economic status[26]
4 Barriers to access to primary care and other outpatient services[23,27,49]
5 Significant mental and physical disease burden[26,49]
6 Other barriers specific to the Medicaid population[28]

The ACA has achieved much-needed reform of the U.S. healthcare system,[29] but more is needed. The current state of the U.S. national healthcare system, particularly the EDs, is not robust enough to meet the future needs of an aging population, growing racial and ethnic diversity, a mounting income gap, and increasing chronic health problems.

ENA Position

It is the position of the Emergency Nurses Association that:

1 All people, regardless of geographical locale or socio-economic status, need equal access to comprehensive healthcare services for critical, acute, and chronic medical conditions, including mental health and substance use disorders.

2   The definition of comprehensive healthcare includes preventive healthcare, wellness promotion, palliative and end-of-life care, and illness and injury prevention.

3   There is compelling evidence that gender, race, ethnicity, and socio-economic class are correlated with persistent and often increasing health disparities that impact and are impacted by diminished access to healthcare.

4   ED staff be knowledgeable about fee reduction programs offered by their facility so that they can refer their patients to support staff and resources that will help them to navigate payment for their care.

5   The use of EDs for primary care and for non-urgent needs can be decreased by expanding primary, preventive, and community healthcare services through a variety of proven strategies, including those listed at the end of this document.

6   Access to primary, preventive, and community healthcare services can be increased by allowing Advanced Practice Registered Nurses (APRNs) to practice to the full extent of their educational preparation, in addition to allowing them equitable reimbursement for services provided.

7   Primary care and non-urgent ED return visits can be reduced through the use of nurse navigators, case managers, and clinical social workers in the ED who assist patients in accessing preventative, primary care, and follow-up resources.

8   Emergency departments and hospital systems can implement evidence-based approaches that increase throughput and reduce patient wait times along with their associated adverse events.

9   Public education and social media initiatives can be implemented to increase public awareness of preventive, community, and primary care resources in an effort to reduce the impact of non-urgent needs on EDs.

10 Our understanding of the ACA's impact on access to quality healthcare is still evolving; therefore, a commitment to ongoing research and review of the ACA's impact on access is critical for the future of the healthcare system.

11 Health insurance companies, by virtue of the human object of their business, have an obligation to responsibly balance commercial profit with the thoughtful and innovative provision of affordable healthcare plans that promote wellness, prevention, and the management of chronic conditions.

Background

Over the past half century the utilization of EDs in the U.S. healthcare system has shifted from treating patients with emergent conditions to one of primarily providing care for non-emergent needs. The rate of ED visits over the past 15 years has outpaced population growth, increasing at double the expected rate between 1997 and 2007.[30–32] In addition, a retrospective study of more than 241,000 ED visits from 1997–2009 concluded that 70% were for primary-care-treatable conditions, [33] and the most recent data from the CDC's National Hospital Ambulatory Medical Care Survey found that 86% of ED visits in 2011 were triage levels 3, 4, or 5 (i.e., urgent, semi-urgent, or non-urgent).34 Patients without insurance accounted for more than 21 million of those visits, and only 11.9% of the total visits resulted in admission.[35]

These problems are worse in non-metropolitan areas, where there are lower odds that seriousness of the medical problem will be the reason for an ED visit. Indeed, non-metropolitan ED patients are almost twice as likely as metropolitan ED patients to indicate that the reason for their visit is that their doctor's office was not open.49 Perhaps unsurprisingly, multiple studies have found decreased rates of hospital admission from ED visits in rural and non-metropolitan areas, as compared to hospitals in metropolitan areas.34,53 These problems are often magnified by the budget and staffing challenges that many rural and community hospitals face, which impede the implementation of technological and specialized solutions.

The ACA was anticipated to provide solutions to these problems by increasing the number of patients with healthcare insurance, thereby allowing patients to have their non-emergent healthcare needs met by PCPs, while at the same time also providing insurance payment for those patients who still utilize the ED. However, many studies predicted that the ACA would likely cause a slight long-term decrease in ED visits, but would increase ED visits by up to 21% among some patient populations in the first three years after its implementation.7,41 A nationwide survey of emergency physicians concluded that ED visits were still on the rise as of March 2015.40

The majority of patients receiving new healthcare insurance under the ACA did so under Medicaid, and although multiple studies have shown an increased use of preventive care among Medicaid recipients,36,37 early studies also revealed that Medicaid patients visited EDs up to 46% more frequently than patients with other types of insurance or with no insurance at all.33,38,39 The most recent data from the CDC's National Health Interview Study, which looked at ED visits in 2013-2014, found that adults with Medicaid had the highest prevalence of both a single ED visit and multiple ED visits in the previous 12 months, when compared with patients with private insurance and patients without insurance, and almost four times the odds of having one or more ED visits in the previous 12 months when compared with privately insured adults.49

One of the ways that the ACA pays for itself is by offering tiered plans that trade lowered monthly premiums for cost-sharing approaches to payment.43 Such health plans and their high out-of-pocket costs are a burden for households with incomes between 100% and 250% of the Federal Poverty Limit (FPL), 80% of which do not have the assets to meet the high deductibles required by their healthcare plans.42 They are also a burden for households with incomes between 250% and 400% of the FPL, which do not benefit from the ACA's provisions for subsidized insurance.42 HDHPs are particularly prevalent in the private healthcare market, in part because this cost-sharing approach allows employers to reduce their portion of their employees' coverage. In 2013, 58% of companies with fewer than 200 workers offered insurance that had an average annual deductible of at least $1,000.43 Some studies have found that the ACA's elimination of out-of-pocket costs for preventative services has improved screening among patients with HDHPs;44 however, HDHPs also force patients to stop essential treatment,45 decrease the dosage of or cease taking prescribed medications to reduce costs,46 and schedule expensive diagnostic procedures late in the calendar year in order to minimize out-of-pocket costs.47 Many are simply unable to pay their medical bills.46

As mentioned above, the problem is compounded by insurance companies' established track record of decreasing competition through consolidation and driving down healthcare costs through the power of volume bargaining, while at the same time increasing premiums and deductibles rather than passing those savings on to the patient.60 The degree of consolidation within the healthcare industry can be appreciated by comparing it with the airline industry. In 2014 the market share of the top four insurance companies was 83%, while the market share of the top four airlines was only 62%.60 The consequences of HDHPs and insurance company consolidation for hospitals and providers include decreased reimbursement from insured patients who are nevertheless unable to pay their portion and increased acuity and number of comorbidities in patients who have avoided treatment to cut costs.

Some of the changes brought about by the ACA improved benefits to Medicare patients (e.g., closing the gap in Part D prescription drug coverage by 2020), but many patients with Medicare still struggle to pay for needed services and medications. In 2016, Part B premiums and deductibles for 16 million Americans rose by 16% and 13%, respectively, and both premiums and deductibles are projected to rise by up to 8% per year between 2016-2024.56,57 Perhaps more problematic, the Medicare system can be incredibly complex and difficult to navigate, and an inability to understand it can lead to poor decisions and lost healthcare access.58 The potential for insolvency of the program, increased eligibility age, and increasing numbers of eligible Americans constitute future potential barriers to access to quality healthcare that are yet to be solved.

The use of EDs for primary care and non-urgent needs can be decreased by expanding primary, preventive, and community healthcare services through a variety of proven strategies, including:

- Increasing access to local community health centers, neighborhood and specialty chronic disease clinics, and nurse-managed health clinics

- Expanding evidence-based community prevention and wellness programs

- Increasing the use of mobile integrated health and community paramedicine programs

- Increasing the use of advanced practice nurses and allowing them full practice authority in all states

- Eliminating barriers that prevent triaging of patients from the ED to primary care health facilities

- Collaborating with community-based programs to build and maintain a coordinated system of services that advance a continuum of quality care for patients with mental illnesses and substance use disorders

- Increasing the use of case managers and clinical social workers in the ED who can help patients access non-ED resources whenever possible[52,53]

EDs can also help combat the problem of overcrowding by adopting practices that more efficiently treat all patients, including those requiring specialized care,22 thereby improving ED patient flow.[48] .

Resources

Claxton, G., Cox, C., & Rae, M. (2015, February 1). *The cost of care with marketplace coverage*. The Henry J. Kaiser Family Foundation.

Emergency Nurses Association. (2013). *White paper: Care of the psychiatric patient in the emergency department.*

Emergency Nurses Association. (2014). *Topic brief: Care of behavioral health patients in the emergency department.*

Emergency Nurses Association. (2014). *Topic brief: Collaborative care of the older adult.*

Emergency Nurses Association. (2015). *Position statement: Emergency nursing interface with mobile integrated health (MIH) and community paramedicine (CP) programs.*

Gindi, R. M., Black, L. I., & Cohen, R. A. (2016). Reasons for emergency room use among U. S. adults aged 18-64: National Health Interview Study, 2013 and 2014. *National Health Statistics Reports*, 90, 1-15.

Health Insurance Industry Consolidation: What Do We Know From the Past, Is It Relevant in Light of the ACA, and What Should We Ask?: Hearings before the Committee on the Judiciary, Senate, 114th Cong. 1 (2015) (Testimony of Leemore S. Dafny).

Heisler, E. J., & Tyler, N. L. (2014). *Hospital-based emergency departments: Background and policy considerations*. Washington, DC: Congressional Research Service.

Medford-Davis, L. N., Eswaran, V., Shah, R. M., & Dark, C. (2015). The Patient Protection and Affordable Care Act's effect on emergency medicine: A synthesis of the data. *Annals of Emergency Medicine*, 66(5), 496–506. doi:10.1016/j.annemergmed.2015.04.007

Shenkin, B. N., & the American Academy of Pediatrics Committee on Child Health Financing, 2013–2014. (2014). Policy Statement: High-Deductible Health Plans. *Pediatrics* 133(5), e1461–1470.

U.S. Department of Health and Human Services, Centers for Disease Control and Prevention. (2016). *National Center for Health Statistics.*

U.S. Department of Health and Human Services, Centers for Disease Control and Prevention, National Center for Health Statistics. (2015). *Health insurance and access to care.*

References

1 The Affordable Care Act is made up of the Patient Protection and Affordable Care Act of 2010 (Pub. L. No. 111–148) and the Health Care and Education Reconciliation Act of 2010 (Pub. L. 111–152), retrieved from https://www.gpo.gov/fdsys/pkg/PLAW-111publ152/pdf/PLAW-111publ152.pdf and https://www.gpo.gov/fdsys/pkg/PLAW-111publ148/pdf/PLAW-111publ148.pdf

2 Uberoi, N., Finegold, K, & Gee, E. (2016, March 3). *ASPE issue brief: Health insurance coverage and the Affordable Care Act, 2010-2016.* Washington, DC: U. S. Department of Health and Human Services Office of the Assistant Secretary for Planning and Evaluation, Figure 4, p. 6. Retrieved from https://aspe.hhs.gov/sites/default/files/pdf/187551/ACA2010-2016.pdf

3 The Henry J. Kaiser Family Foundation. (2016, March 14). *Status of state action on the Medicaid expansion decision.* Retrieved from http://kff.org/health-reform/state-indicator/state-activity-around-expanding-medicaid-under-the-affordable-care-act/

4 Garfield, R., & Damico, A. (2016, January 21). *The coverage gap: Uninsured poor adults in states that do not expand Medicaid – An update.* Retrieved from the Henry J. Kaiser Family Foundation website: http://kff.org/health-reform/issue-brief/the-coverage-gap-uninsured-poor-adults-in-states-that-do-not-expand-medicaid-an-update/

5 Wharam, J. F., Zhang, F., Landon, B. E., Soumerai, S. B., & Ross-Degnan, D. (2013). Low-socioeconomic-status enrollees in high-deductible plans reduced high-severity emergency care. *Health Affairs*, 32(8), 1398-1406. doi:10.1377/hlthaff.2012.1426

6 Internal Revenue Service. (2015). *Publication 969.* Washington, DC: Author. Retrieved from https://www.irs.gov/publications/p969/ar02.html

7 Medford-Davis, L. N., Eswaran, V., Shah, R. M., & Dark, C. (2015). The Patient Protection and Affordable Care Act's effect on emergency medicine: A synthesis of the data. *Annals of Emergency Medicine*, 66(5), 496–506. doi:10.1016/j.annemergmed.2015.04.007

8 Department of Labor, Employee Benefits Security Administration. (2015). *FAQs about Affordable Care Act implementation (part XXVII).* Retrieved from http://www.dol.gov/ebsa/pdf/faq-aca27.pdf

9 Claxton, G., Cox, C., & Rae, M. (2015, February 11). *The cost of care with marketplace coverage.* Retrieved from The Henry J. Kaiser Family Foundation website: http://kff.org/health-costs/issue-brief/the-cost-of-care-with-marketplace-coverage/

10 Claxton, G., Rae, M., Long, M., Panchal, N., Damico, A., Kenward, K., & Whitmore, H. (2015). *Employer health benefits: 2015 annual survey.* Chicago, IL: The Henry J. Kaiser Family Foundation & the Health Research & Educational Trust. Retrieved from http://files.kff.org/attachment/report-2015-employer-health-benefits-survey

11   Hamel, L., Norton, M., Pollitz, K., Levitt, L., Claxton, G., & Brodie, M. (2016, January 5). *The burden of medical debt: Results from the Henry J. Kaiser Family Foundation/New York Times Medical Bills Survey. Section 2: The role of health insurance.* Retrieved from The Henry J. Kaiser Family Foundation website: http://kff.org/report-section/the-burden-of-medical-debt-section-2-the-role-of-health-insurance

12   Galbraith, A. A., Ross-Degnan, D., Soumerai, S. B., Rosenthal, M. B., Gay, C., & Lieu, T. A. (2011). Nearly half of families in high-deductible health plans whose members have chronic conditions face substantial financial burden. *Health Affairs*, 20(2), 322–331. doi:10.1377/hlthaff.2010.0584

13   Hamel, L., Norton, M., Pollitz, K., Levitt, L., Claxton, G., & Brodie, M. (2016, January 5). *The burden of medical debt: Results from the Kaiser Family Foundation/New York Times Medical Bills Survey. Section 4: Patients as consumers.* Retrieved from The Henry J. Kaiser Family Foundation website: http://kff.org/report-section/the-burden-of-medical-debt-section-4-patients-as-consumers

14   Collins, S. R., Gunja, M., Doty, M. M., & Beutel, S. (2015). *How high is America's health care cost burden? Findings from the Commonwealth Fund Health Care Affordability Tracking Survey, July–August 2015.* Washington, DC: The Commonwealth Fund. Retrieved from http://www.commonwealthfund.org/~/media/files/publications/issue-brief/2015/nov/1844_collins_how_high_is-americas_hlt_care_cost_burden_tb_v1.pdf

15   Singer A. J., Thode, H. C., Viccellio, P., & Pines, J. M. (2011). The association between length of emergency department boarding and mortality. *Academic Emergency Medicine*, 18(12), 1324–1329. doi:10.1111/j.1553-2712.2011.01236.x

16   Sun B. C., Hsia, R. Y., Weiss, R. E., Zingmond, D., Liang, L. J., Han, W. . . . Asch, S. M. (2013). Effect of emergency department crowding on outcomes of admitted patients. *Annals of Emergency Medicine*, 61(6), 605–611. doi:10.1016/j.annemergmed.2012.10.026

17   Liu, C., Srebotnjak, T., & Hsia, R. Y. (2014). California emergency department closures are associated with increased inpatient mortality at nearby hospitals. *Health Affairs*, 33(8), 1323–1329. doi:10.1377/hlthaff.2013.1203

18   Emergency Medical Treatment and Labor Act of 1986, Pub. L. 42 U.S.C. § 1395dd.

19   U.S. Department of Health and Human Services, Centers for Medicare and Medicaid Services (2003). 42 CFR Parts 413, 482, and 489: Medicare program; Clarifying policies related to the responsibilities of Medicare-participating hospitals in treating individuals with emergency medical conditions. *Federal Register*, 68(174). Retrieved from https://www.gpo.gov/fdsys/pkg/FR-2003-09-09/pdf/03-22594.pdf

20   Petterson, S. M., Liaw, W. R., Phillips, R. L., Rabin, D. L., Meyers, D. S., & Bazemore, A. W. (2012). Projecting US primary care physician workforce

needs: 2010–2025. *Annals of Family Medicine*, 10(6), 503–509. doi:10.1370/afm.1431

21 U.S. Department of Health and Human Services, Health Resources and Services Administration Bureau of Health Professions, National Center for Health Workforce Analysis. (2013). *Projecting the supply and demand for primary care practitioners through 2020*. Rockville, MD: U.S. Department of Health and Human Services. Retrieved from http://bhpr.hrsa.gov/healthworkforce/supplydemand/usworkforce/primaryc are/projectingprimarycare.pdf

22 Weiss, A. P., Chang, G., Rauch, S. L, Smallwood, J. A., Schechter, M., Kosowsky, J., . . . Orav, E. J. (2012). Patient- and practice-related determinants of emergency department length of stay for patients with psychiatric illness. *Annals of Emergency Medicine*, 60(2), 162–171.e5. doi:10.1016/j.annemergmed.2012.01.037

23 Cheung, P. T., Wiler, J. L., Lowe, R. A., & Ginde, A. A. (2012). National study of barriers to timely primary care and emergency department utilization among Medicaid beneficiaries. *Annals of Emergency Medicine*, 60(1), 4–10e2. doi:10.1016/j.annemergmed.2012.01.035

24 Geissler, K. H., Lubin, B., & Marzilli Ericson, K. M. (2016). Access is not enough: Characteristics of physicians who treat Medicaid patients. *Medical Care*, 54(4), 350–358. doi:10.1097/MLR.0000000000000488

25 Decker, S. L. (2012). In 2011 nearly one-third of physicians said that they would not accept new Medicaid patients, but rising fees may help. *Health Affairs*, 31(8), 1673–1679. doi:10.1377/hlthaff.2012.0294

26 Capp, R., Kelley, L., Ellis, P., Carmona, J., Lofton, A., Cobbs-Lomax, D., & D'Onofrio, G. (2016). Reasons for frequent emergency department use by Medicaid enrollees: A qualitative study. *Academic Emergency Medicine*, 23(4), 476–481. doi:10.1111/acem.12952

27 Capp, R., Rooks, S. P., Wiler, J. L., Zane, R. D., & Ginde, A. A. (2014). National study of health insurance type and reasons for emergency department use. *Journal of General Internal Medicine*, 29(4), 621–627. doi:10.1007/s11606-013-2734-4

28 Jiang, H. J., Boutwell, A. E., Maxwell, J., Bourgoin, A., Regenstein, M., & Andres, E. (2016). Understanding patient, provider, and system factors related to Medicaid readmissions. *The Joint Commission Journal on Quality and Patient Safety*, 42(3), 115–121.

29 Bernardi, B, & Wright, G. (2012, June 28). *Press release: ENA applauds Supreme Court decision upholding healthcare reform law*. Retrieved from the Emergency Nurses Association website: https://www.ena.org/about/media/PressReleases/2012/Pages/HealthCare Law.aspx

30 The Henry J. Kaiser Family Foundation. (2015). *Hospital emergency room visits per 1,000 population by ownership type*. Retrieved from http://kff.org/other/state-indicator/emergency-room-visits-by-ownership/#graph

31 Pitts, S. R., Pines, J. M., Handrigan, M. T., & Kellermann, A. L. (2012).

National trends in emergency department occupancy, 2001 to 2008: Effect of inpatient admissions versus emergency department practice intensity. *Annals of Emergency Medicine*, 60(6), 679–686. doi:10.1016/j.annemergmed.2012.05.014

32   Tang, N., Stein, J., Hsia, R. Y., Maselli, J. H., & Gonzales, R. (2010). Trends and characteristics of U.S. emergency department visits, 1997–2007. *Journal of the American Medical Association*, 304(6), 664-670. doi:10.1001/jama.2010.1112.

33   Pukurdpol, P., Wiler, J. L., Hsia, R. Y., & Ginde, A. A. (2014). Association of Medicare and Medicaid insurance with increasing primary care-treatable emergency department visits in the United States. *Academic Emergency Medicine*, 21(10), 1135–1142. doi:10.1111/acem.12490

34   U.S. Department of Health and Human Services, Centers for Disease Control and Prevention. (2014). *National Hospital Ambulatory Medical Care Survey: 2011 emergency department summary tables*. Retrieved from http://www.cdc.gov/nchs/data/ahcd/nhamcs_emergency/2011_ed_web_tables.pdf

35   U.S. Department of Health and Human Services, Centers for Disease Control and Prevention, National Center for Health Statistics. (2016). *Emergency department visits*. Retrieved from http://www.cdc.gov/nchs/fastats/emergency-department.htm

36   Kreider, A. R., French, B., Aysola, J., Saloner, B., Noonan, K. G., & Rubin, D. M. (2016). Quality of health insurance coverage and access to care for children in low-income families. *JAMA Pediatrics*, 170(1), 43–51. doi:10.1001/jamapediatrics.2015.3028

37   Baicker, K., Taubman, S. L., Allen, H. L., Bernstein, M., Gruber, J. H., Newhouse, J. P., . . . Finkelestein, A. N. (2013). The Oregon experiment — effects of Medicaid on clinical outcomes. *New England Journal of Medicine*, 368(18), 1713–1722. doi:10.1056/NEJMsa1212321

38   Taubman, S. L., Allen, H. L., Wright, B. J., Baicker, K., & Finkelstein, A. N. (2014). Medicaid increases emergency-department use: Evidence from Oregon's Health Insurance Experiment. *Science, 343*(6168), 263–268. doi:10.1126/science.1246183

39   DeLeire, T., Dague, L., Leininger, L., Voskuil, K., & Friedsam, D. (2013). Wisconsin experience indicates that expanding public insurance to low-income childless adults has health care impacts. *Health Affairs*, 32(6), 1037-1045. doi:10.1377/hlthaff.2012.1026

40   Marketing General Incorporated. (2015). 2015 *ACEP poll Affordable Care Act research results*. Retrieved from https://www.heartland.org/sites/default/files/2015acepacapollreportfinal1.pdf

41   Lo, N., Roby, D. H., Padilla, J., Chen, X, Salce, E. N., Pourat, N., & Kominski, G. F. (2014). *Increased service use following Medicaid expansion is mostly temporary: Evidence from California's Low Income Health Program*. Retrieved from the UCLA Center for Health Policy

Research website:
http://healthpolicy.ucla.edu/publications/Documents/PDF/2014/Demand_P
B_FINAL_10-8-14.pdf

42   Claxton, G., Rae, M., & Panchal, N. (2015, March 11). *Consumer assets and patient cost sharing*. Retrieved from The Henry J. Kaiser Family Foundation website: http://kff.org/health-costs/issue-brief/consumer-assets-and-patient-cost-sharing/

43   Oberlander, J. (2014). Between liberal aspirations and market forces: Obamacare's precarious balancing act. *Journal of Law, Medicine, & Ethics*, 42(4), 431–441. doi:10.1111/jlme.12166

44   Wharam, J. F., Zhang, F., Landon, B. E., LeCates, R., Soumerai, S., & Ross-Degnan, D. (2016). Colorectal cancer screening in a nationwide high-deductible health plan before and after the Affordable Care Act. *Medical Care*,54(5), 466–473. doi:10.1097/MLR.0000000000000521

45   Dusetzina, S. B., Winn, A. N., Abel, G. A., Huskamp, H. A., & Keating, N. L. (2014). Cost sharing and adherence to tyrosine kinase inhibitors for patients with chronic myeloid leukemia. *Journal of Clinical Oncology*, 32(4), 306–311.

46   Hamel, L., Norton, M., Pollitz, K., Levitt, L., Claxton, G., & Brodie, M. (2016, January 5). *The burden of medical debt: Results from the Kaiser Family Foundation/New York Times Medical Bills Survey* (Section 3: Consequences of medical bill problems). Retrieved from The Henry J. Kaiser Family Foundation website: http://kff.org/report-section/the-burden-of-medical-debt-section-3-consequences-of-medical-bill-problems/

47   Hunter, W. G., Zhang, C. Z., Hesson, A., Davis, J. K., Kirby, C., Williamson, L. D., Barnett, J. A., Ubel, P. A. (2016). What strategies do physicians and patients discuss to reduce out-of-pocket costs? Analysis of the cost-saving strategies in 1755 outpatient clinic visits. *Medical Decision Making*, 30, 1–11. doi:10.1177/0272989X15626384

48   Zocchi, M. S., McClelland, M. S., & Pines, J. M. (2015). Increasing throughput: Results from a 42-hospital collaborative to improve emergency department flow. *The Joint Commission Journal on Quality and Patient Safety*, 41(12), 532–541.

49   Gindi, R. M., Black, L. I., & Cohen, R. A. (2016). Reasons for emergency room use among U. S. adults aged 18-64: National Health Interview Study, 2013 and 2014. *National Health Statistics Reports*, 90, 1-15. Retrieved from http://www.cdc.gov/nchs/data/nhsr/nhsr090.pdf

50   Kippenbrock, T., Lo, W-J., Odell, E., & Buron, B. (2015). The Southern states: NPs made an impact in rural and healthcare shortage areas. *Journal of the American Association of Nurse Practitioners* 27, 707-713.

51   Institute of Medicine Committee on the Robert Wood Johnson Foundation Initiative on the Future of Nursing, at the Institute of Medicine. (2011). *The future of nursing: Leading change, advancing health*. Washington, D.C.: National Academies Press, Part II, Chapter 3. Retrieved from http://www.ncbi.nlm.nih.gov/books/NBK209871/

52   Kim, T., Mortensen, C., & Eldridge, B. (2015). Linking uninsured patients

treated in the emergency department to primary care shows some promise in Maryland. *Health Affairs, 34*(5), 796-804. doi: 10.1377/hlthaff.2014.1102

53   Pourat, N., Davis, A. C., Chen, X., Vrungos, S., & Kominski, G. F. (2015). In California, primary care continuity was associated with reduced emergency department use and fewer hospitalizations. *Health Affairs, 34*(7), 1113-1120.

54   Hines, A., Fraze, T., & Stocks, C. (2011). Emergency department visits in rural and non-rural community hospitals, 2008. *Healthcare Cost and Utilization Project (HCUP) Statistical Briefs #116*. Rockville, MD: Agency for Healthcare Policy and Research. Retrieved from http://www.hcup-us.ahrq.gov/reports/statbriefs/sb116.pdf

55   APRN Consensus Work Group & National Council of State Boards of Nursing APRN Advisory Committee. (2008). *Consensus model for APRN regulation: Licensure, accreditation, certification & education.* Chicago, IL: National Council of the State Boards of Nursing. Retrieved from https://www.ncsbn.org/Consensus_Model_for_APRN_Regulation_July_2008.pdf

56   Cubanski, J., & Neuman, T. (2015). *What's in store for Medicare's Part B premiums and deductible in 2016, and why?* Retrieved from The Henry J. Kaiser Family Foundation: http://kff.org/medicare/issue-brief/whats-in-store-for-medicares-part-b-premiums-and-deductible-in-2016-and-why/

57   The Henry J. Kaiser Family Foundation. (2016). *Total number of Medicare beneficiaries.* Retrieved from http://kff.org/medicare/state-indicator/total-medicare-beneficiaries/

58   The Henry J. Kaiser Family Foundation. (2012). *Seniors' knowledge and experience with Medicare's open enrollment period and choosing a plan: Key findings from the Kaiser Family Foundation 2012 National Survey of Seniors.* Retrieved from The Henry J. Kaiser Family Foundation website: http://kff.org/medicare/issue-brief/seniors-knowledge-and-experience-with-medicares-open/

59   Jacobsen, G., Swoope, C., & Neuman, T. (2015). *Income and assets of Medicare beneficiaries, 2014-2030.* Retrieved from The Henry J. Kaiser Family Foundation website: http://kff.org/medicare/issue-brief/income-and-assets-of-medicare-beneficiaries-2014-2030/

60   U.S. Senate. (2015). *Health insurance industry consolidation: What do we know from the past, is it relevant in light of the ACA, and what should we ask*: Hearings before the Committee on the Judiciary, Senate, 114th Cong. 1 (Testimony of Leemore S. Dafny). Retrieved from: http://www.judiciary.senate.gov/imo/media/doc/09-22-15%20Dafny%20Testimony%20Updated.pdf .

61   UnitedHealth Group. (2015, January 21). *UnitedHealth Group reports 2014 results, highlighted by strength in growth markets.* [Press release]. Retrieved from http://www.unitedhealthgroup.com/~/media/2B5EEC6F00F446AC9051674E259BA80B.ashx

Authors

Authored by
Justin Winger, PhD, MA, BA
Reviewed by the Position Statement Committee
E. Marie Wilson, MPA, RN, Chair
Katie Bush, MA, RN, CEN, SANE-A
Melanie Crowley, MSN, RN, CEN
Kathy Dolan, MSHA, RN, CEN, CPHRM
Ellen Encapera, RN, CEN
Elizabeth Stone, MSN, RN, CPEN
ENA 2016 Board of Directors Liaison
Sally Snow, BSN, RN, CPEN, FAEN
ENA Staff Liaisons
Dale Wallerich, MBA, BSN, RN

Developed: 2016.
Approved by the ENA Board of Directors: 1988.
Revised and Approved by the ENA Board of Directors: 1990.
Revised and Approved by the ENA Board of Directors: September 1992.
Revised and Approved by the ENA Board of Directors: September 1994.
Revised and Approved by the ENA Board of Directors: May 1996.
Revised and Approved by the ENA Board of Directors: July 1998.
Revised and Approved by the ENA Board of Directors: September 2000.
Revised and Approved by the ENA Board of Directors: September 2002.
Revised and Approved by the ENA Board of Directors: February 2006.
Revised and Approved by the ENA Board of Directors: December 2010.
Revised and Approved by the ENA Board of Directors: July 2016.
©Emergency Nurses Association, 2016.

Position Statement of the Emergency Nurses Association

Telephone Triage

Since the 1970's there has been an almost 400% increase in ED visits while the US population has increased by approximately 10% per decade.[3] Telephone triage, telephone advice counseling (Sabin) or telehealth nursing, as it is sometimes called today, became a popular method used by managed care and other private physician and health maintenance organization (HMO) groups in the 1970's to provide an entry into the healthcare system for an increasingly large number of patients.[1,2]

Today these formal commercial telephone triage programs function with specific physician-approved policies, protocols, staff education, patient documentation requirements, and quality improvement programs in order to function safely.[2,4-5] The chief advantage of telephone triage systems to the patient is timely access to a healthcare professional.[6] Successful systems of telephone triage have also been reported to make a positive difference in the appropriate use of the emergency department, patient satisfaction, and nurse/provider satisfaction.[7,8] By reducing unnecessary visits to a physician's office or an emergency department, the use of telephone triage may save time, patient costs and emotional trauma.[4,9] Although the goal of telephone triage is to provide the right level of care with the right provider at the right location at the right time there are challenges with the system.[6]

Identified concerns include: nurses, in spite of these protocols and decision-tree algorithms, may employ their own clinical judgment;[10] legal liability issues may put not only the nurse, but the physician and facility at risk of a lawsuit;[2] the inability to review the medical record or past medical history of the caller;[10] language barriers;[10] incomplete documentation issues;[10] lack of patient compliance and evaluating the appropriateness of decision-making algorithms.[6] When nurses were surveyed, they cited challenges assessing patients without visual cues and the demands of being the gatekeeper for large numbers of patients without a corresponding supply of available services.[11]

The Netherlands recently implemented a large scale, country-wide research intervention using the same five-level urgency markers for both physical and telephone triage in a primary care setting. Compliance to triage was good; safety was acceptable, however, as in other cases, further research is recommended to validate tool performance, compliance, decision-making and continued competence.[1,5,6,9]

ENA Position

It is the position of the Emergency Nurses Association that:

1 Emergency nurses do not give advice or clinical management recommendations over the telephone.
2 Formal commercial telephone triage nurses require specialized education; follow pre-established and physician-approved policies and protocols, complete patient documentation, and participate in quality improvement programs for safe and quality patient care.
3 Further research is recommended to determine if commercial telephone triage programs improve the use of available health services within the community.

Background

In 2010, the American College of Emergency Physicians (ACEP) and the Emergency Nurses Association (ENA) Joint Five-Level Triage Task Force approved a joint position statement stating "the quality of patient care benefits from implementing a standardized emergency department triage scale and acuity categorization process."[12] They went on to support the use of a reliable, valid five level triage scale such as the Emergency Severity Index (ESI)." Telephone triage is not addressed as a function of that process.

The Emergency Nursing Scope and Standards of Practice, Standard 1a Triage, approved and endorsed by the both the ENA and American Nurses Association (ANA), states, "the emergency registered nurse triages each health care consumer utilizing age, developmentally appropriate and culturally sensitive practices to care, prioritize and optimize health care consumer flow, expediting those health care consumers who require immediate care."[13, pg21] Telephone triage is not included within the scope of emergency nursing practice.

Giving advice over the phone outside of a formal telephone triage system can put the nurse, physician, and facility at risk.[2]

In a policy statement approved in 2013, ACEP recommends that "emergency department personnel not attempt medical assessment or management by telephone."[14] They further explain that callers with a mental health or limb- or life-threatening emergency are an exception and recommended they be instructed to access emergency medical services. As for patients recently discharged from the ED, ACEP recommends they be managed according to pre-determined protocols.[14] Emergency nurses are advised not to give advice or clinical management recommendations over the telephone.[10] However, if patients call with questions regarding ED discharge instructions and the chart is readily available, follow facility policy if clarifying instructions and notify the concerned patient to return to the emergency department, since the nurse may be liable for miscommunication.[10] Instruct patients to dial 911 in cases of a mental health, life or limb threatening emergency after determining if they need assistance to make the call. And as always, observe common courtesy and handle these matters in a respectful, caring manner.

Resources

Briggs, J.K. (2012) *Telephone Triage Protocols for Nurses (4th Edition)*.

Philadelphia, PA: Wolters Kluwer/Lippincott Williams & Wilkins.

References

1 Sabin, M. Telephone Triage Improves Demand Management Effectiveness. *Health Finance Management*. 1998;52(8):49-51. Retrieved from http://www.ncbi.nlm.nih.gov/pubmed/10182276

2 American College of Physicians–American Society of Internal Medicine: Telephone Triage. Philadelphia: American College of Physicians–American Society of Internal Medicine; 2000: White Paper. (Available from American College of Physicians–American Society of Internal Medicine, 190 N. Independence Mall West, Philadelphia, PA 19106.

3 Pines, J, Abualenain, J, Scott, J, Shesser, R. ed, *Emergency Care and the Pubic's Health*, Wiley Blackwell, 2014.

4 Dent, R.L. (2010). The effect of telephone nurse triage on the appropriate use of the emergency department. *Nursing Clinics of North America*. 45(1): 65-69.

5 Van Ierland, Y., van Veen, M., Huibers, L., Giesen, P. and Moll, H.A. (2011). Validity of telephone and physical triage in emergency care: The Netherlands Triage System. *Family Practice*. 28:334-341.

6 National Capital Poison Center. Retrieved from http://www.poison.org/about-us

7 Blank, L., Coster, J., O'Cathain, A., Knowles, E., Tosh, J., Turner, J., and Nicholl, J. (2012) The appropriateness of, and compliance with, telephone triage decisions: a systematic review and narrative synthesis. *Journal of Advanced Nursing*. 68(12): 2610-2621.

8 Bunn, F., Byrne, G., & Kendall, S. The effects of telephone consultation and triage on healthcare use and patient satisfaction: a systematic review. *The British Journal of General Practice*. 2005: 55(521): 956-961.

9 Hertz, A.& Schmitt, B. Decreasing ER Utilization with Nurse Telephone Triage and Establishing a National Network of Medical Call Centers. *American Academy of Pediatrics*. July 2011. Retrieved from http://www2.aap.org/sections/telecare/Decreasing%20ER%20Utilization%20with%20Nurse%20Telephone%20Tri.pdf

10 Huibers, L., Keizer, E., Geisen, P., Grol, R. and Wesing, M. (2012). Nurse telephone triage: good quality associated with appropriate decisions. *Family Practice*. 29:547-552.

11 Austin, S. Are you liable for telephone advice? *Nursing*. 2008;38:6-7. Retrieved from http://journals.lww.com/nursing/fulltext/2008/09001/are_you_liable_for_telephone_advice_.2.aspx

12 Purc-Stephenson, R.J. and Thrasher, C. (2010). Nurses' experiences with telephone triage and advice: A meta-ethnography. *Journal of Advanced Nursing*. 66(3): 482-494

13 American College of Physicians (ACEP) and Emergency Nurses Association (ENA) joint position statement on Standardized ED Triage Scale and Acuity Categorization. ENA. July 2010. Retrieved from

https://www.ena.org/SiteCollectionDocuments/Position%20Statements/ST ANDARDIZEDEDTRIAGESCALEANDACUITYCATEGORIZATION.pdf

14   Emergency Nurses Association. (2011). Emergency Nursing Scope and Standards of Practice. 1st edition. Des Plaines, IL.

15   ACEP Policy Statement "*Providing Telephone Advice from the Emergency Department.*" Retrieved from http://www.acep.org/Clinical---Practice-Management/Providing-Telephone-Advice-from-the-Emergency-Department/

Authors

Authored and Reviewed by the Position Statement Committee
Diane Gurney, MS, RN, CEN, FAEN, Chair
Katie Bush, MA, RN, CEN, SANE-A
Melanie Crowley, MSN, RN, CEN
Gordon Gillespie, PhD, DNP, RN, CEN, CPEN, CNE, PHCNS-BC, FAEN
Steven Jewell, BSN, RN
Robin Walsh, MS, BSN, RN
E. Marie Wilson, MPA, RN
ENA 2015 Board of Directors Liaison
Sally Snow, BSN, RN, CPEN, FAEN
ENA Staff Liaisons
Dale Wallerich, MBA, BSN, RN

Developed: 2015.
Approved by the ENA Board of Directors: April 1991.
Revised and Approved by the ENA Board of Directors: September 1992.
Revised and Approved by the ENA Board of Directors: September 1994.
Revised and Approved by the ENA Board of Directors: September 1996.
Revised and Approved by the ENA Board of Directors: September 1998.
Revised and Approved by the ENA Board of Directors: December 2001.
Revised and Approved by the ENA Board of Directors: July 2010.
Revised and Approved by the ENA Board of Directors: December, 2015.
©Emergency Nurses Association, 2015.

Telephone Triage of Elderly Populations

NOTE FROM THE AUTHOR: Some experts feel that the elderly, like pediatric populations, are different from healthy adult populations. While I agree that "the elderly are a different animal" from the healthy adult, the comparison stops there. We need to ask ourselves, are the symptom presentation and diseases (content of symptom complexes) of the elderly different enough, and yet sufficiently consistent (within the elderly group) to warrant creating a completely separate set of protocols?

While diseases such as Paget disease, decubitus ulcers, polymyalgia rheumatica, cataracts, prostatic carcinoma are common only in old age, disease presentation of other more acute illnesses is so variable that developing a classic picture for ordinary diseases would be nearly impossible. What is consistent is the constant challenge of how to accurately assess atypical, silent, or late presentation of symptoms, complicated by multiple chronic diseases and further compounded by communication difficulties.

In an effort to address this challenge, this section addresses problems and concerns specific to the elderly (chronic disease, depression, polypharmacy), with methodologies to facilitate communications and more sophisticated assessments on this population. Indeed, the elderly are "a different animal"—so unique in some ways, that no text can adequately capture the myriad possibilities of symptomatology. However, there are some general guideposts that will facilitate the process of assessing this most complex of client populations.

THE ELDERLY AND HEALTH CARE TRENDS

Recent studies indicate that we are living longer. Projections for the year 2020 indicate that 17% of the population will be made up of people over 55 years of age (Nobles-Knight 1995). However, longer lives do not always translate into healthier long lives. The elderly are a high-risk population. In the elderly, risks are commonly linked to decreased function of the immune system, increased accidents, and increased risk of fracture caused by osteoporosis. The elderly have more disease. According to one expert, 80% of persons over 65 years of age have at least one chronic illness and over 40% have multiple chronic diseases (Nobles-Knight 1995). The implications for telephone triage are that the volume and acuity of calls from this high-risk group will increase as this "demographic bulge" ages.

Several trends are projected which will impact the elderly in the near future. According to Finley (1995), there will be increased telephone triage—a major link between clients and health care providers. The major trend in health care away from the acute care setting to the ambulatory care setting will continue. As a result, there will be increased emphasis on drug therapy and ambulatory clients who are sicker, will be treated at home with drugs with less margin for error.

ELDERLY CLIENTS AND TELEPHONE TRIAGE: UTILIZATION PATTERNS

Studies of telephone triage demonstrate that the elderly have a high utilization pattern of telephone triage services. As a group, the elderly tend to use telephone triage more and for different reasons than other age groups. Telephone triage may be more valued by the elderly. One study found that nearly 30% of all calls were from callers over the age of 65 (Daugird & Spencer, 1989). The authors also found that the elderly call more frequently about chronic complaints and were more likely to be on long-term or psychotropic drugs.

In some cases, the phone serves as an irreplaceable, cost-effective "lifeline." According to one author (Guy 1995), for the elderly, travel by car or other means may be difficult or impossible because of their homebound status. The elderly seem to have more reasons to call: they actually have more health problems than younger patients. Because many elderly live on fixed incomes, they use "telephone visits" as a substitute for an office visit, to save money.

The elderly may even use the phone differently. More than any other group (with the possible exception of the inexperienced mother of a newborn), they use the phone for "hand holding" or reassurance. The elderly feel vulnerable and may fear abandonment following early discharge, for example. Old age is a period of heavy loss—loss of friends and spouse through death, retirement, and relinquishing home ownership and the loss of physical health. Because some elderly are isolated and lonely, they use the phone to simply make contact. For example, nurses relate the story of the elderly women who called the ED daily at 7:15 "to see if everything was okay" (Wheeler 1993). The nurses finally invited her to come for a visit and a cup of coffee. The motivation for such calls may be a way of "testing the system," reassurance or simple human contact—factors that reinforce the need for compassion and formal "warm lines" for this age group.

HEALTH RISKS OF THE ELDERLY

How much at risk are the elderly? The rapidly growing population of "frail" or "vulnerable elderly" are most at risk. Characteristics of this group include: Age > 75; suffering from multiple, chronic diseases; functional disability; psychosocial problems. Functional ability is the ability to carry out basic activities of daily living, eating, toiling, and walking, dressing, and bathing. Psychosocial problems may include risk factors such as poverty, living alone, and recent bereavement.

There are three categories of problems that differentiate the aged from healthy adult populations—chronic disease management, depression, and adverse drug reactions (ADRs). First, the elderly often have chronic diseases that need monitoring and management by phone. Second, the elderly are more prone to depression and suicide. In the elderly, depression may present as multiple physical complaints. White, retired males over the age of 65 have a suicide rate four times the national average (Osgood, 1985). Finally, and most important, the elderly are at risk for problems with ADRs—typically preceded by polypharmacy, defined as "the concurrent use of several different drugs (Fletcher, 1995). She goes on to point out several disturbing statistics:

1. While the elderly "comprise only 12% of the population, they take 25% of all prescriptions and 40% of all OTC drugs."
2. Three out of every five ED visits by the elderly are a result of ADRs.
3. 10.5% of all elderly hospital admissions are precipitated by medication problems.

Fletcher defines ADRs as "any unintended response to a drug that occurs at doses usually used for prophylaxis, diagnosis, or therapy of disease or for the modification of psychological function." Factors related to excessive drug use include:

1. Use of medications with no apparent indications
2. Drug duplication
3. Drug interaction
4. Contraindicated medications
5. Inappropriate dosage
6. Use of drugs to treat ADRs
7. Symptom improvement after medication discontinuation

Exactly why are the elderly so much at risk for ADRs? As a group, they have more disease——thus use more medications. They suffer from decreased functions: drugs are absorbed, distributed, metabolized, excreted, and affect target tissues differently. In general, they take more drugs and "the more drugs ingested, the greater the risk for ADR." For example, if two drugs are used, the risk is 6%; if five are taken, the risk is 50%; and if eight are taken, the risk is 100%. When assessing the patient, be alert to risk factors for ADRs: frail elderly, polypharmacy, polydisease, compliance problems, or inappropriate prescriptions (Fletcher, 1995). When assessing the patient's medication history, remain alert to the following categories of drugs— known to be the riskiest categories for ADRs:

- Analgesics
- Anticoagulants
- Cardiovascular
- Gastrointestinal
- Flypoglycemics
- Psychotropics (Fletcher 1995)

Drugs that require monitoring due to narrow therapeutic range:

- Antineoplastic preparations
- Ethosuximide
- Phenobarbital
- Phenytoin
- Primidone
- Theophylline
- Thyroid preparations
- Valproic acid (Fletcher, 1995)

SYMPTOM PRESENTATION IN THE ELDERLY

As with young children, symptoms in the elderly are often generalized or subtle rather than specific. If it is true that "ruling out urgency is more difficult than identifying it," this "rule of thumb" is especially true for the elderly client. In general, when acute illness arises, the healthy immune system usually sends out clear-cut, predictable signals of distress. In the aged, these messages become blunted, garbled, and nonspecific, requiring painstaking triage.

Typical symptom and disease presentations are derived from a medical model based on younger, healthy clients with well-functioning immune systems. According to Horan (1992), symptom presentation in the elderly may be atypical, silent, or late. Because they often have multiple diseases, they may present with multiple complaints but no chief complaint and are thus often atypical in presentation. In addition, deteriorating function of several systems make it very difficult to sort out symptoms, and concurrent disease in the lungs may lead to cardiovascular failure.

Silent presentation has been defined by Horan as "the absence of typical (or key) features." Thus, the elderly may present with painless MI (pain being a key symptom) or infection without fever (fever being a key symptom of infection). Horan defines late presentation of disease as a "tendency of disease to present in an advanced form." Thus, the elderly may quietly develop serious illness before being intercepted by a health care provider, making the task of the "first responder" the advice nurse, extremely difficult.

HEAT RELATED ILLNESS AND THE ELDERLY

The callers with elderly relatives or neighbors, advise them to avoid heat-related stress in the following ways:

- Visit older adults at risk at least twice a day when it is very hot
- Watch them for signs of heat exhaustion or heat stroke
- Bring elderly adults to air-conditioned places
- Make sure that the elderly have electric fans whenever possible

CHALLENGES IN ASSESSING THE ELDERLY CALLER

Common presenting symptom complexes found in most protocol content and descriptions are based on an adult model—not the elderly. Developing a model based on the elderly is not feasible because presenting symptoms in the elderly are often atypical and the possibilities are endless. Thus, the user must be judicious in the interpretation and matching of "common presenting symptom complexes" with patient's symptomatology. Rules of Thumb related to the elderly in Guidelines for Adult Populations in the User's Guide will facilitate assigning acuity. However, in large measure, the quality of the initial assessment may be the most critical element in determining the disposition.

This process will be facilitated through sophisticated use of the acronyms SAVED, SCHOLAR, PAMPER and ADL. These tools may be "fine tuned" to be more sensitive to the risks of the elderly. Sensitivity takes the form of "Red flags"—information that should stand out in the nurse's mind as possible indicators of acuity, if no explanation for presenting symptoms.

As mentioned before, SAVED (severe symptoms, age, veracity, emotional distress, debilitation/distance) is a "gross sort" tool, used to quickly identify high-risk callers. Since many elderly have nearly every risk factor (with the exception of severity), they should be triaged with care. For example, the frail elderly have many of the following characteristics: advanced age (age >75), unreliable, incomplete, confused communications (veracity); anxiety and depression (emotional distress); multiple diseases (debilitation); and inability to drive or be easily transported to the office or hospital (distance).

The SCHOLAR may not be as useful as with younger patients since the elderly caller may not present with major presenting symptom. Nevertheless, it is still useful to elicit standardized data about any "chief complaint," however subtle or generalized. In the case of the elderly, as with children, PAMPER and ADL may give a more accurate picture of the caller's history and current state of health compared to the normal.

Red Flags and PAMPER: Allergies, Medications, Previous Medical History and Emotional State, Recent Injury, Illness, Ingestion.

Medications: Always elicit a careful medication history, including OTC and prescription as well as alcohol and recreational drugs, remaining alert to the potential for ADRs. Common presenting symptoms such as confusion, hypotension and falls, anxiety, depression, insomnia, and constipation are often related to adverse drug reactions. Chemical restraints may include overmedication with prescription drugs, OTC or alcohol, leading to confusion and severe lethargy.

Previous medical history: Take note of histories of chronic or multiple diseases—a red flag associated with frailty and ADRs.

Injury: Falls and accidents are common in the elderly and may be more serious. The aged suffer fractures more easily because of osteoporosis. Be alert to the potential for elder abuse or neglect (See Abuse) when considering any trauma with a suspicious explanation. Remember that the elderly are more susceptible to heat and cold exposure.

Illness: Because the elderly may have depressed immune responses to infections, the presentation may be atypical. Look for subtle signs of infection rather than fever.

Ingestion/Emotional State: Depression in the elderly may take the form of multiple physical complaints. The elderly are not only more prone to suicide and the possibility of intentional ingestions but may also be victims of "chemical restraints"—a form of elder abuse (See Abuse).

Red Flags and ADL: In the absence of any chief complaint, the client's activities of daily living (ADL) might prove the most useful assessment tool—because it provides a picture of the client's current health as compared with his/her normal baseline. Because the elderly are at greater risk for dehydration, ADL is a good way to determine hydration status as well. Assess in detail the client's intake (food and fluids), output (urine, BM, emesis). Remain vigilant about major changes in the client's mood, color, and sleep pattern—a useful indicator of illness in the elderly.

COMMUNICATING WITH THE ELDERLY BY PHONE

As with the low literacy caller (see Appendix D), the elderly require simple, consistent, concrete, and conversational instruction and communications. In addition, since hearing impairment and aphasia of the caller may complicate the interaction and data gathering process, nurses should use the following guidelines (Guy 1995):

1. Allow enough time to receive, interpret, and respond to information.
2. Tune in to literacy level and cultural cues.
3. Let the patient know about communication problems during interaction.
4. Give positive feedback for communication efforts.
5. Elongate communications by using redundant and revised utterances.
6. Simplify by using short expressions as in Supplemental Information sections.
7. Use familiar terms and lay language.

Many health care providers find elderly callers to be "long-winded" or rambling when they call. One technique suggested by Guy, is to let the caller "tell their story" once in order to experience the relief of having the nurse "hear them out". Other ways to support the elderly include "warm" lines, support groups, visiting programs, and daycare.

The elderly present the greatest challenges to the telephone triage nurse, most of which can be overcome not by more detailed protocols, but by more sophisticated use of protocols and assessment tools and the therapeutic use of "self" in triage: patience, persistence, attention to unique "red flags," and adequate "talk time."

Telephone Triage of Low Literacy Populations

These guidelines were designed to address the informational needs of low literacy populations as well as college educated callers. Thus, the home treatment instructions and disease descriptions are written at the fifth- to eighth-grade literacy level. This step facilitates communications by "preprocessing the information, translating it into lay language at the most basic literacy level." This accomplishes two important functions: 1) Patients can quickly process the information, and 2) the nurse is spared those tasks, while she/he is performing the arduous intellectual task of critical thinking.

As a teaching and assessment tool, these protocols are designed to be user friendly. The true "end user" is the patient. For the caller with low literacy skills, questions and instructions must be clear, detailed and specific. Since the nurse often does not know when she/he is speaking to someone with low literacy skills, it is best to write instructions to the broadest possible literacy level—that of the fifth-grade reading level.

According to some experts, "23 million American adults may not be able to comprehend what health professionals are talking about." Communication is a complex process. While the low literacy client's listening comprehension may be better than reading comprehension, low literacy clients have special communication barriers. Common barriers to communication include: Patient overcompliance, anxiety, and masking.

Over-compliance is a common coping mechanism of low literacy clients. They tend to agree to whatever is asked of them, perhaps out of embarrassment. It is best to explore the situation further when clients seem overcompliant.

A second barrier is patient anxiety. Patients may have difficulty processing information when they are worried or anxious about not understanding. We can help reduce anxiety by establishing trust and showing warmth, and writing protocols in language, which is easily understandable.

A third barrier to comprehension is "masking." "Masking" occurs when the client is very concrete or misunderstands the meaning of a word, which has many meanings. We can help to overcome this barrier by realizing that sometimes low literacy clients are very concrete or literal. We can ask the caller to repeat back our instructions to clarify their understanding.

In order to achieve strong patient understanding and reliable compliance, we must link already known information with new ideas—creating a frame of reference. There are two ways to do this: One is to make a point as vivid as possible and to teach the smallest amount of information to do the job.

Methods to make information vivid include:
1. Writing at fourth or fifth grade reading level— avoid multisyllable words.
2. Using detailed, concrete, specific information.
3. Using a conversational style—short, precise, natural sounding sentences.
4. Using terminology consistently.

Teach the smallest amount possible to do the job. Organize information into chunks: "Advance organizers," tells the patient what you are about to tell them. Like explaining the "facts of life," don't overwhelm the listener with too much information or details. Think about what the client needs to know to "survive"—what, when, how and which complications to watch for. Finally, telling the caller "why" they are doing a certain treatment will help to get caller "buy in" and facilitate compliance. Examples of these can be found in the Supplemental Information Sections:

1. Signs/symptoms/cause
2. Possible complications
3. Prevention
4. Treatment goal (why) and activities

REFERENCES

Daugird, A. J., & Spencer, D. C. (1989). Characteristics of patients who highly utilize telephone medical care in a private practice. *The Journal of Family Practice, 27,* 420-421.

Finley, R. (1995). *Polypharmacy and the elderly.* Presented at the Contemporary Forums Conference, Telephone Triage: Essential for Expert Practice, Dublin, CA.

Fletcher, K. (1995). *Polypharmacy in the elderly.* Presented at the Contemporary Forums Conference, Telephone Triage: Essential for Expert Practice, Dublin, CA.

Guy, D. H. (1995). Telephone care for elders. *Journal of Gerontological Nursing, 12,* 27-34.

Nobles-Knight, D. (1995). *Polypharmacy in the elderly.* Lecture presented at the Contemporary Forums Conference, Telephone Triage: Essential for Expert Practice, Dublin, CA.

Osgood, N. J. (1985). *Suicide in the elderly.* Richmond, VA: Aspen.

Wheeler, S. Q. (1993). *Telephone triage: Theory, practice and protocol development.* Albany, NY: Delmar.

APPENDIX C
Miscellaneous Supplemental Information

BIOTERRORISM INFORMATION

PLEASE NOTE: It is advisable to establish a policy related to bioterrorism calls. Calls that arouse suspicions must be treated as emergent or urgent. Nurses should *always contact 911 first* to arrange for paramedic transport. In cases where there is suspicion of biochemical exposure, contact or transfer the call to 911 and Hazardous Materials teams to manage the call. Generally speaking, EMDs are more expert and have better access to resources than nurses do.

The telephone triage nurse may unwittingly be thrust into the role of first responder to initial or ongoing outbreaks of bioterrorism-related illness. The term "first responder" refers to the nurse's role in *identifying* suspicious-sounding symptoms. The nurse should use this information any time there are unusual symptom presentations or patterns. Assess all suspicious symptoms described by callers who may have, *unknowingly*, been exposed to biological or chemical weapons.

The list below was developed by the CDC and further adapted and modified for telephone triage nurse use. The Global pattern of biological or chemical terrorism is as follows:

- ® Symptoms: Sudden onset
- Patients: In large numbers
- ® Patients: Not normally affected (i.e., young, previously healthy adults and children)
- Patient presentation: Acutely ill
- Patient presentation: Rapid disease progression, i.e., from upper respiratory symptoms and bronchitis to life-threatening pneumonia and systemic infections

BIOTERRORISM RED FLAGS

Review the Red Flags below frequently and remain alert for the following patterns, which may be indicators of bioterrorist events:

- » Large numbers of ill persons calling with similar disease or syndrome
- Large numbers of unexplained disease, syndromes, or deaths
- Unusual increases in illness in a population (e.g., an increase in influenza-like illness that might be anthrax in disguise or an increase in poxlike illness that might be smallpox)
- Atypical geographic or seasonal distribution of a disease (e.g., Tularemia in a nonendemic area, influenza in the summer)
- Atypical patient distribution (e.g., several adults with unexplained rash, previously healthy populations)
- 111 persons presenting near the same time (unusual surges in call volumes)
- Reports of death or illness among animals, which may be unexplained or attributed to a bioterrorist agent, that precedes or accompanies illness or death in humans
- Unusual disease presentation (e.g., pulmonary versus cutaneous anthrax)
- Unexplained increase in incidence in endemic disease (e.g., Tularemia, plague)
- Simultaneous clusters of similar illness in noncontiguous areas (neither adjacent nor bordering), domestic or foreign disease transmitted through aerosols, food, or water suggestive of sabotage

In the case of confirmed bioterrorism diagnoses, EDs must inform the State Health Department, CDC, and FBI. For the latest information, refer to CDC Web site at www.bt.cdc.gov.

Herbal Supplements Associated with Illnesses and Injuries

Quick Reference: Frequently Asked Questions   Further Information

Risk Factors for   Herbal Ingredients

Supplemental Use   Vitamins and Essential

How to Decide to   Minerals

Use Supplements   Other Supplements

How to Identify Fraud   Federal Agencies

How to Identify High-Quality   Health Professional

Products   Organizations

Reporting Side Effects

FREQUENTLY ASKED QUESTIONS

Who Should Not Use Supplements?

- Before starting a dietary supplement, check with your doctor. This is extremely important for people who
  —Are pregnant or breastfeeding.
  —Have chronic illness like HIV, heart problems, high blood pressure, diabetes.
  —Are over the age of 50 or under the age of 18.
  —Are taking any prescription or over-the-counter medicines. Certain supplements can raise blood levels of certain drugs to dangerous levels.
- For example, garlic and the supplement ginkgo biloba both thin the blood, which can be dangerous for people taking prescription medicines that also thin the blood.

Who Can Help Me Make Decisions?

- In addition to medical doctors, other health care professionals, such as registered pharmacists, registered dietitians and nutritionists, also can be sources of information about dietary supplements.

How Can I Tell if a Product Is Fraudulent?

- Fraudulent products are products that don't do what they say they can or don't contain what they say they contain. They waste consumers' money, and they may cause physical harm. You can tell which ones are fraudulent products by the types of claims made on labels and in advertising. Some possible signs of fraud are
  —Words like "secret cure," "breakthrough," "magical," "miracle cure," and "new discovery." If the product were a cure for a serious disease, it would be widely reported in the media and used by health care professionals.
  —Medical sounding words such as "detoxify," "purify," and "energize" to describe the way the product works. These claims are vague and hard to measure. So, they make it easier for the product makers to claim success, even though nothing has actually been accomplished.
  —Claims that the product can cure a lot of different diseases. No product can do that.
  —Claims that a product is backed by scientific studies that have no list of references (medical studies). In some cases, the references are incomplete, the citations cannot be traced, or if they are traceable, the studies are out-of-date, irrelevant, or poorly developed.
  —Claims that the supplement has only benefits—and no side effects. A product strong enough to help people will be strong enough to cause side effects.
  —Claims that the medical profession, drug companies, and the government are stopping information about it.
- Though it may be hard, consumers also can protect themselves from economic fraud. Economic fraud is the act of using inferior, cheaper ingredients and then passing it off as the real thing but at a lower cost. Avoid products sold for considerably less money than competing brands. If it's too cheap, the product is probably not what it's supposed to be.

How Can I Know if a Product Is High Quality?

- Poor manufacturing practices are not unique to dietary supplements, but the growing market for supplements in a less restrictive regulatory environment creates the potential for supplements to be prone to quality-control problems. For example, the FDA has identified several problems where some manufacturers were buying herbs, plants, and other ingredients without first adequately testing them to determine whether the product they ordered was actually what they received or whether the ingredients were free from contaminants. To help protect themselves, consumers should note the following:

—Look for ingredients in products with the U.S. Pharmacopoeia notation, which indicates the manufacturer followed standards established by the U.S. Pharmacopoeia.

—Realize that the label term "natural" doesn't guarantee that a product is safe. "Think of poisonous mushrooms," says one expert, "They're natural."

—Consider the name of the manufacturer or distributor. Supplements made by a nationally known food and drug manufacturer, for example, have likely been made under tight controls because these companies already have in place manufacturing standards for their other products.

—Write to the supplement manufacturer for more information. Ask the company about the conditions under which its products were made.

What Should I Do if I Have Side Effects?

• Consumers who use dietary supplements should always read product labels, follow directions, and heed all warnings. Supplement users who suffer a serious harmful effect or illness that they think is related to supplement use should call a doctor or other health care provider. He or she in turn can report it to FDA MedWatch by calling 1-800-FDA-1088 or going to http://www.fda.gov/medwatch/ report/hcp.htm on the MedWatch Web site. Patients' names are kept confidential.

• Consumers also may call the toll-free MedWatch number or go to http://www.fda.gov/medwatch/ report/consumer/consumer.htm on the MedWatch Web site to report an adverse reaction. To file a report, consumers will be asked to provide

—Name, address, and telephone number of the person who became ill.

—Name and address of the doctor or hospital providing medical treatment.

—Description of the problem.

—Name of the product and store where it was bought.

• Consumers also should report the problem to the manufacturer or distributor listed on the product's label and to the store where the product was bought.

How Do I Get More Information?

The list of herbal supplements below is based on the 1998 list issued by the Food and Drug Administration Web site. For the most up-to-date information, visit http://www.fda.gov.

HERBAL INGREDIENTS

• Chaparral (a traditional American Indian medicine). Possible health hazards: Liver disease, possibly irreversible.

• Comfrey. Possible health hazards: Obstruction of blood flow to liver, possibly leading to death.

• Slimming/dieter's teas. Possible health hazards: Nausea, diarrhea, vomiting, stomach cramps, chronic constipation, fainting, possibly death (See Dieter's Brews Make Tea Time a Dangerous Affair in the July-August 1997 *FDA Consumer*).

• Ephedra (also known as Ma huang, Chinese Ephedra, and epitonin). Possible health hazards: Ranges from high blood pressure, irregular heartbeat, nerve damage, injury, insomnia, tremors, and headaches to seizures, heart attack, stroke, and death.

• Germander. Possible health hazards: Liver disease, possibly leading to death.

• Lobelia (also known as Indian tobacco). Possible health hazards: Ranges from breathing problems at low doses to sweating, rapid heartbeat, low blood pressure, and possibly coma and death at higher doses.

• Magnolia-Stephania preparation. Possible health hazards: Kidney disease, possibly leading to permanent kidney failure.

• Willow bark. Possible health hazards: Reye syndrome, a potentially fatal disease associated with aspirin intake in children with chickenpox or flu symptoms; allergic reaction in adults. (Willow bark is marketed as an aspirin-free product, although it actually contains an ingredient that converts to the same active ingredient in aspirin.)

• Wormwood. Possible health hazards: Neurological symptoms, characterized by numbness of legs and arms, loss of intellect, delirium, and paralysis.

VITAMINS AND ESSENTIAL MINERALS

• Vitamin A (in doses of 25,000 or more International Units a day). Possible health hazards: Birth defects, bone abnormalities, and severe liver disease.

• Vitamin B_6 (in doses above 100 mg a day). Possible health hazards: Balance difficulties, nerve injury causing changes in touch sensation.

- Niacin (in slow-released doses of 500 mg or more a day or immediate-release doses of 750 mg or more a day). Possible health hazards: Range from stomach pain, vomiting, bloating, nausea, cramping, and diarrhea to liver disease, muscle disease, eye damage, and heart injury.
- Selenium (in doses of about 800 meg to 1000 meg a day). Possible health hazards: Tissue damage.

OTHER SUPPLEMENTS

- Germanium (a nonessential mineral). Possible health hazards: Kidney damage, possibly death.
- L-tryptophan (an amino acid). Possible health hazards: Eosinophilia myalgia syndrome, a potentially fatal blood disorder that can cause high fever, muscle and joint pain, weakness, skin rash, and swelling of the arms and legs.

FEDERAL AGENCIES

Food and Drug Administration

Food Information Line
1-888-723-3366
(202)205-4314 in the Washington, D.C., area
FDA Web site: http://www.cfsan.fda.gov/dms/
supplmnt.html. Accessed 8/2008.

HEALTH PROFESSIONAL ORGANIZATIONS

You're Free to Reproduce the Information on the FDA Web Site

Unless otherwise noted, the contents of the FDA Web site (http://www.fda.gov), both text and graphics, are *not* copyrighted. They are in the public domain and may be republished, reprinted, and otherwise used freely by anyone without the need to obtain permission from FDA. Credit to the U.S. Food and Drug Administration as the source is appreciated but not required. The *FDA also appreciate being informed about use of materials.* Contact FDA, HFI-40, Rockville, MD 20857 or E-mail: webmail@oc.fda.

APPENDIX E
TELEPHONE TRIAGE STANDARDS MANUAL

OVERVIEW OF TELEPHONE TRIAGE STANDARDS

A major goal of the Telephone Triage service is to optimize safe, timely access for patients and reduce decision error by the following means:

- Hire high quality RNs.
- Provide excellent training.
- Provide excellent protocols and documentation forms.
- Provide adequate staff (60 calls/8hr/RN).
- Provide feedback mechanism where possible.
- Provide for rotation of phone work and frequent breaks where possible.
- Support the reasonable, prudent approach where possible.

Secondarily, a goal for Telephone Triage services is to include the client population as part of the solution. Clients will not use services that they know nothing about. Therefore, it is reasonable to support the pretriage of calls through the mechanism of a patient brochure, which fosters patient independence and provides for a partnership which supports appropriate, timely access.

Overall management of the service is the responsibility of the program coordinator under the direction of the director of Ambulatory Care Services with the direction and support of upper management. Medical staff and associated departments will collaborate quarterly through Steering Committee meetings.

LINE MANAGEMENT

- The telephone triage program coordinator (PC) is a practitioner with appropriate clinical and managerial experience and/or the potential for it. The PC is selected by Ambulatory Care Administration to assume responsibility for the effective functioning of staff, including collaborating with clinic managers on their development and evaluation. The PC is responsible for the efficient functioning of telephone triage and the quality of telephone triage provided in this setting.
- The clinic manager assigns a shift coordinator to oversee the 8 (10 or 12) hr shift in order to facilitate service communication, coordination, and delivery of patient care.
- Nursing standards will be reviewed and updated annually by the Steering Committee. After approval from nursing and medical administration, these standards will outline additional nursing functions and responsibilities within telephone triage.

MEDICAL ADMINISTRATION

- The chiefs of the various medical, surgical, and special services shall be available to the PC, clinic managers, and shift coordinators for the purpose of resolving conflicts and/or providing medical direction in the case of unavailability of a primary care physician.
- The director of Ambulatory Care Services shall be available to the PC and clinic managers regarding nurse-physician communications, adequacy of direction provided to the nursing staff, and general working relationships.

STEERING COMMITTEE

This committee is an ad hoc group consisting of representatives from Poison Control, Medicine, Emergency Department, Education and Professional Development, Marketing Ambulatory Care Administration, and Nursing Staff and Management. This committee meets quarterly to discuss matters related to the Telephone Triage Program. The Director of Ambulatory Care Services selects members.

HOURS OF OPERATION

Telephone Triage is a telephone management system, which provides adult triage during clinic hours and after hours (all day, year round).

USE OF TELEPHONE TRIAGE SERVICES

Criteria

- All callers are considered clients for Telephone Triage services, whether they are experiencing acute, or potentially acute illness or injury in single or multiple body systems, or are seeking education, information, counseling, advocacy or referral.
- Telephone recordings will be available in three languages, notifying clients that they are on hold and will be helped soon. Callers will be advised to call 911 for life-threatening emergencies and to call Poison Control for poisoning information and assistance.
- Other client populations served include
  —Clients seeking medical advice and education for home treatment.
  —Clients seeking health-related information including hospital approved written reference materials, community resources, and hotlines.

—Clients seeking referrals, i.e., physician, pharmacist, community resource, support groups, hotlines, hospital services, and in-house self-care and self-help programs.

—Clients seeking emotional support and counseling.

—Clients seeking information and support as health consumer or self-advocate (patients' rights, second opinions, living wills, etc.)

Limitations

- Telephone Triage is not designed as a message-answering service for physicians.
- Telephone Triage will not fill prescriptions at client request.
- AIDS related questions would be referred directly to the AIDS hotline.
- Drug-related questions will be referred directly to the pharmacist.
- Poison related questions will be transferred directly to Poison Control.
- Crisis level calls will be managed per the appropriate crisis intervention protocol.

Demand for Information/Service Beyond Capacity (Call Volume)

- The capacity of Telephone Triage is 60 calls per 8 hr per practitioner (7 calls/hr). When call volume is in excess of budgeted daily call volume, it is the responsibility of the shift coordinator to notify the clinic manager for staffing consideration.
- Nursing staff (shift coordinator) will collaborate as needed with clinic manager to validate call acuity, volume, and peak volume times, including
  —"Flu season"
  —Weekends, Holidays
  —Peak hours
  —Disaster

Call Duration (Talk Time)

- General guidelines. Client and problem acuity and need for emotional/informational support determines the amount of time spent on each call.
- Average duration of call. The *average duration* of call is 8.5 min. Generally, this time period allows for safe, effective interactions for all populations, including elderly, high risk, low income, and multicultural populations.
- Timely disposition. All available resources will be used to facilitate timely disposition of all calls, i.e., crisis intervention, referral, informational, educational, and counseling.

- Chronic callers. Chronic callers shall be noted by shift coordinators and referred to Department of Social Services or Public Health Nurses as necessary.

Disposition

- Information. All disposition information will be documented.
- Disposition (When, where, and by whom client will be seen/treated). Clients will be classified according to one or more of the following criteria:
  —Emergent ("Immediate"—0 min—1 hr)
  —Urgent (1 hr—8 hr)
  —Acute (8—24 hours)
  —Nonacute/Appt (24+ hr)
  —Advice

GOVERNING RULES OF AREA

General Safety

- Traffic/visitor control. Telephone Triage is not to be used by hospital personnel as a thoroughfare. Traffic is limited to physicians and staff conducting the business of client service.
- Students. The management staff of Telephone Triage will adhere to the Department of Nursing Policy regarding institutional affiliation as well as specific role of nursing students as described in Addendum B.

Confidentiality and HIPAA

- Client information. All client information is highly confidential and is protected by the Health Insurance Portability and Accountability Act of 1996 (HIPAA) and Hospital Patient Bill of Rights.
- Discussion of client information in areas of public traffic is a violation of hospital policy and is considered a major disciplinary offense.
- Client records are to be in the hands of the appropriate employee at all times. Clients requesting to see own records may do so in the presence of medial record staff.
- Media request for information. Telephone Triage staff may not give out information by phone to any media representative unless prior arrangements have been made with administration (See Hospital Policy on Confidentiality).
- Duplication of client records. No client record may be copied except that which is for transfer or educational activity (See Hospital Policy on Client Records).
- Regulations governing AIDS testing: Knows and adheres to current AIDS confidentiality laws.

STAFFING

Quantity

- Staffing. Telephone Triage is staffed with sufficient number of professional personnel to provide established minutes of nursing care to an average daily call volume as outlined in the annual budget. Staffing will always provide for no less than 75% regular service staff.
- Acuity levels. Changing acuity levels and/or increased call volume demanding increased nursing coverage shall be met via intervention of the shift coordinator and/or PC. Additional staff is provided via (1) approved overtime by full-time employees (double shifts), (2) additional hours by part-time employees, and (3) use of per diem ambulatory care float personnel. Appropriate records of staff utilization are maintained by the service.
- The program manager/clinic manager in cooperation with the shift coordinator makes staffing adjustments.
- Regular scheduling. The clinic manager defines and has responsibility for adhering to the Telephone Triage staffing pattern. This pattern is based on staffing parameters outlined above as well as Personnel Policy regarding staffing.
- Clinic manager is responsible for scheduling nursing staff to provide adequate Telephone Triage services to clients and adhering to policy that all clients have access to an RN staff member (See Addendum A, Scheduling Policies).
- Management coverage. The clinic manager will designate a responsible person to manage in their absence.
- Assignments and protocols will be addressed as outlined in Delivery of Care Methodology of these policies.

Delivery of Care Methodology

- The method of patient care delivery of Telephone Triage is consistent with the goals and philosophy of the Ambulatory Care Health Services.
- See Addendum C for "Delivery of Care Methodology" on Telephone Triage.

Preparation

- Selection:
  - The program/clinic manager in collaboration with the director of Ambulatory Care Services will hire staff for Telephone Triage service. Staff selection will be based on current vacancies, educational and experiential background, and the interview process.
  - See Addendum D.

- Orientation
  - All Telephone Triage staff will participate in hospital and service orientation programs, which are structured, formalized, and individualized.
  - See Addendum D.
- Basic preparation/internship
  - All staff will have an additional period of review at the end of the 3-wk orientation period based on Telephone Triage standards, nursing responsibilities for the specific client population, and identified learning needs of the new staff member.
  - Orientation schedule is as follows:
    - c Week 1, 2, 3: Meet weekly with the preceptor to set goals for the next week,
    - o Weeks 4,8, and 12: Meet with preceptor, clinic manager, and AHN and Education and Professional Development person to set goals for the following month.
    - o Month 6 and 9: Meet with above people for written evaluation and goals.
- Continuing education
  - All staff will participate in continuing education related to the Telephone Triage service. These educational activities will be based on routine and new responsibilities of nursing staff, patient care review activities.
  - Staff will be expected to attend all mandatory events dealing with the following issues:
    - ° CPR and Emergency Measures
    - o Safety (general, electrical, fire, and disaster)
    - o Infection control review
    - ° AIDS update
    - ° General hazardous materials
  - Educational records will be maintained within the Telephone Triage service. It is the responsibility of each staff member to maintain her/his own record. This record will be updated quarterly. Participation in continuing education is an essential component of the employee appraisal process and Telephone Triage quality improvement plans.
- Maintaining/assuring competency
  - All staff will be expected to participate in periodic evaluation to determine learning needs. This will include surveys, questionnaires, and unsolicited suggestions for continuing education programs.
  - Staff will also be expected to participate in competency evaluations, which will be conducted as

joint activity by Clinical Educations, Clinical Specialist, and Telephone Triage management team. Annual testing will be conducted to validate cognitive and skill knowledge base relative to the work and client population.

—Finally, staff will be expected to participate in ongoing quality improvement activities for the ongoing purpose of assuring compliance to Telephone Triage standards, identifying learning needs and identifying/resoling staff/unit/patient-care problems.

RESPONSIBILITIES—ADVICE NURSES

- Demonstrates knowledge of and use of nursing process in carrying out Telephone Triage services to include triage, crises intervention, and client education.

- Demonstrates knowledge of and use of physical/psychosocial assessment skills as specified in protocols.

- Acts as public relations representative for the hospital.

- Markets hospital services and programs, as appropriate.

- Identifies need for protocol and forms update and revisions as necessary. Submits suggestions to PC.

Organization Chart Narrative

Telephone Triage is a patient service that facilitates appropriate and timely access, while enhancing system cost effectiveness.

The success of Telephone Triage depends on quality service. It is therefore recommended that a steering committee meet on a regular basis to guide this project, but maintain a direct reporting system to one department to ensure program effectiveness.

The organizational charts reflect the optional reporting system, but they both include a Steering Committee made up of the following departments: Nursing, ED, Marketing, Administration, and Medicine.

TELEPHONE ORGANIZATION CHART

DIRECTOR, AMULATORY CARE SERVICES

↓

TELEPHONE TRIAGE
STEERING COMMITTEE

↓

TELEPHONE TRIAGE
PROJECT COORDINATOR

↓

CLINIC MANAGERS

↓

SHIFT COORDINATOR

↓

TELEPHONE TRIAGE NURSES

Job Description

Position Title: Program Coordinator, Telephone Triage
Reports to: Director of Ambulatory Care Services
Summary: The *program coordinator* is a first line manager designated as the leader for Telephone Triage service, its patient population, and assigned staff. He/she has responsibility and accountability for all Telephone Triage activities, service operation, and staff function.

SPECIAL CHARACTERISTICS

- The program coordinator is a skilled communicator who is experienced in maintaining communication mechanisms among professional staff, outside agencies, patients, and family.
- o The program coordinator demonstrates leadership skills to include delegation, organization, and problem identification/solving skills.
- Functions as a role model in his/her clinical specialty.

DUTIES AND RESPONSIBILITIES

The program coordinator will

- Demonstrate competency in clinical knowledge of Telephone Triage, judgment, and technical skills. Provide clinical direction to staff. Evaluate the level of care provided by the nursing staff.
- Demonstrate awareness of hospital and departmental policies, participate in their development as appropriate, and use these as a basis for decision making for both clinical and management issues.
- Demonstrate awareness of and adherence to safety and legal requirements established at the hospital and department level with emphasis on those pertinent to the Telephone Triage service.
- Participate in budgetary planning and implementation for the department.
- Serve on committees, task forces, and work groups on a voluntary and appointed basis at the department and hospital level. Participate actively, and complete follow-up activities in a consistent manner.

- Participate in the development of criteria-based job descriptions as directed. Write performance standards for employees of Telephone Triage service.
- ° Actively develop standards for the Telephone Triage service to define service function, staff performance, and patient care activities.
- Actively participate in licensing and accreditation process.
- Plan and implement service-based quality improvement activities. Share results for integration at the department level.
- Participate in personnel functions to include (1) annual and ongoing performance appraisal on employees; (2) engage in annual licensure validation for employees; (3) recruit, interview, select and hire nursing employees. Endeavor to maintain stable staff and minimize staff turnover.
- Independently and in conjunction with others, plan and participate in the clinical and leadership development of employees in the Telephone Triage service. Maintain accurate records and evaluate effectiveness of activities.
- Assess self-learning needs. Seeks ways to meet those needs and to maintain current competency and respond to new clinical and management demands.
- Remain aware of current nursing research and implement relevant findings as appropriate.

QUALIFICATIONS

- Current State License
- BSN required
- Prior proven experience and medical surgical nursing (minimum 3-5 yr)
- Prior proven experience and expertise in management • Excellent verbal and written communication skills
- Strong pediatric and OB/GYN background preferred
- Telephone Triage experience or formal training
- Demonstrates computer literacy
- Meets requirements of employee physical

Job Description

Position Title: Telephone Triage Nurse
Reports to: Clinic Manager

JOB SUMMARY

The telephone triage nurse is a health care professional that assumes responsibility and accountability for a group of clients for a designated time frame. The triage nurse provides Telephone Triage services to clients via therapeutic use of self, protocols, the environment/instrumentation, and other telephone triage and crises intervention team members.

- Demonstrates knowledge of and use of nursing process in carrying out Telephone Triage.
- Demonstrates knowledge of and use of physical/ psychosocial assessment skills as specified in key questions and protocols.
- Acts as public relations representative for facility services and programs, as appropriate.
- Acts as an information broker and referral agent, using approved references and referrals.
- Identifies need for protocol and forms update and revisions as necessary. Submits suggestions to manager.

SPECIAL CHARACTERISTICS

- Demonstrates an awareness of own responsibility and accountability for professional practice.
- Demonstrates strong communication skills. Uses lines of authority appropriately. Delegates tasks and duties appropriately when directing and coordinating health care team members, client care, and department activities.
- Demonstrates effective problem identification and resolution skills as a method of sound decision making.

DUTIES/RESPONSIBILITIES:

The telephone triage nurse will

- Demonstrate a sound knowledge base and decision making for a diverse client population with a wide range of problems and acuity.
- Perform effectively in crisis intervention, follow established protocols, remaining calm, informing appropriate persons, and documenting events.
- Perform assessment/data collection in an ongoing and systematic manner, focusing on physiological, psychological, educations, resource referral, and cognitive status.
- Document in timely, accurate, comprehensive and concise manner.

- Formulate sound working diagnosis.
- Select protocols appropriately.
- Instruct patients in an articulate, skillful, consistent and professional manner.
- Base client care on expressed needs and available resources of time, personnel, and equipment.
- Evaluate effectiveness of client self-care as appropriate.
- Identify client/significant other learning needs and implement appropriate measures to meet these.
- Demonstrate awareness and sensitivity to rights of client, as identified within the institution.
- Demonstrate awareness of legal issues in all aspects of Telephone Triage service function. Strive to manage situations to reduce legal risks.
- Seek validation of knowledge base, skill level, and decision making as necessary. Assertively seek guidance in areas of question. Participate in continuing education to meet own professional development.
- Participate in peer review, and Telephone Triage service and department quality improvement activities as well as standards development.
- Be aware of safety issues as identified by the institution.
- Participate actively as preceptor for staff development activities for Telephone Triage service personnel.
- Participate in nursing research activities as requested.
- Remain flexible in staffing patterns and resolution of staffing conflicts; perform related duties as required.

TELEPHONE TRIAGE NURSE—JOB QUALIFICATIONS

All attempts will be made to employ staff with previous medical/surgical experience compatible with the Telephone Triage population of clients and surrounding community. If this is not possible, applicant learning ability, motivation, or leadership potential will be carefully considered at the time of the interview. The ideal candidate will be a trained, mature, and experienced RN with good judgment.

Personal Qualifications

- Ability to make good medical decisions under conditions of uncertainty and urgency
- Ability to set priorities
- Good judgment
- Excellent written and spoken communications skill
- Excellent interpersonal skills

In addition, applicants with the following life/work experience are preferred:

- Applicants who are parents or possess pediatric experience
- Applicants who possess OB/GYN experience. Generally, applicants will have
  - A minimum of 5 yrs recent experience in medical/surgical nursing or clinic setting
  - Recent experience in Critical Care or Emergency Department desirable
- Triage experience (walk-in or telephone)—Preferred
- Case management skill—Preferred
- Bilingual (preferred)—Spanish
- Current BLS certification
- Demonstrates good judgment and problem solving skills

- Demonstrates a caring manner with clients
- Works well independently
- Functions well under pressure
- Works effectively with
  - Culturally diverse populations
  - Educationally diverse and illiterate populations
  - Non-English speaking populations
  - High-risk populations
- Able to serve as resource/liaison for clients, clerical staff, physicians, nurses, telephone triage nurses, medical assistants,_____ ED staff,_____poison control, and clinic administrators.

Applicants lacking the above experience are required to take refresher courses as part of the conditions of employment

Sample Performance Standards

Title: RN Performance Standards for the Telephone Triage function

Clinic:_____

Purpose: To define the daily expectation of this employee category

CONTENT

Nursing Process

Assessment

- Performs client assessment for all callers to Telephone Triage services
- Documents required data on triage form (per triage form directives and guidelines) or electronic medical record (EMR) (per EMR guidelines)
- Obtains specific data (physical, psychosocial, and cultural) from patient and family, significant others, other health care providers and medical record(s) as appropriate
- Assesses and interprets client symptoms
- Able to assess clients within an average of 7-10 min, as appropriate, using the appropriate guidelines and protocol(s)
- Documents working diagnosis and states to client
- Performs follow-up assessment, as appropriate, 1-24 hr after initial call

Plan

- Selects and implements the appropriate protocol(s) (plan of care) utilizing assessment information
- Implements protocol directives (per protocol directives and guidelines)
- Modifies and/or individualizes plan as appropriate and documents all modifications to protocol plan
- Establishes priorities for care based on
  —Presenting symptoms/chief complaint
  —Appointment availability
- Includes patient/family/significant others in the development of nursing care
- Collaborates with other health disciplines as necessary (Pharmacy, Poison Control, 911, Suicide Prevention, Community Resources and others)

Intervention

- Appropriately implements crisis intervention for life-threatening symptoms.
- Advises (and/or schedules) same day and future appointments appropriately
- Initiates referrals with appropriate agencies
- Provides advice from protocols or approved texts
- Offers counseling and emotional support as appropriate

Evaluation/Teaching for Client Self-Evaluation

- Evaluates the effectiveness of advice as appropriate by
  —For advice only clients: Follow up call(s) as appropriate
  —For appointment clients: Chart (EMR) review within 1 wk
- Evaluates client's ability and resources available to effectively carry out self-care measures at home. Determines availability of home treatment materials (OTC meds, thermometer, specific diet, etc.).
- Demonstrates ability to quickl and effectively assess client's learning needs and carry out teaching/advice segment for basic protocols. 15.
- Evaluates client response to protocols in areas specified in protocol and documents as appropriate.
- Judges the effectiveness of current protocol(s) on patient.
- Judges the effectiveness of comfort measures including all nonprescription medications taken within 2-8 hr as appropriate.
- Evaluates client's response to physical and psychological self-care procedures as appropriate
- Evaluates client's/significant other's (SO) ability to carry out self-care, home treatment, and teaching. Modifies teaching as appropriate.
- Evaluates protocol advice effectiveness as appropriate related to
  —OTC and approved prescription medications
  —First aid measures/home treatment
  —Client advocacy
  —Referral

EDUCATION

Patient, Family, Significant Others

- Maintains adequate amount of client brochures as well as other patient education literature. Ensures that each caller is aware of client brochure.
  - Identifies needed education literature that is needed for clinic managers.
- Refers/schedules patient, family and significant others to appropriate educational classes within the hospital/community, based on identified learning needs.
- Documents actions taken.

- Demonstrates cultural sensitivity in regard to client's learning needs and literacy level. Observes principles of cultural sensitivity when carrying out teaching related to all protocols.
- Uses "layman's language" in communicating with client.
- Acts as patient advocate as appropriate
  - Demonstrates working knowledge and endeavors to meet client needs in the following items:
    - HIPAA
    - Patient's Bill of Rights
    - Informed consent
    - Second medical opinions
  - Client Dissatisfaction. Refers dissatisfied clients to_____
  - Referrals. Makes appropriate and timely referrals to appropriate self help and support groups, community agencies, and in-house programs and meetings.

Staff and Students

- Functions as a preceptor for new staff as part of orientation programs.
- Acts as a resource for
  - Nursing staff
  - Medical staff
  - Clerical staff
- Provides learning opportunities for students/staff based on identified needs within legal guidelines.
- Evaluates competency level of staff in relation to the learning objectives.

Self-Growth and Development

- Assesses own knowledge, skill, and function on an ongoing basis. Seeks on-going high practice level. Verifies knowledge and practice constantly. Sets high standards of practice and constantly seeks to fulfill them.
- Participates in formal credentialing mechanism annually. Pursues identified follow-up activities assertively in a timely manner.
- Maintains own records of professional practice. Documents strengths and weaknesses and evidence of professional practice.
- Participates in self-evaluation at performance appraisal by completing evaluation tool, providing documentation of practice, and mutually setting goals for achievement with PC.
- Participates in quarterly coaching and counseling sessions with PC to review accomplishments and short-term goal development.

- Participates in peer review at performance appraisal time.
- Demonstrates willingness to critique own daily practice for errors.
- Documents errors from problem sheets or occurrence reports, and pursues corrective action.
- Demonstrates willingness to critique the practice of coworkers and report inappropriate actions on a timely basis.
- Attends minimum of three in-services per year (given by other staff).
- Reports back on all outside conferences within period of next staff meeting or six weeks, whichever is appropriate.
- Attends all annual mandatory educational and licensure sessions.
- Engages in daily, informal teaching of other staff members. Documents these activities on own practice record. Communicates general needs to PC for planning purposes.

Practice Management

Orientation:

- Actively participates in staff orientation by
  - Accepting coach/mentor position as requested
  - Using *Service Orientation Manual* as designed
  - Maintaining Orientation Evaluation Tool
  - Giving weekly feedback to clinic manager re: orientee performance and progress
  - Participating in orientation evaluation conference

Licensure:

- Maintains current licensure and provides assistant head nurse with copies of
  - RN license
  - State/national certificates
  - Hospital required certifications

Shift Coordinator:

- Each shift will have a shift coordinator assigned by the clinic manager. There will be a back up assigned in case of illness.
- In summary, this role includes but is not limited to
  - Assignments of duties and breaks
  - Coordination of emergency situations as necessary
  - Maintaining contact with the (nurse supervisor) regarding unit problems and staffing
  - Supervision and direction of new staff members
  - Handling of complaints from clients, physicians, and staff, as well as interdepartmental problems

—Preparation and submission of daily log

—Completion of "shift report" for submission to clinic manager; facilitation of nursing office report at end of shift.

—Planning, coordination, and presentation of educational programs in collaboration with PC

—Charge responsibilities (as noted in site-specific manual)

Goal Setting/Attainment:

• Actively commits self to goal accomplishment. Reviews goals as a staff member weekly and participates in quarterly goal summary with clinic manager and staff. Contributes suggestions for new goals.

• Actively volunteers or accepts assignment for projects to achieve Telephone Triage Department goals.

Communications/Meetings (as per site specific standards)

• Documentation. Documents appropriately, using approved terminology and abbreviations. Follows guidelines for use of triage form.

• Bulletin board update. Utilizes bulletin board as communication support.

• Shift report. Gives shift report to shift coordinator as appropriate.

• Communications. Demonstrates effective verbal communication skills in following areas:

—Telephone

—Concise report

• Medical consultation. Calls primary MD (after hours-ED/MD on Call) in a timely and appropriate manner to

—Report client incidents

—Report abnormal lab work that is likely to require immediate intervention

—Report changes in client's condition relative to deteriorating vital signs or negative response to home treatment

• Effectively elicits information relative to client needs, comfort and concerns.

• Report. Adheres to report activities by timely and regular attendance as outlined in Delivery of Care Methodology.

• Staff meetings. Attends 75% of service staff meetings; reads minutes when not able to attend; reads posted agenda before meeting; actively participates in discussions of problem identification and resolution.

• Emergency department. Calls ED as appropriate to notify of impending arrival of emergent and urgent level acuity clients.

• Crisis intervention. Communicates effectively and appropriately with members of Crisis Intervention Team (911, Poison Control, Drug Crisis, etc).

Technical Computer Skills

• Is computer literate

• Able to type 50 wpm.

• Competently operates required software programs and EMR.

Safety

• Demonstrates appropriate use of occurrence reports with

—All unusual calls (homicide, suicide, rape, drug-related, child/spousal/elder abuse)

—Medication errors

—All lawsuit threats

Emergency Situations:

e Demonstrates effective response to the following service/client crisis situations as outlined in the telephone advice protocols:

—Symptoms of shock

—Symptoms of cardiac arrest

—Symptoms of respiratory crisis

—Trauma related symptoms

—Symptoms of hemorrhage

—Neurologic complications (seizures, unconsciousness)

—Symptoms of severe emotional disturbance

—Symptoms of drug-related problems

—Documents essential data and disposition for all crisis level calls

Quality Improvement

Poiicy/Procedures/Protocois

• Complies with current applicable standards

• Actively participates in protocol development and review process

• Participates on task forces/quality teams/clinical practice groups as needed and/or requested by clinic manager

• Maintains competency for protocols and support materials contained in protocol book

Knowledge Base

• Is aware of location of, possesses working knowledge of, and ability to use following manuals/references on the unit:

—Telephone Triage protocols in hard copy and electronic versions

- —Standards Manual
- —Quality Improvement Manual
- —Infection Control Manual
- —Hazardous Substance Program Manual
- —Occupational Injury and Illness Prevention Program Manual
- —Emergency Preparedness Manual
- Accesses and utilizes the following reference manuals/ Telephone Triage reference books including, but not limited to
- —Formulary or Drug Reference
- —Merck Manual
- —Telephone Triage Approved Reference Library
- —Communicable Diseases in Man
- Demonstrates ability to locate and use other reference manuals and books on the nursing unit:
- —County Phone Book
- —Directory of Human Services
- —Hospital library
- Demonstrates working knowledge of the following agencies and departments:
- —Public health
- —Home care
- —Hospice management
- Demonstrates ability to interpret lab values and report abnormalities to the physicians.
- Demonstrates the ability to provide Telephone Triage services for clients requiring the following interventions:
- —Crisis intervention (medical and emotional)
- —Telephone Triage (assessment and advice for medical problems)
- —Physician referral
- —Health education
- —Community resource referral (self-help and support groups)
- —Hospital programs and services referral
- —Hotline referral
  - ° Parental stress
  - ° AIDS
  - ° Sexual assault
  - o Poison control
- —Advocacy, health consumerism
- Demonstrates working knowledge of the following major classification of medications as well as current knowledge of new medications and pharmacological trends. Uses drug references as needed.
- —Analgesics
- —Anti-inflammatory drugs
- —Anesthetics
- —Antiasthmatic drugs
- —Antibiotics
- —Anticonvulsants
- —Antifungal drugs
- —Antiviral drugs
- —Cardiovascular drugs: cardiac glycosides, calcium channel blockers, Ace inhibitors, antidysrhythmics, antihypertensive, diuretics, vasodilators, anticoagulants, thrombolytics, antihyperlipidemics
- —Immunosuppressants, immunomodulators
- —Chemotherapy
- —Contraceptive medications and devices
- —Hormone replacement therapy
- —Psychotropic drugs
- —Steroids
- Demonstrates ability to modify protocol advice after clearly considering implications of appropriateness for client, relationship to current therapy, and integration with nursing standards.

Standards

- Standards/protocol development. Actively identifies new areas for standards/protocol development and communicates these to PC.
- Protocol update/review. Reviews and critiques current protocols and standards for areas of obsolescence or ineffectiveness; participates in annual review.
- Continuous quality improvement. Participates in CQI sessions.
- Analysis of present problems. Uses past experiences and results to analyze present problem situations for effective decision making. Demonstrates ability to transfer information from one situation to another.
- Minor problem solving. Assertively attempts to solve minor problems of care, relationships, equipment, supplies, environment prior to PC intervention; documents actions and communicates actions to PC.

Delegation/Coordination

- Carries out shift coordinator role when assigned that duty.
- Participates in Delivery of Care Methodology defined in service structure (Addendum C—Delivery of Care Methodology) with regard to
  - —Assignment mechanism of clients and unit duties
  - —Use of nonprofessional personnel

- Actively supervises other members of his/her assignment team via verbal interaction to validate call volume, acuity, and problems.
- Functions as dependable team member, assisting when requested and volunteering when need is obvious. Perceived by other team members as a helpful team member.
- Accepts assignment willingly or discusses concerns appropriately with shift coordinator, keeping continuity and quality of care uppermost in mind.
- Delegates assigned "follow-up clients" to responsible team member in report when going off duty.
- Demonstrates priority setting ability and organizational skills by
  —Completing assignment in allotted time
  —Maintaining clean and orderly work area
  —Minimal use of overtime and obtaining approval ahead of time when possible
  —Taking scheduled breaks and dinner times
  —Integrating care conferences and in services into work schedule
  —Preparing for and attending meetings
  —Utilizing clerk for clerical tasks and phone calls
  —Timely notification of physician as to client's condition
  —Appropriate use of the PC and shift coordinator for problem resolution

Working Relationships/Behaviors

Working Relationships

- Cultivates and maintains effective working relationships with professional staff, coworkers, physicians, and members of Crisis Intervention Team.
- Cultivates and develops working relationships characterized by mutual support, open communication, trust, and respect.
- Separates personal biases and private life from work setting.
- Participates as desired in planning and conducting service social activities (approved by PC in advance) to celebrate personal events for the purpose of maintaining staff morale. Takes into considerations hospital policy governing appropriate and safe social activities.
- Reports irreconcilable differences among coworkers to PC for intervention and possible assignment considerations.
- Gives criticism to others in a private, constructive manner.

- Accepts criticism in a positive manner.
- Demonstrates ability to appropriately challenge questionable protocol treatment and advice.
- Demonstrates appropriate use of colleagues (clinical specialists, medical librarian, physicians, other RNs, dietitian, social worker, pharmacist, hospice, and home health care nurse). Effectively collaborates and coordinates with these resources in planning and delivering service.
- Demonstrates ability to work effectively with the following Crisis Intervention agencies:
  —Medical Dispatchers (911)
  —Suicide Prevention
  —Sexual Assault
  —Poison Control
- Demonstrates collaboration and coordination skills in planning and giving telephone advice.

Behaviors

- Is punctual in reporting to work and required meeting.
- Maintains good attendance record. Uses sick time sparingly; adheres to call-in policy defined by Telephone Triage.
- Adheres to facility dress code.
- Maintains positive public relations image with clients/visitors at all times by phone, in rooms, on elevator, and in public places.
- Responds to client request with promptness, empathy, and genuine interest as perceived by clients and coworkers.
- Participates in Telephone Triage annual needs assessment to identify new topics for continuing education.
- Volunteers to teach minimum of two 20-min in services per year to service staff on selected Telephone Triage topics.

Staffing/Flexibility

- Time schedules. Checks and records posted time schedules on a weekly basis to remain up to date with changes.
- Schedule changes. Demonstrates flexibility in requesting and time changes.
- Floating. Floats to other areas as requested following policy on temporary reassignment.
- Staffing adjustments. Works with shift coordinator in conjunction with PC when staffing assistance is required. Works with shift coordinator to adjust assignments and set priorities to complete assignments.

TELEPHONE TRIAGE ADDENDA

ADDENDUM A
Staffing and Scheduling Policies

MODEL-STAFFING PATTERN FOR TELEPHONE TRIAGE

Weekdays

- Day Shift (trained Telephone Triage RNs)
  —Preferred Staff_____
  —Minimum Staff_____
- Evening Shift (trained Telephone Triage RNs)
  —Preferred Staff_____
  —Minimum Staff_____
- Night Shift (trained telephone triage RNs)
  —Preferred Staff_____
  —Minimum Staff_____

Weekends and Holidays

- Day Shift (trained telephone triage RNs)
  —Preferred Staff_____
  —Minimum Staff_____
- Evening Shift (trained Telephone Triage RNs)
  —Preferred Staff_____
  —Minimum Staff_____
- Night Shift (trained Telephone Triage RNs)
  —Preferred Staff_____
  —Minimum Staff_____

Scheduling is the responsibility of the PC. Time schedules will be written for 6-wk time periods. The draft will be

- Written in the first week of the month (schedule posted)
- Approved in the second week of the month (schedule posted)
- Posted in the third week of the month (schedule posted)

All staff may be scheduled on a rotating basis.

- A request form is used for staff requests for special time on or off. Every effort is made to honor reasonable requests. Request must be submitted in writing at least 6 wk in advance.
- Vacations will be handled as outlined in department policy.
- Staff may trade shifts only after receiving approval from management and completing change request form.

ADDENDUM B
Nursing Students' Observations of Telephone Triage

Students from various university settings often affiliate with the Department of Nursing. Nursing students will be limited in responsibilities to observation only when working within the Telephone Triage system. Nursing instructors will be responsible for establishing orientation dates for themselves and the student groups.

ADDENDUM C
Delivery of Care Methodology for Telephone Triage

METHOD

The method of client care delivery for Telephone Triage is compatible with current goals and philosophy of ambulatory nursing.

- Call volume. Nurses are assigned to provide Telephone Triage for all incoming calls not to exceed more than 10/hr. Nurses are to perform with consistency and maintain patient continuity.
- Level of urgency. All nurses are assigned to answer all levels of calls from routine to crisis level.
- Staffing. Nurses will deliver care over an 8-, 10-, or 12-hr period.
- Supervision. The RN is responsible for supervision of all other staff that works with Telephone Triage area when management is not available.
- The nurse will always perform the initial assessment on all new callers.
- Telephone Triage means carrying out all aspects of the nursing process for those tasks that cannot be delegated to nonprofessional staff including:
  —Assessment (data collection and analysis)
  —Problem identification ("working diagnosis" or "impression")
  —Formulation of a client plan of action and disposition
  —Instruction for client self-evaluation of effectiveness of nursing intervention(s) or home treatment
  —Closure and disclaimer
  —Use of appropriate Protocols
  —Medication/treatment advice
  —Documentation
  —Interaction with physician, family, client, Crisis Intervention Team
  —Carrying out teaching from prescribed Protocols and approved books
  —Counseling for emotional or psychological stress
  —Regular shifts are traditionally 8 hr long

ASSIGNMENTS

- Assignments are made by the Clinic Manager.
  —Assignments are based on
    o Client acuity
    ° Staff availability
    ° Staff learning needs, interest, variety
    ° Continuity of client care
    o Limiting the call volume to the maximum projected number of 60 calls per nurse per 8-hr shift
    o Seasonal increases in call volume (i.e., "flu season")
    o Weekly increases in call volume (weekends, holidays)
    ° Predictable patterns of peak call volume (peak times)
  —Assignments may be changed during or after report as deemed necessary by the Shift Coordinator

Report

- Shift report will be written on a shift report form and given orally to the oncoming staff. Routine report will cover:
  —The current status of call volume and acuity
  —Review of current problem calls
  —Review of needed "follow-up" calls. All relevant calls will be reviewed as follows:
    ° Name
    ° Phone number
    ° Age
    ° Symptoms
    ° "Working diagnosis"
    ° Plan
    ° Disposition
    o Immediate needs relevant to next 8 hours
    ° Significant changes in plan for nursing care
    ° Significant emotional, communications, psychological, educational needs or problems
- All staff will give report, remain attentive to client status, and take notes as appropriate.
- Immediately after report, all oncoming staff RNs will make verbal contact with off going staff to validate report information, clarify any questions, and update any changes.
- Immediately following this routine, the oncoming staff will begin answering calls.

ADDENDUM D
Staffing Policies

The following policies are designed to augment current and future staffing policies established by the Nursing and Personnel Departments. They are found in the *Standards Manuals of the Telephone Triage Service* and are shared with new staff. Reviews and updates are preformed on an annual basis.

ORIENTATION

- All new staff in the Telephone Triage service shall receive the general hospital, Department of Nursing, and Ambulatory Services orientation before independent assignment within the Telephone Triage service.
- In Addition, each staff member will receive an additional orientation to the nursing standards and responsibilities of the Telephone Triage service. This orientation period will have written objectives, and structured content. It will consist of a 1-day formal class. This class will consist of a Telephone Triage "core program" and protocol and standards review. During the 4-wk orientation period, calls will be supervised.
- The above Telephone Triage service orientation may be extended as appropriate if the PC feels that the additional time will result in safe, effective, knowledgeable staff members.
- During the additional orientation, educational content may be modified according to the employee's self-evaluation and demonstrated learning needs.

HIRING

- Staff may be recruited from outside the hospital or in-house. The PC will interview all staff after their resume is reviewed for education and nursing experience. All interviewees will be given a tour of the Telephone Triage service. The PC will review the appropriate job description and performance standards with the applicant as well as the Standards Manual. Specific issues discussed will be nursing responsibilities, scheduling, and participative style of unit management.
- All attempts will be made to employ staff with previous medical/surgical experience compatible with the Telephone Triage population of clients and surrounding community. If this is not possible, applicant learning ability, motivation or leadership potential will be carefully considered at the time of the interview.

- Generally, applicants will have
  —At least 3-yr recent experience in medical/surgical nursing or
  —At least 1- to 3- yr recent experience in Critical Care or Emergency Department or in addition, applicants with the following life/work experience are preferred:
    o Applicants who are parents or possess pediatric experience
    o Applicants who possess OB/GYN experience

Applicants lacking the above experience are required to take refresher courses as part of the conditions of employment.

- Generally, contingent staff will not be utilized unless extreme staffing shortages exist.
- Part-time staff hired for Telephone Triage will be expected to participate in the general and service orientation schedule on a full-time basis before beginning their part-time schedule.
- Staff members transferring into the Telephone Triage service will be expected to go through the Telephone Triage orientation.
- Regular part-time status is limited to 4 shifts per 2-wk period in order for telephone advice nurse staff to maintain nursing skills, contribute to telephone Triage projects, and keep abreast of communication and changes in the Department and within the Telephone Triage service.

STAFF PREPARATION AND RESPONSIBILITY

- New staff are expected to meet minimum requirements for continued employment by the end of the probationary (3 mo) period to include (but not limited to) the following:
  —Demonstrated clinical competency in basic Telephone Triage assessment and communication skills, plan of action, intervention, and evaluation of education (application of nursing process).
  —Communication skills with peers, physicians, supervisory staff, clients/families, Crisis Intervention Team, pharmacologist.
  —Appropriate documentation according to hospital/department requirements (standards).
  —Demonstrated knowledge of Telephone Triage policy, procedure, and all written standards.
  —Minimum crisis level intervention competency (mock call practicums, Appendix D).

- Staff will perform self-evaluation methods during orientation to identify learning needs; staff will collaborate with PC to need educational deeds by taking advantage of Telephone Triage service continuing education.

- Staff will participate in review of calls at monthly staff meetings. This responsibility is assigned to meet specific learning needs, refine techniques, increase sophistication of work habits, and enhance overall knowledge.

Role-Playing Practicum

Using the scripts, the protocols, a copy of the documentation form and the QA score sheet, three participants take turns role-playing nurse, patient, and evaluator.

- In the nurse role, that participant will use the protocol and documentation form, while interviewing the caller.

- In the patient/caller role, that participant will use the mock call scripts to present the symptoms. "Patients" should neither volunteer too much information initially, nor make it unduly difficult for the nurse to collect information. If information is not included in the script, it is acceptable to "make it up" during the interview process.

- In the evaluator role, that participant should assess whether the nurse is collecting the information listed on the QA score sheet. Listen for key questions and evaluate the documentation as well. Each item collected counts for 2 points. Each item that is volunteered by the patient also counts for 2 points.

Items that don't apply (such as questions regarding breastfeeding/pregnancy, inappropriate for males) still count as 2 points. A perfect score is 100 points. A passing score is 70. Failure to obtain the caller's age, be helpful, or ask open-ended questions initially will result in a loss of 10 points for those three reasons. That is because these criteria are so critically important in the history-taking process.

- Each "call" should take no longer that 15 minutes initially, and time efficiency should improve with practice.

- Participants should each take a turn as patient, nurse, or evaluator.

- Feel free to make up your own "mock calls" for ongoing training.

- Ideally, it would be best if the patient calls the nurse from another room, thereby making the call more realistic.

QA AUDIT

ROLE (*7,10, 15 16)	Call 1	Call 2	Call 3	Call 4
Helpful Manner: Warm, Friendly, "Business-like"				
Inquisitive, Investigative, timely decisionmaking				
Teaching: Uses Effective, Lay Language				
Crisis Management: Proficiently management of life-threatening & emergent calls. Proficient Warm Transfers				
COMMUNICATION (*11 Communication)				
Call Management is Confident, Timely, Professional				
Performs Preliminary Assessment prior to Selecting Guideline & before using "Smart Phrases"				
Consistently inquires about & documents *repeat Calls*				
Inquires & Rules out Symptoms of Sepsis & Dehydration				
States Impression (Working Diagnosis) in Lay Terms				
States Disposition (When, Where, Why) As Appropriate				
Verbalizes Precautions				
Provides Informed Consent: Understanding & Agreement				
ASSESSMENT (* 1 Systematic Data Collection)				
SAVED + 1 or more Assessment Tools				
1. Severe, Strange, Suspicious Symptoms				
2. Age				
3. Veracity				
4. Emotional Distress				
5. Red Flag Symptoms & Populations				
6. SCHOLAR (6-8 items)	#			
7. RAMP (4-5 items)	#			
8. ADL (6-8 items)	#			
9. A DEMERIT (6-8 items)	#			
DECISION MAKING & DISPOSITION (*2 Data Analysis)				
Selects Appropriate Guideline				
Uses Guideline Correctly				
Uses Master Guideline Appropriately				
Able to Estimate Symptom Urgency (5-Tier Triage)				
DOCUMENTATION (*11 Communication)				
Guideline Title				
Impression with acuity level				
Disposition using 5-Tier Triage Method				
Documents in "real time"				
CONTINUITY: (*4 Continuity, Coordination)				
Provides for safe, timely, 5-Tier Triage Dispositions				
SCORE:				

Score 1 point per question, except Assessment tools. NA- 1 for Not Applicable. O for errors.
Total Possible Score: 25-29 . Acceptable Score: 25
*Related 2011 AAACN Standards noted in parentheses
Related Measures to Avoid Root causes of Error (Joint Commision)

Mock call practicum

Adult/Geriatric Problems

Mock Cain

71-year-old female
Noted chest tightness when walking
Stopping makes it better
Has had it 2-4 weeks, 3-4 times per week
Feels like she sometimes has sore throat
Denies shortness of breath, dizziness, sweating, nausea
Medical history—hypertension
Medication—Atarax
Allergies—salicylates, tomatoes, green peppers

Impression: Chest tightness: *Mild, > w exertion; elderly female*

Protocol: Chest Pain

Acuity Level: Urgent

Mock Call 2

61-yr-old male
History of hypertension
Feet and ankles look like "balloons"
Fatigue for 2 days
Taking Theodur, Prednisone, Wytension, Valium
4 plus pitting edema
Seems worse today than yesterday
Ankles 11 $\frac{1}{2}$ in circumference on left, 127_4 on right
History of emphysema, colitis
Hypertension for 3 yr

Identify: Red Flags
           Red Herrings

Apply: Rules of Thumb

Impression: Swollen ankles/feet, *mod.-sev., CHF Hx*

Protocol(s): Extremities Problem 3

Acuity Level: Urgent

Mock Call 3

21-year-old female
Generalized abdominal pain x 3-4 days, *moderate*
Lying on back helps
Lying on stomach makes it worse
Slight nausea
Vomited 2 hr ago
Diarrhea
No medications
No allergies
No vaginal discharge
No sexual activity

Identify: Red Flags
           Red Herrings

Apply: Rules of Thumb

Impression: Abdominal Pain: *Generalized, mod.*

Protocol(s): Abdominal Problem 1

Acuity Level: Nonacute w advice

Mock Call 4

44-year-old woman
Severe stomach pains
Temp— 103°F (39.4°C)
Became ill 28 hours ago
Sweating
No diarrhea
Bowel movement today looked like pellets
Pain is 4 in below umbilicus
No history of previous pain like this
Earlier felt constipated—now has dull tender spot in left
    lower pelvis
Medical history—kidney stone
Allergies—none
Medications—none
No appetite/drinking poorly

Identify: Red Flags
           Red Herrings

Apply: Rules of Thumb

Impression: Abdominal Pain: *Severe, LLQ*

Protocol(s): Abdominal Problem 2

Acuity Level: Urgent

Mock Call 5

Daughter calling regarding mother
Mother has Hx of minor stroke, incontinence
Now appears extremely lethargic, confused
Daughter gives evasive and confused history of problem
Daughter is sole caregiver
They live alone—no other family

Identify: Red Flags
           Red Herrings

Apply: Rules of Thumb

Impression: Confusion: Etiology unknown

Protocol(s): Confusion, Abuse

Acuity Level: Urgent

Mock Call 6

22-yr-old female student
c/o "bad headache"
Awoke this AM with throbbing headache
Had headache like this several times over past 10 years
Fatigue, chills, diarrhea, severe nausea
Denies any visual disturbances
Headache is on left side, made worse by bright light and noise
Family history of migraines
Recently started on birth control pills

Identify: Red Flags
               Red Herrings

Apply: Rules of Thumb

Impression: Headache: *Severe*

Protocol(s): Head Problem 2

Acuity Level: Urgent

Advice: Headache Tx per protocol

Mock Call 7

Daughter calling regarding father
Elderly male, 67 yr old
Recently retired—a "loner"
Wife just died—they were very close
Husband has no pets or hobbies
Lost interest in watching TV and gardening
Sleeping a lot
Not eating well

Identify: Red Flags
               Red Herrings

Apply: Rules of Thumb

Impression: Emotional Problem: *Apparent* depression, *severe*

Protocol(s): Emotional Problem 1 and 2, Supplemental Information

Acuity Level: Urgent

Ob/Gyn Problems

Mock Call 1

35-year-old female, unmarried
c/o "flu symptoms"
BC method IUD x 2 yr (Copper T)
Pelvic pain, fever, chills, muscle aches
Headache
Vaginal discharge—foul smelling
Recent STI exposure
Menses late x 2 months
Sexually active

Identify: Red Flags
               Red Herrings

Apply: Rules of Thumb

Impression: Pelvic Pain: *Fever/IUDHx, Vaginal Discharge*

Protocol(s): Abdomen Problem 2

Acuity Level: Urgent

Mock Call 2

35-year-old mother of newborn twins (has three other children)
6 wk postpartum
Recent C-section following prolonged labor
c/o breastfeeding problem: Sore cracked nipples, possible inadequate milk supply
Requesting information about vitamins and iron pills
c/o "feeling dizzy and exhausted, depressed and overwhelmed"
Passing clots x 3 days

Identify: Red Flags
               Red Herrings

Apply: Rules of Thumb

Impression: Postpartum vaginal bleeding: *mod. amt., postpartum*

Protocol(s): Postpartum Problem

Acuity Level: Urgent

Mock Call 3

40-yr-old multipara, 8 mo pregnant
Recent refugee to this country from Nicaragua (language barrier)
c/o headache, "stomach pain," "feels dizzy"
Thinks face and hand look puffy
c/o "blind spot" in vision

Identify: Red Flags
               Red Herrings

Apply: Rules of Thumb

Impression: Headache: *severe, pregnancy*

Protocol(s): Breastfeeding problem; Pregnancy Problem 2

Acuity Level: Emergent

Mock Call 4

20-yr-old female, sexually active
Painful intercourse
Pelvic pain, LLQ
Left shoulder pain
History of endometriosis
c/o nausea, vomiting, "feels like the flu"
Frequency of urination

"Pulled shoulder muscle playing tennis yesterday"
LMP was "normal" 1 mo ago

Identify: Red Flags
Red Herrings

Apply: Rules of Thumb

Impression: Abdominal pain: *Severe, LLQ*

Protocol(s): Abdominal Problem 2

Acuity Level: Emergent

Mock Call 5

21-yr-old student
Unprotected intercourse
No symptoms
Has questions regarding STIs

Identify: Red Flags
Red Herrings

Apply: Rules of Thumb

Impression: Poss. std exposure

Protocols): Vaginal Problem, STI Supplemental Information

Acuity Level: Acute; advice

WALL CHART

SAVED: RED FLAG POPULATIONS

Severe/Strange/Suspicious Symptoms:

Severe pain, bleeding, trauma, etc.

Age

Sexually active adolescents (male or female)
All women of childbearing age
All frail elderly

Veracity

Second-party calls
Low literacy
Language barrier
In Elderly: Suspected substance abuse: Incoherent or slurred speech in patient/caretaker
In Elderly: Caretaker unfamiliar w patient

Emotional Status (Caretaker and/or Child)

Hysteria or denial; inappropriate affect in caretaker
Parent or caretaker with history of abuse (physical or sexual), psychiatric problems, or substance abuse

Debilitation

In general, debilitation refers to chronic illness. Chronic illnesses may include but are not limited to the following:

All Populations
AIDS
Asthma
Diabetes
Sickle Cell

Immunocompromised
Lack of adequate immunizations
Chemotherapy
HIV
Splenectomy
Steroid therapy/chronic
Transplants
Nephrotic Syndrome

Adult/Frail Elderly
Cardiac Problems
COPD
Dementia

Distance

Parent/caretaker calling from remote location over 1 hr from hospital.

In emergent situation: Unable to arrive by car within 1 hr because of traffic or lack of available car. Must take public transportation that is sporadic or nonexistent after certain hours at night.

SCHOLAR: PROBLEM HISTORY

Symptoms and associated symptoms
    Is it an isolated symptom or a complex of symptoms?
    Course of symptoms: Is it better? Worse? The same?

Characteristics (aids in precise description)
    Quantitative (scale of 10)
    Qualitative (sharp, dull, pounding)

History of complaint in past
    What was done? By whom?
    When? Results?

Onset of symptoms
    When started? How long present?
    Sudden or gradual? (Sudden = Higher acuity)

Location of symptoms
    Strive for precision.
    Radiation? (Localized = Higher acuity)

Aggravating factors: What makes it worse?

Relieving factors: What makes it better?

PAMPER: PATIENT HISTORY

Pregnancy/breastfeeding?
Ask all women between ages of 12-50:
    "Is there any chance you might be pregnant?
    "Have you used birth control consistently and correctly?

Allergies
    Food, chemical, drugs, insect bites, cosmetics?

Medications
    Current OTC, Rx, and BCP, recreational drugs, alcohol

Previous chronic illness
    Recurrent illness, multiple surgeries, family history

Emotional state
    Psychiatric history, current reaction to illness

Recent injury, illness, ingestion
    Recent accident or child/elder/spouse abuse/neglect
    Exposure to communicable disease
    Possible ingestion

STRESS BUSTER PROGRAM

Stress Reduction

Hackman and Oldham's Job Characteristics Model

Stress reduction and job satisfaction can be increased by developing the following job characteristics. The more skill variety, task identity and significance, autonomy and feedback that managers can build into the task of telephone triage, the higher will be job satisfaction and stress reduction.

1. Skill variety—the degree to which the job requires a variety of different activities so the worker can use a number of different skills and talents
2. Task identity—the degree to which the job requires completion of a whole and identifiable piece of work
3. Task significance—the degree to which the job has a substantial impact on the lives or work of other people
4. Autonomy—the degree to which the job provides substantial freedom, independence, and discretion to the individual in scheduling the work, and in determining the procedures to be used in carrying it out
5. Feedback—the degree to which carrying out the work activities required by the job results in the individual obtaining direct and clear information about the effectiveness of his or her performance

Why is Telephone Triage So Stressful?

"Telephone Triage is ... high stakes activity ... making decisions under conditions of uncertainty and urgency ... like work of air traffic controller, fire captain, emergency medical dispatcher" (Patel 1995).

1. High-volume systems
2. Lack of training/knowledge
3. Sensory deprivation
4. Lack of acknowledgment/status
5. Angry callers
6. High-stress work
7. Uncertainty: Lack of feedback about outcome and QA

Job satisfaction can be increased by managing the volume, knowledge deficits, sensory deprivation, lack of status, caller hostility, and uncertainty to any degree that is reasonably possible.

"STRESS BUSTER" PROGRAM

The cumulative effect of several stressors can result in burnout and high levels of stress. Conversely, certain activities and remedies can also have a cumulative effect of stress reduction. Create a workspace and mental attitude that is rich in stress reduction triggers as illustrated below:

The External Environment

1. Clear your desk: Uncluttered, pleasant workspaces are restful and calming. Clutter is visually tiring.
2. Personalize your workspace: Pictures of places and people and/or things (plants, stones, icons, and goldfish) can calm and center you between calls.

   Visual vacations: Posters of scenes you won't tire of, like vacation spots or nature.
3. Workstation: Ergonomic/head set/light/air/quiet/ sense of repose/openable window looking onto nature.
4. Dim, warm light: Pink light bulbs, neither too bright nor too low; nonglare screen on your computer.
5. Paint your office soft green or blue.
6. Sound and music resources: Most relaxing: Classical, light jazz, new age, or nature sounds (ocean, rain, birds).

   Music can actually trigger relaxation response.

   Low-level volume just above level of awareness.
7. Aroma therapy: A few drops of lavender, rosemary, or mint oil on warm light bulb.

The Internal Environment

Stress is inevitable. We cannot remake the world, but according to most experts and spiritual leaders, we can change our attitudes. Anything that "stills the mind" can help.

1. Clear your mind: Like clearing your desk, clearing your mind helps reduce stress.

   Take allotted breaks.

   Use your breaks to clear your mind and emotions, NOT as "catch up" time on work.

   Leave your workstation completely. Take a brisk walk outdoors.

   Take a mental vacation—Read a short story, magazine, poetry, inspirational readings.

   Meditate/mindfulness.

   Emphasize your desire to serve.
2. Workstation exercises: Create a short exercise to mentally "clear your mind between calls."

   Breathe: Diaphragmatic breathing: Count as you breathe in, or recite an affirmation. Breathe deeply and smile.

Shoulder: Shoulder lifts and rolls.

Back: Stand, bend forward and shake out neck and shoulders.

Arms/hands: Lace fingers together, lift, palms to ceiling, and stretch.

3. Mental preparation: Decide who you would be, then develop a repertoire or package of consumer friendly, but effective responses (Nordstrom's/ED/car talk). Be ready for the inevitable "difficult call": Mentally rehearse or write down statements to use to handle certain predictable difficult situation. After difficult calls: Debrief as needed.

4. Develop tools of communication as a way to manage stress. Practice communication techniques to reduce stress by diffusing anger, setting limits, or managing conflicts. Share your experience and expertise through "war stories," tales of difficult but successfully managed calls.

5. Create and implement a realistic exercise program: The best antidotes to stress are moderate exercise three times a week, three balanced meals daily, and good friends.

6. Monitor and adjust: Are you at risk for burn out? Danger signs include: prolonged fatigue, insomnia, lack of appetite, loss of libido, inability to concentrate, or feeling your life is out of control.

General References

- Baumeister & Tierney (2011) Will Power
- Donabedian (2003) An Introduction to Quality Assurance in Health Care
- Donabedian A. Quality assurance. Structure, process and outcome. Nursing Standard (Royal College Of Nursing (Great Britain). 1992;7(11 Suppl).
- Gawande (2009) The Checklist Manifesto
- Institute of Medicine. To Err is Human: Building a Safer Health System. . In: Institute of Medicine Committee on the Quality of Health Care in America, editor. Washington DC: Institute of Medicine; 1999.
- Kahneman (2011) Thinking Fast and Slow
- Joint Commission. Sentinel Event Data: Root Causes by Event Type 2004-2Q 2012. In: Commission TJ, editor. Washington, DC: The Joint Commission, Office of Quality Monitoring; 2012.
- Johns Hopkins Research, 5/4/16. BMJ http://www.hopkinsmedicine.org/news/media/releases/study_suggests_medical_errors_now_third_leading_cause_of_death_in_the_us
- Lephrohon, J. & Patel, V. (1995). Decision Strategies In Emergency Telephone Triage. Medical Decision-Making. 15 (3): 240 -253.
- Mahlmeister, L, & Van Mullen, C. (2000). The Process Of Triage In Perinatal Settings: Clinical And Legal Issues. J Perinatal Neonatal Nurse 2000 Mar; 13(4): 13-30
- Perrin EC, Goodman HC. Telephone management of acute pediatric illnesses. The New England Journal of Medicine 1978;298(3):130-5 , Washington,
- Wachter (2015) The Digital Doctor: Hope, Hype and Harm Medicine's Computer Age
- Wheeler, et al. (2015) Safety of Clinical & Non-Clinical Decision Makers in Telephone Triage. Journal of Telemedicine & Telecare, Sep;21(6):305-22.
- Wheeler, S. Q. (2009). Telephone Triage Guidelines For Adult Populations with Women's Health, TeleTriage Systems Publishers, San Anselmo, CA
- Wheeler, S.Q. (2017) Telephone Triage: Essentials for Expert Practice. Preceptor Workbook. TeleTriage Systems Publishers(teletriage.com)

Safety References

- Huibers L, Smits M, Renaud V, Giesen P, Wensing M. Safety of telephone triage in out-of-hours care: a systematic review. Scandinavian Journal of Primary Health Care. 2011 Dec;29(4):198-209.
- Wheeler SQ. Telephone triage protocols for adult populations. New York City: McGraw Hill Publishers; 2009.
- The Lancet. Nurse-telephone triage. The Lancet. 2001;357(9253):323.

- Perrin EC, Goodman HC. Telephone management of acute pediatric illnesses. The New England Journal of Medicine 1978;298(3):130-5.

- Blank L, Coster J, O'Cathain A, Knowles E, Tosh J, Turner J, et al. The appropriateness of, and compliance with telephone triage decisions: a systemic review and narrative synthesis. . Journal of Advanced Nursing 2012;68(12):2610–21.

- Bunn F, Byrne G, Kendall S. Telephone consultation and triage: effects on health care use and patient satisfaction (Review). The Cochrane Library. 2009;1:1-36.

- Carrasqueiro S, Oliveira M, Encarnacao P. Evaluation of Telephone Triage and Advice Services: a Systematic Review on Methods, Metrics and Results. Fairfax, VA: IOS Press; 2011 [cited.

- Donabedian A. Quality assurance. Structure, process and outcome. Nursing Standard (Royal College Of Nursing (Great Britain). 1992;7(11 Suppl).

- Flannery M, Moses G, Cykert S, Ogden P, Keyserling T, Elnicki M, et al. Telephone management training in internal medicine residencies: a national survey of program directors. Academic Medicine 1995;70(12):1138-41.

- Brown JL. Pediatric telephone medicine: principles, triage, and advice. Philadelphia: Lippincott Williams & Wilkins; 1994.

- Katz H, Telephone Manual of Paediatric Care, Wiley, 1982

- Schmitt B. Pediatric Telephone Advice. Boston, MA: Little Brown & Co; 1980.

- Wheeler, S & Windt, J. Telephone Triage: Theory, Practice and Protocol Development, Delmar Publishers, Albany, NY. 1993

- Leprohon J, Patel V. Decision-making Strategies for Telephone Triage in Emergency Medical Services. Medical Decision Making. 1995;15:240-53.

- Reisman AB, Brown KE. Preventing communication errors in telephone medicine: A case based approach. Journal of general internal medicine. 2005 Oct;20:959-63.

- Mahlmeister, 2012, Affordable Care Act and Telephone Triage, Online CE Course available through TeleTriage Systems, In press TeleTriage Systems,

- Smith, 2005, Telephone Triage Risk Management, Online CE Course available through TeleTriage Systems teletriage.com

- 1Dahlberg CP. State probes whether Kaiser call centers endanger patients. The Kaiser Papers, A Public Service Page Sacramento, CA: Sacramento Bee; 2009.

- Greatbatch D, Hanlon G, Goode J, O'Caithain A, Strangleman T, Luff D. Telephone triage expert systems and clinical expertise. Sociology of Health & Illness. 2005;27(6):802-30.

- Rutenberg C, Greenberg L. The Art and Science of Telephone Triage. Consulting TT, editor. Hot Springs, Arkansas: Telephone Triage Consulting; 2012.

- Deakin CD, Alasaad M, King P, Thompson F. Is ambulance telephone triage using advanced medical priority dispatch protocols able to identify patients with acute stroke correctly? Emergency Medicine Journal. 2009 Jun;26(6):442-5. (NOTED IN TABLE 3 Decision Maker Frame work)

- Institute of Medicine. To Err is Human: Building a Safer Health System. . In: Institute of Medicine Committee on the Quality of Health Care in America, editor. Washington DC: Institute of Medicine; 1999.

- Norman GR, Eva KW. Diagnostic error and clinical reasoning. Medical Education 2010;44:94-100.

- The Joint Commission. Sentinel Event Data: Root Causes by Event Type 2004-2Q 2012. In: Commission TJ, editor. Washington, DC: The Joint Commission, Office of Quality Monitoring; 2012.

- Deakin CD, Sherwood DM, Smith A, Cassidy M. Does telephone triage of emergency (999) calls using Advanced Medical Priority Dispatch (AMPDS) with Department of Health (DH) call prioritisation effectively identify patients with an acute coronary syndrome? An audit of 42,657 emergency calls to Hampshire Ambulance Service NHS Trust. Emergency medicine journal : EMJ. 2006 Mar;23(3):232-5.

- Kempe A, Bunik M, Ellis J. How safe is triage by an after-hours telephone call center? . Pediatrics 2006;118:457-63.

- Kempe A, Luberti A, Belman S, Hertz A, Sherman H, Amin D, et al. Outcomes Associated With Pediatric After-Hours Care by Call Centers: A Multicenter Study. Ambulatory Pediatrics. 2003;3:211-7.

- Lee TJ, Baraff LJ, Guzy J, Johnson D, Woo H. Does telephone triage delay significant medical treatment? Archives of Pediatrics and Adolescent Medicine. 2003;157:635-41., 32

- Andrews J, Armstrong K, Fraser J. Professional telephone advice to parents with sick children: time for quality control! Journal of paediatrics and child health. 2002;38:23-6.

- Katz H, Kaltsounis D, Halloran L, Mondor M. Patient safety and telephone medicine: some lessons from closed claim case review. Journal of general internal medicine. 2008;23:517-22.

- Killip S, Ireson CL, Love MM, Fleming ST, Katirai W, Sandford K. Patient Safety in After-hours Telephone Medicine. Family Medicine. 2007;39:404-9.

- Fourny M, Lucas AS, Belle L, Debaty G, Casez P, Bouvaist H, et al. Inappropriate dispatcher decision for emergency medical service users with acute myocardial infarction. The American journal of emergency medicine. 2011 Jan;29(1):37-42.

- Hildebrandt DE, Westfall JM, Fernald DH, Pace WD. Harm resulting from inappropriate telephone triage in primary care. . The Journal of the American Board of Family Medicine. 2006;19(5):437-42.

- Hildebrandt DE, Westfall JM, Smith PC. After hours telephone triage affects patient safety. Journal of Family Practice. 2003;52(3):222-7.

- Klasner A, King W, Crews T, Monroe K. Accuracy and response time when clerks are used for telephone triage. Clinical Pediatrics. 2006;45:267-9.

- Derkx HP, Rethans J-JE, Muijtjens AM, Maiburg BH, Winkens R, van Rooij HG, et al. Quality of clinical aspects of call handling at Dutch out of hours centres: cross

- North F, Odunukan O, Varkey P. The value of telephone triage for patients with appendicitis. Journal of Telemedicine and Telecare. 2011;17:417-20.

- Ernesäter A, Engstrom M, Holmstrom I, Winblad U. Incident reporting in nurse-led national telephone triage in Sweden: the reported errors reveal a pattern that needs to be broken. Journal of Telemedicine and Telecare. 2010 Jul;16(5):243-7.

- Ernesäter A, Winblad U, Engstrom M, Holmstrom IK. Malpractice claims regarding calls to Swedish telephone advice nursing: what went wrong and why? Journal of Telemedicine and Telecare. 2012 Aug 24.

- Hirsh DA, Simon HK, Massey R, Thornton L, Simon JE. The host hospital 24-hour underreferral rate: an automated measure of call-center safety. Pediatrics. 2007;119:1139-44.

- Giesen P, Ferwerda R, Tijssen R, Mokkink H, Drijver R, van den Bosch W, et al. Safety of telephone triage in general practitioner cooperatives: do triage nurses correctly estimate urgency? Quality and Safety in Health Care. 2007;16:181–4.

- Huibers L, Giesen P, Smits M, Mokkink H, Grola R, Wensing M. Nurse telephone triage in Dutch out-of-hours primary care: the relation between history taking and urgency estimation. European Journal of Emergency Medicine 2012;19:309-15.

- Marklund B, Ström M, Månsson J, Borgquist L, Baigi A, Fridlund B. Computer-supported telephone nurse triage: an evaluation of medical quality and costs. Journal of Nursing Management 2007;15:180-7.

- Hannan TJ, Celia C. Are doctors the structural weakness in the e-health building? Internal Medicine Journal 2013;43:1155-64.

Patient Brochure

Please take the opportunity to customize this brochure for your individual practice.

TELEPHONE ADVICE SERVICES

We now offer telephone advice services 24 hours a day, 365 days a year. Call the advice nurse if you have symptoms, questions, need advice about any health problem, information about counseling, and referrals to community resources. They have had special training to help you. If your symptoms are not serious, you may not need an appointment; the advice nurse will tell you how to treat the problem at home. We can help you decide whether the problem needs an appointment right away or whether your symptoms can be safely treated at home.

Thank you in advance for taking the time to read this brochure. Please keep and use this list of important phone numbers. Attach it to the wall close to your telephone. Please tell others about this service. This pamphlet is available in English, Spanish, Vietnamese, and Cambodian at all clinics. You can get more pamphlets by calling:

HOW TO HELP THE ADVICE NURSE TO HELP YOU

There are many ways you can help the advice nurse. First, unless it is an emergency, please call the advice nurse *before* you come in. Also, if you can't keep your appointment, please call the clinic and let us know, so we can give that appointment to someone else. You can also help the advice nurse by providing a current address and phone number, so the nurse can call you back later. Also, let the nurse know if you do not have the medicine we advise or the home-treatment materials needed to follow the advice given.

WHAT TO TELL THE ADVICE NURSE

The advice nurse will want to talk directly with the sick person if that person is old enough and well enough to give good information. The information you give us helps us decide whether the symptoms are serious and whether an appointment is necessary. Please be ready to answer the following questions, if at all possible:

When did the symptom(s) start?

Is it getting worse?

If there is pain? Where is it?

Have you had this symptom before?

What makes it better?

What makes it worse?

How have you treated it?

Are you taking any medicines?

Are you pregnant or breastfeeding?

Do you have any allergies?

Have you had any recent injury, surgery, infection, illness?

Has there been any possible ingestion of toxic material or poisons?

Do you have any chronic disease?

HELP BY PHONE FOR EMERGENCIES

Problems like suicide or poisoning need quick help from hotlines like Suicide Prevention or Poison Control. The hotlines listed here are free and will give you fast help by telephone, 24 hr a day to all callers:

HOTLINES

- Poison Control (24 Hour/day)
- Suicide Prevention
- Parental Stress
- Spousal Abuse/Crisis Care
- "Warm Line" for Kids

HELP BY PHONE FOR CHRONIC EMOTIONAL OR PHYSICAL PROBLEMS

You can get help by phone for chronic emotional and physical problems, such as depression, AIDS, or drug and alcohol abuse. Learn about the groups listed in this brochure. Use them, and tell others about them.

- AIDS
- Drug/Alcohol Help Line
- Alcoholics Anonymous, AlAnon, Alateen
- Emotional Problems
- Seniors
- Teens

IMPORTANT PHONE NUMBERS

Clinic Hours/Days: Phone No.:

PRESCRIPTION REFILLS 24-HOUR NUMBER (Please call at least a week before your medication runs out):

MEDICATION QUESTIONS: Pharmacist

TRANSPORTATION:

MEDICARE INFORMATION:

MEDICAL INFORMATION:

LAB TEST RESULTS

Directory of Hotlines/Web Sites for Support Groups

QUICK REFERENCE:

Abuse: Physical, Sexual, Emotional, Spousal, Elder
AIDS/HIV: Education; Women and Children; Others

Bioterrorism

Cancer: Breast; Chemotherapy; Hospice; Leukemia; Lymphedema; Ovarian; Prostate, Skin; Support Groups; Others

Disease-Specific: Allergy; Alzheimer Disease; Arthritis; Asthma; Communication Disorders; Diabetes; Disabilities: Learning, Physical; Eye Care; Hearing Impairment; Heart Disease; Infectious Disease; Kidney; Multiple Sclerosis; Parkinson Disease; Psoriasis; Rehabilitation; Scleroderma; Sexually Transmitted Infections; Spinal Cord Injuries; Visual Impairment; Others

Emotional Problems (Mental Health): Anxiety; Autism; Bipolar; Depression and Schizophrenia; Eating Disorders; Obsessive-Compulsive Disorder; Social Phobia; Panic Disorder; Others

Pain Management

Parent's Help: Parenting; Attention Deficit Disorder; Birth-Related Disorders; Others

Reproductive Health: General; Infertility; Pregnancy; Others; Postpartum

Seniors

Sexuality Issues

Sleep Disorders

Substance Abuse—Drug/Alcohol

Teens

Women's Health: Menopause; Others

Miscellaneous Hotlines

HOTLINES/WEB SITES

Abuse: Physical, Sexual, Emotional, Spousal, Elder

Abuse Hotlines

Canadian Clearinghouse on Family Violence Information
1-800-FYI-3366

Childhelp USA Hotline
1-800-4-A-CHILD

National Domestic Violence Hotline
1-800-799-SAFE

Abuse Web Sites

Elder Abuse
www.elderabusecenter.org

Emotional Abuse
www.safechild.org

Physical Abuse
www.preventchildabuse.com/physical.htm

Sexual Abuse
wvw.rainn.org

Spousal Abuse
wvw.ndvh.org

AIDS/HIV

Education Hotlines

AIDS ETC (Education and Training Centers) Program
(301) 443-6364

AIDS Info
1-800-HIV-0440

Education Web Sites

AIDS Education Global Information System
www.aegis.com

New England AIDS Education and Training Center
www.neaetc.org

Women and Children Hotlines

Health Information Network—Women and AIDS
(206) 784-5655

National Resource Center on Women and AIDS
(202) 872-1770

Women and Children Web Sites

International Community of Women Living with HIV/AIDS
www.icw.org

Other Hotlines

AIDS Action Council
(202)530-8030

AIDS Health Project
(415) 476-3902

AIDS Health Service Program
(415)476-3902

AIDS National Hotline
1-800-342-4636

Canadian AIDS Society
(613)230-3580

CDC National Prevention Information Network
1-800-458-5231

CDC National STD Hotline
1-800-227-8922

Churches AIDS Task Force, National Council of
(212) 870-2228

Gay Men's Health Crisis Line
(212) 807-6655

People With AIDS, National Association of (NAPA)
(240) 247-0880

Protection and Advocacy—HIV/AIDS Advocacy Project
1-800-432-4682

Public Health Service AIDS Hotline
1-800-342-AIDS
1-800-232-4136
(Same as AIDS National Hotline)

Social Security Administration HIV/AIDS
1-800-772-1213

Teachers, American Federation of, HIV/AIDS Education Project
(202) 879-4490

Other Web Sites

AIDS Treatment News
www.aids.org

International AIDS Society
www.aidsonline.com

Johns Hopkins AIDS Service
www.hopkins-aids.edu

The Body: HIV/AIDS Information Resource
www.thebody.com

Bioterrorism

Bioterrorism Hotlines

CDC Bioterrorism Hotline
1-888-246-2675

Bioterrorism Web Sites

CDC Public Health Emergency Preparedness and Response
www.bt.cdc.gov

Center for the Study of Bioterrorism
www.bioterrorism.slu.edu

Cancer

Breast Cancer Hotlines

Komen Alliance (Breast Cancer Research)
1-800-IM-AWARE

Y-Me National Organization for Breast Cancer
1-800-221-2141

Breast Cancer Web Sites

National Alliance of Breast Cancer Organizations
www.nabco.org

National Breast Cancer Coalition
www.natlbcc.org

Susan G. Komen Breast Cancer Foundation
www.komen.org

Y-Me National Breast Cancer Organization
www.y-me.org

Chemotherapy Hotlines

Chemotherapy Foundation
(212) 213-9292

Chemotherapy Web Sites

Antimicrobial Agents & Chemotherapy
aac.asm.org

National Cancer Institute
www.cancer.gov

Hospice Hotlines

Foundation for Hospice and Homecare
(202) 547-7424

National Hospice Organization
1-800-658-8898

Hospice Web Sites

Hospice Foundation of America
www.hospicefoundation.org

Hospice Net
www.hospicenet.org

National Hospice & Palliative Care Organization
www.nhpco.org

Leukemia Hotline

Leukemia and Lymphoma Society of America
(914)949-5213

Leukemia Web Sites

Leukemia 8< Lymphoma Society
www.leukemia-lymphoma.org

Leukemia Links
www.acor.org/leukemia

Leukemia Research Foundation
www.leukemia-research.org

Lymphedema Hotline

National Lymphedema Network
1-800-541-3259

Lymphedema Web Sites

Circle of Hope Lymphedema Foundation
www.lymphedemacircleofhope.org

National Lymphedema Network
www.lymphnet.org

Ovarian Cancer Hotlines

Gilda Radner Familial Ovarian Cancer Registry
1-800-OVARIAN

Ovarian Cancer Web Sites

Gilda Radner Familial Ovarian Cancer Registry
www.ovariancancer.com

National Ovarian Cancer Coalition
www.ovarian.org

Ovarian Cancer National Alliance
www.ovariancancer.org

Prostate Cancer Hotlines

National Prostate Cancer Coalition
1-888-245-9455

Prostate Cancer Research Institute
(310)743-2110

Prostate Cancer Web Sites

National Prostate Cancer Coalition
www.4npcc.org

Prostate Cancer Research Institute
www.prostate-cancer.org

Skin Cancer Hotline

Skin Cancer Foundation
1-800-SKIN-490

Skin Cancer Web Sites

CDC Skin Cancer Page
www.cdc.gov/ cancer/nscpep/skin.htm

Melanoma ABC's
www.melanoma.com

Skin Cancer Foundation
www.skincancer.org

Cancer Support Group Hotlines

Exceptional Cancer Patients
(203)865-8392

National Coalition for Cancer Survivorship
(301) 650-9127

Reach to Recovery
1-800-4-CANCER

Cancer Support Group Web Sites

Cancer Information Network—Support Links
www. cancerlinksusa. com/support

Cancer News Support Group Links
www.cancernews.com/support.html

National Cancer Institute—Support Groups
http://cis.nci.nih.gov/fact/8_8.htm

Other Cancer Hotlines

AMC Cancer Information and Counseling Line
1-800-525-3777

American Cancer Society
1-800-227-2345

Cancer Control Society
(323) 663-7801

Cancer Information Service (Weekdays 9-4:30)
1-800-4-CANCER

Physician's Data Query (National Cancer Institute)
1-800-4-CANCER

R.A. Bloch Cancer Foundation
1-800-433-0464

Other Cancer Web Sites

American Cancer Society
www.cancer.org

Cancer Care
www.cancercare.org

National Cancer Institute
www.cancer.gov

OncoLink
www.oncolink.com

Disease Specific

Allergy Hotlines

Allergy & Asthma Network/Mothers of Asthmatics
1-800-878-4403

Allergy and Infectious Disease, Institute of
(301) 496-5717
(866)284-4107

Asthma and Allergy Information Hotline
1-800-7-ASTHMA

Allergy Specific Web Sites

American Academy of Allergy, Asthma, and Immunology
www.aaaai.org

Food Allergy and Anaphylaxis Network
www.foodallergy.org

Alzheimer Disease Hotlines

Alzheimer's Association
1-800-272-3900

Alzheimer's Disease Education and Referral Center
1-800-438-4380

Alzheimer Disease Web Sites

Alzheimer's Association
www.alz.org

Alzheimer's Disease Education and Referral Center
www.alzheimers.org

Alzheimer's Disease International
www.alz.co.uk

Arthritis Hotlines

Arthritis Foundation
1-800-283-7800

Juvenile Arthritis Foundation, American (AJAO)
(800) 283-7800

Arthritis Web Sites

Arthritis Foundation
www.arthritis.org

National Institute of Arthritis
http://catalog.niams.nih.gov

Online Arthritis Resource
www.arthritis.com

Asthma Hotlines

Allergy & Asthma Network/Mothers of Asthmatics
1-800-878-4403

American Lung Association
(212) 315-8700

Asthma and Allergy Foundation of America
1-800-822-2762

Asthma and Allergy Information Hotline
1-800-7-ASTHMA

Asthma Hotline
1-800-222-LUNG

Asthma Web Sites

Allergy & Asthma Network/Mothers of Asthmatics
www.aanma.org

American Academy of Allergy, Asthma and Immunology
www.aaaai.org

Asthma and Allergy Foundation of America
www.aafa.org

Communication Disorders Hotlines

Deafness and Other Communication Disorders, Institute on
1-800-241-1044

Neurological and Communicative Disorders, Institute of
(301) 496-9746

Speech-Language-Hearing, American Association of
1-800-638-8255

Stuttering, Center for
1-800-221-2483

Stuttering Foundation of America
(901) 452-0995
(800) 992-9392

Communication Disorders Web Sites

National Institute on Deafness and Other Communication Disorders
www.nidcd.nih.gov

Stuttering Foundation of America
www.stuttrsfa.org

Diabetes Hotlines

American Diabetes Association
1-800-342-2383

Diabetes Research Foundation, JFK International
1-800-223-1138

Juvenile Diabetes Foundation International
1-800-223-1138

Diabetes Web Sites

American Diabetes Association
www.diabetes.org

Children with Diabetes Online
www.childrenwithdiabetes.com

National Institute of Diabetes
www.niddk.nih.gov

Disabilities, Learning Hotlines

International Dyslexia Association
1-800-222-3123

Learning Disabilities, National Center for
(212) 545-7510

Disabilities, Learning Web Sites

LDOnline
www.ldonline.org

Learning Disabilities Association of America
www.ldantal.org

National Center for Learning Disabilities
www.ncld.org

Disabilities, Physical Hotlines

Amputee Foundation, American
(501)835-9290

Devereux Foundation-Treatment of the Handicapped
1-800-345-1292

Disabled Sports USA
(301) 217-0960

Orthotics and Prosthetics, American Academy of
(703)836-0788

Paralyzed Veterans of America
(202)872-1300

Disabilities, Physical Web Sites

Amputees in Motion
www.aimny.org

Disability Resources Online
www.disabilityresources.org

Medline Plus Amputee Information
www.nlm.nih.gov/medlineplus/amputees.html

National Organization on Disability
www.nod.org

Eye Care Web Sites

American Academy of Ophthalmology
www.aao.org

Eye Care Foundation
www.eyecarefoundation.org

Eye Care Info
www.eyecareinfo.com

Hearing Impairment Hotlines

Better Hearing Institute
(703)684-3391

Deaf, Association of the
(301) 587-1788

Deafness and Other Communication Disorders, Institute on
1-800-241-1044

Hearing and Speech Action, Association for
1-800-638-8255

International Hearing Society
1-800-521-5247

Self-Help for Hard of Hearing People
(301) 657-2248

Speech-Language-Hearing, American Association for
(301) 897-5700

Hearing Impairment Web Sites

Deafness/Hard of Hearing Links
http://deafness.about.com/mbody.htm

Deafness Research Foundation
www.drf.org

National Institute on Deafness and other Communication Disorders
www.nidcd.nih.gov

Heart Disease Hotlines

American Heart Association
1-800-242-8721

Heart Disease Research Foundation
(718) 649-6210

Heart Disease Web Sites

American Heart Association
www.americanheart.org

Congenital Heart Information Network
www.tchin.org

Nutrition, Health 8t Heart Disease
www.heart-health.org

Infectious Disease Hotline

Centers for Disease Control and Prevention (CDC)
1-888-246-2675

Infectious Disease Web Sites

CDC Emerging Infectious Diseases
www.cdc.gov/ncidod/eid

Infectious Diseases Society of America
www.idsociety.org

National Institute for Allergy & Infectious Diseases
www.niaid.nih.gov

Kidney Hotlines

Kidney Foundation
1-800-622-9010

Kidney Foundation Hotline
1-800-ACT-GIVE

Kidney Fund, American
1-800-638-8299

Kidney Patients, American Association of
1-800-749-2257

Polycystic Kidney Research Foundation
1-800 PKD-CURE

Urologic Disease, Inc., American Foundation for
(866) 746-4282

Kidney Web Sites

Kidney Foundation of Canada
www.kidney.ca

National Institute of Diabetes/Digestive/Kidney Disorders
www.niddk.nih.gov

National Kidney Foundation
www.kidney.org

Multiple Sclerosis Hotlines

Multiple Sclerosis Information
1-800-FIGHT-MS

Multiple Sclerosis Society
1-800-FIGHT-MS

Multiple Sclerosis Web Sites

Multiple Sclerosis Foundation
www.msfacts.org

Multiple Sclerosis International Federation
www.msif.org/language_choice.html

National Multiple Sclerosis Society
www.nmss.org

Parkinson Disease

Parkinson's Disease, American Association
1-800-223-2732

Parkinson's Disease Foundation
1-800-457-6676

Parkinson's Foundation
1-800-327-4545

Parkinson Disease Web Sites

American Parkinson's Disease Association
www.apdaparkinson.org

National Parkinson Foundation
www.parkinson.org

Parkinson's Disease Foundation
www.pdf.org

Psoriasis Hotline

Psoriasis, National Foundation
1-800-723-9166

Psoriasis Web Sites

American Academy of Dermatology
www.aad.org

National Psoriasis Foundation Homepage
www.psoriasis.org

Rehabilitation Hotlines

American Counseling Association
(703) 823-9800

Rehabilitation Association
(703)836-0850

Rehabilitation Web Sites

American Academy of Physical Medicine and Rehabilitation
www.aapmr.org

National Rehabilitation Information Center
www.naric.com

Scleroderma Hotlines

Scleroderma Foundation
1-800-722-4673

Scleroderma Research Foundation
1-800-441-CURE

Scleroderma Web Sites

International Scleroderma Network
rvww.sclero.org

Scleroderma Foundation
www.scleroderma.org

Sexually Transmitted Diseases Hotlines

CDC National STD Hotline
1-800-227-8922

National Sexually Transmitted Diseases Hotline
1-800-227-8923

Sexually Transmitted Diseases Web Sites

CDC STD Information
www.cdc.gov/std

Spinal Cord Injuries Hotlines

Christopher Reeve Paralysis Foundation
1-800-225-0292

Spinal Cord Injury Association
1-800-962-9629

Spinal Cord Injury Hotline
1-800-526-3456

Spinal Cord Society
(218) 739-5252

Spinal Cord Injuries Web Sites

Foundation for Spinal Cord Injury Prevention
www.fscip.org

National Spinal Cord Injury Association
www.spinalcord.org

Spinal Cord Injury Information Network
www.spinalcord.uab.edu

Visual Impairment Hotlines

American Foundation for the Blind
1-800-232-5463

Blind Veteran's Association
(202) 371-8880

Prevent Blindness American Information Center
1-800-331-2020

Visually Impaired, Association for Parents of the
1-800-562-6265

Visual Impairment Web Sites

American Foundation for the Blind
www.afb.org

Foundation Fighting Blindness
www.blindness.org

Prevent Blindness America
www.preventblindness.org

Other Disease-Specific Hotlines

ADD Warehouse Catalogue
1-800-233-9273

Alopecia Areata Foundation
(415) 456-4644

Amyotrophic Lateral Sclerosis Association
1-800-782-4747

Brain Injury Association, Family Helpline
1-800-444-6443

Cleft Palate-Craniofacial Association, American
(919) 933-9044

Craniofacial, Children's Association
1-800-535-3643

Crohn's and Colitis, Foundation for
1-800-932-2423

Cystic Fibrosis Foundation
1-800-FIGHT-CS

Digestive Disease National Coalition
(202) 544-7497

Down Syndrome, National Society
1-800-221-4602

Epilepsy Foundation of America
1-800-EFA-1000

False Memory Syndrome Foundation for
(214)940-1040

Fibromyalgia Network
1-800-853-2929

Fracture, American Association for
(602)254-9646

Headache Foundation
1-800-843-2256

Hemophilia, National Foundation (NHF)
1-800-42-HANDI

Hepatitis Foundation
1-800-891-0707

High Blood Pressure Information Line
1-800-575-WELL

Huntington's Disease Society of America
1-800-345-4372

Immunology and Respiratory Medicine, Jewish Center for
1-800-222-5864

Jaw Joints and Allied Musculoskeletal Disorders
(617)266-2550

Laryngectomies, International Association of
(404) 320-3333

Lupus Foundation of America
1-800-558-0121

Meniere's Network
1-800-545-4327

Muscular Dystrophy Association
1-800-572-1717

Neurofibromatosis Foundation
1-800-323-7938

Neurological Disorders and Stroke, Institute of
1-800-352-9424

Osteogenesis Imperfecta Foundation
1-800-981-2663

Osteoporosis Foundation
(202)223-2226

Ostomy, United Association for
1-800-826-0826

Pain, International Association for the Study of
(206) 547-6409

Rare Disorders, National Association for
1-800-999-NORD

Rheumatology, American College of
(404)633-3777

Shy-Drager Syndrome Support Group
(866) SDS-4999

Spondylitis Association of America
1-800-777-8189

Texas Back Institute
1-800-247-BACK

Thyroid, American Association
1-800-THYROID

Tourette's Syndrome Support/Information
1-800-237-0717

Emotional/Mental Health

Anxiety Disorders Hotlines

Anxiety Disorders Association of America
(240) 485-1001

National Mental Health Association
800-969-6642

Anxiety Disorders Web Sites

Anxiety Self-Help
www.anxietyselfhelp.com

Anxiety Disorders Association of America
wrvw.adaa.org

National Institute of Mental Health
www.nimh.nih.gov/anxiety/anxietymenu.cfm

Autism Hotlines

Autism Society of America
301-657-0881

Center for the Study of Autism
619-563-6840

Cure Autism Now Foundation
888-8AUTISM

Families for Early Autism Treatment
916-843-1536

National Alliance for Autism Research
888-777-NAAR

Unlocking Autism
225-665-7270

Autism Web Sites

Autism-PDD Resources Network
www.autism-pdd.net

Autism Society of America
www.autism-society.org

Center for the Study of Autism
www.autism.org

Families for Early Autism Treatment
www.feat.org

National Alliance for Autism Research
www.naar.org

Unlocking Autism
www.unlockingautism.org

Bipolar Disorder Hotline

Depression and Bipolar Support Alliance
800-826-3632

Bipolar Disorder Web Sites

Bipolar Significant Others (BPSO)
www.bpso.org

Child & Adolescent Bipolar Foundation (CABF)
www.bpkids.org

Depression and Bipolar Support Alliance
www.dbsalliance.org

Peer to Peer Support
www.harbor-of-refiige.org

Depression and Schizophrenia Hotlines

Depression After Delivery
(908)575-9121

Depression Awareness Recognition & Treatment (D/ART)
(301) 443-4140

Depressive and Bipolar Support Alliance
1-800-826-3632

National Alliance for Research on Schizophrenia and Depression
(516) 829-0091

National Foundation for Depressive Illness
1-800-248-4344

Phobias, Anxiety, National Center for the Treatment of
(202)363-7792

Depression and Schizophrenia Web Sites

Depression Alliance
www.depressionalliance.org

National Foundation for Depressive Illness
www.ifred.org

National Mental Health Association
www.depression-screening.org

Eating Disorders Hotlines

American Anorexia/Bulimia Association
(212) 575-6200

Bulimia Anorexia Self-Help (B.A.S.H.)
1-800-762-3334

Center for the Study of Anorexia and Bulimia
(212)595-3449

National Institute of Mental Health Eating Disorders
Program
(301) 496-1891

Eating Disorders Web Sites

Eating Disorders Association
www.edauk.com

National Eating Disorders Association
www.nationaleatingdisorders.org

Obsessive-Compulsive Disorder Hotlines

National Institute of Mental Health Obsessive Compulsive
Foundation
301-443-4513

Nations Voice on Mental Illness
800-950-6264

Obsessive Compulsive Foundation
203-315-2190

Obsessive-Compulsive Disorder Web Sites

Mental Health Channel
www.mentalhealthchannel.net/ocd

Nations Voice on Mental Illness
www.nami.org

Obsessive Compulsive Foundation
www.ocfoundation.on.org

Social Phobia Hotlines

Face to Face Online
www.socialanxiety.org

Social Phobia/Social Anxiety Association
www.socialphobia.org

Panic Disorder Hotlines

American Psychiatric Association
703-907-7300

American Psychological Association
212-336-5700

National Institute of Mental Health Panic Campaign
800-64-PANIC

Panic Disorder Web Sites

American Academy of Child & Adolescent Psychiatry
www.aacap.org

American Psychiatric Association
www.psych.org

American Psychological Association
www.apa.org

Panic Campaign
www.nimh.nih.gov

Other Emotional/Mental Health Hotlines

AMEND (Aiding Mothers and Fathers Experiencing
Neonatal Death)
(316) 268-8441

Covenant House (Crisis Hotline for Teens)
1-800-999-9999

Panic Disorder Line
1-800-64-PANIC

Post-Traumatic Stress Disorder, National Center for
(802)296-5132

Pregnancy and Infant Loss Center
(612)473-9372

Schizophrenia and Depression, National Alliance for
Research on
(516) 829-0091

Youth Crisis Hotline, National
1-800-HIT-HOME

Pain Management

Pain Management Hotlines

American Academy of Pain Management
(209) 533-9744

American Chronic Pain Association
800-533-3231

American Pain Foundation
888-615-7246

North American Chronic Pain Association of Canada
866-470-7246

Pain Management Web Sites

American Academy of Pain Management
www.aapainmanage.org

American Chronic Pain Association
www.theacpa.org

American Pain Foundation
www.painfoundation.org

Chronic Pain Foundation
www.nationalpainfoundation.org

Chronic Pain Support Group
www.chronicpainsupport.org

Partners Against Pain
www.partnersagainstpain.com(under construction)

Parent's Help

Parenting Hotlines

Parent Help-Line
800-543-6381

Parenting National Hotline
800-448-3000

Parenting Project
888-PARENTS

Parenting Web Sites

Parenting National Hotline
www.parenting.org

Parenting Project
www.parentingproject.org

Attention Deficit Disorder Hotlines

ADD Warehouse Catalogue
1-800-233-9273

Attention Deficit Disorder Action Group
212-769-2457

Attention Deficit Disorder Association
847-432-ADDA

Children 8c Adults with ADD/ADHD
800-233-4050

Attention Deficit Disorder Web Sites

Attention Deficit Disorder Action Group
www.addgroup.org

Attention Deficit Disorder Association
www.add.org

Children 8c Adults with ADD/ADHD
www.chadd.org

Birth-Related Disorders Hotlines

American Cleft Palate Education Foundation
800-242-5338

Association of Birth Defect Children
800-313-2232

Cystic Fibrosis Foundation
800-344-4823

National Down's Syndrome Society
800-221-4602

Spina Bifida Association of America
800-621-3141

Tay Sachs Foundation
800-672-2022

Birth-Related Web Sites

Birth Defects Research for Children
www.birthdefects.org

March of Dimes
www.modimes.org

National Birth Defects Prevention Network
www.nbdpn.org

Other Parent's Help Hotlines

Allergy 8c Asthma Network/Mothers of Asthmatics
1-800-878-4403

American Academy of Pediatrics
800-433-9016

Behaviorally Different Children, Parents of
1-800-273-PBDC

Child Care Information Service
1-800-424-2460

Child Safety Council (Missing 8c Kidnapped Children)
1-800-222-1464

Child Welfare League of America, Inc.
(202) 638-2952

Covenant House (Crisis Hotline for Teens)
1-800-999-9999

Disabilities, NICCYD-Center for Children with
1-800-695-0285

Exceptional Children, Council for
(703) 620-3660

Families Anonymous
1-800-736-9805

Family of the Americas Foundation
1-800-443-3395

Family Caregiver Alliance
(415) 434-3388

Immunization, National Campaign for
(202)338-7227

"Just Say No" Kids Club International
800-258-2766

March of Dimes
(914) 428-7100

Maternal and Child Health and Resources Development,
Bureau of
(301) 443-2170

Missing Children's Hotline
1-800-THE-LOST

Missing and Exploited Children, National Center for
1-800-843-5678

National Association for the Education of Young
Children
800-424-2460

Parents Without Partners
800-637-7974

Runaway Switchboard, National
1-800-621-4000

Shriner's Hospital Referral Line
800-237-5055

Sudden Infant Death Syndrome, National Foundation
(301) 459-3388

Tough Love International
800-333-1069

Visually Impaired, Association for the Parents of
1-800-562-6265

Reproductive Health

General Reproductive Health Hotlines

American Society for Reproductive Medicine
205-978-3000

CDC Reproductive Health Information Service
770-488-5200

Institute for Reproductive Health
202-687-1392

John Hopkins ReproLine
410-537-1800

General Reproductive Health Web Sites

American Society for Reproductive Health
www.asrm.org

CDC Reproductive Health Information Service
www.cdc.gov/nccdphp/drh

Institute for Reproductive Health
www.irh.org

John Hopkins ReproLine
www.reproline.jhu.edu

Infertility Hotlines

American Infertility Association
888-917-3777

Fertility Research Foundation
212-744-5500

International Council on Infertility Information
703-379-9178

Infertility Awareness Association of Canada
800-263-2929

National Infertility Association
888-623-0744

Infertility Network
416-691-3611

Reproductive Medicine, American Society for
(205) 978-3000

Infertility Web Sites

American Infertility Association
www.theafa.org

Fertility Plus
www.fertilityplus.org

Infertility Network
www.infertilitynetworkuk.org

Infertility Nook (Support)
www.thelaboroflove.com/forum/infertility

Infertility Resources
www.ihr.com/infertility

Infertility Support Network (Support)
www.infertilitynetworkuk.com

International Council on Infertility Information
Dissemination
www.inciid.org

National Fertility Association
www.resolve.org

Urology Channel (Male Infertility)
www.urologychannel.com/maleinfertility/index.shtml

Pregnancy Web Sites

Childbirth.org
www.childbirth.org

Online Birth Center
www.moonlily.com/obc

Parents Place
www.parentsplace.com

Pregnancy Place
www.pregnancyplace.com

Pregnancy Support
www.pregnancy.org

Pregnancy Today
www.pregnancytoday.com

Teen Pregnancy
www.teenpregnancy.org

Other Pregnancy Hotlines

Be Healthy, Inc. Positive Pregnancy and Parenting Fitness
1-800-433-5523

Bradley Method of Childbirth
1-800-4A BIRTH

Childbearing Centers, National Association of (NACC)
(215)234-8068

Childbirth Education, International Association
(952) 854-8660

Depression After Delivery
(908) 575-9121

DES Action
(510) 465-4011

DES Action Canada
1-800-482-1-DES

Easter Seal Society, Inc.
1-800-221-6827

Genetic Support Groups, Alliance of
1-800-336-GENE

Healthy Mothers, Healthy Babies Coalition
1-800-673-8444, Ext. 2458

March of Dimes
(914) 428-7100

Maternal and Child Health Clearinghouse, National
1-888-275-4772

Maternal and Child Health Programs, Association of
(202) 775-0436

Maternal and Child Health Resources Development, Bureau of
(301) 443-2170

Planned Parenthood Federation of America
(212)541-7800

Pregnancy and Infant Loss Center
(952) 473-9372

Safety Council (for information regarding accident prevention and safety suggestions)
1-800-621-7619

Other Pregnancy Websites

Pregnancy and Childbirth Information
www.childbirth.org

Pregnancy Information
www.pregnancy.org

Postpartum Hotlines

Depression After Delivery
800-944-4773

National Institute of Mental Health
301-496-9576

National Women's Health Information Center
800-994-9662

Postpartum Education for Parents
805-564-3888

Postpartum Web Sites

Pacific Postpartum Support Society
wwtv.postpartum.org

Postpartum Education for Parents
www.sbpep.org

Seniors

Seniors Hotlines

Aging, National Council on
1-800-424-9046

Aging, National Institute on (NIA)
(301)496-1752

Aging Research, Alliance for
(202)293-2856

Alzheimer's Support
1-800-272-3900

American Association of Retired Persons (AARP)
1-800-424-3410

Children of Aging Parents (CAPS)
1-800-227-7294

Eldercare Locator Line
1-800-677-1116

Medicare Hotline
1-800-638-6833

Older Women's League
(202)783-6686

Seniors Web Sites

ElderWeb—Online Eldercare Sourcebook
www.elderweb.com

National Council on Aging
www.ncoa.org

U.S. Administration on Aging
www.aoa.gov

Sexuality Issues

Sexuality Issues Hotlines

Gay and Lesbian Population, Pride Institute Treatment Center for
1-800-54-PRIDE

Gay Men's Health Crisis
(212) 807-6655

Sexaholics Anonymous
(615) 331-6230

Sexuality and Disability, Coalition on
(212) 242-3900

Sexuality Information and Education Council of the U.S.
(212) 819-9770

Sexually Transmitted Diseases Hotline, National
1-800-227-8922

Sexuality Issues Web Sites

Pride Institute
www.pride-institute.com

Sexaholics Anonymous
www.sa.org

Sexuality Education & Information Council of the United States
www.siecus.org

Sleep Disorders

Sleep Disorders Hotlines

American Academy of Sleep Medicine
(708)492-0930

Better Sleep Council (for general information about sleep)
(703)683-8371

Sleep Disorders Web Sites

American Academy of Sleep Medicine
www.aasmnet.org

National Center for Sleep Disorders Research
www.nhlbi.nih.gov/about/ncsdr

Sleepnet.com—Tips for Healthy Sleep
www.sleepnet.com

Substance Abuse: Drug/Alcohol

Alcohol Abuse Hotlines

Adult Children of Alcoholics
(310) 534-1815

Alcohol and Drug Helpline
1-800-821-4357

Alcohol and Drug Information, National Clearinghouse for
1-800-729-6686

Alcoholics Anonymous
(212) 870-3400

Alcoholism Center for Women
(213) 381-8500

Alcoholism and Drug Dependence, Inc., National Council on
1-800-622-CALL

Assisted Recovery
1-800-527-5344

Children of Alcoholics, National Association for
(301)468-0986

Drug 8c Alcohol Information Hotline
1-800-662-HELP

Mothers Against Drunk Driving (MADD)
1-800-438-6233

Women for Sobriety
(215) 536-8026

Alcohol Abuse Web Sites

Alcoholics Anonymous
www.alcoholics-anonymous.org

American Council on Alcoholism
www.aca-usa.org

National Institute on Alcohol Abuse and Alcoholism
www.niaaa.nih.gov

Drug Abuse Hotlines

Alcohol and Drug Information, National Clearinghouse for
1-800-729-6686

Alcoholism and Drug Dependence, Inc., National Council on
1-800-622-CALL

Cocaine Anonymous
(310) 559-5832

Co-Dependents Anonymous
(602) 277-7991

Drug 8c Alcohol Information Hotline
1-800-662-HELP

Drug Information Association
(215) 442-6100

Hazelden Center for Youth and Families
1-800-257-7810

Naranon Family Group Headquarters, Inc.
(212)496-4341

Narcotics Anonymous
(818)773-9999

Drug Abuse Web Sites
Narcotics Anonymous
www.na.org

National Clearinghouse for Alcohol and Drug Information
www.health.org

National Institute on Drug Abuse
www.nida.nih.gov

Teens

Teen Hotlines
Children of Alcoholics, National Association for
(301)468-0985

Covenant House (Crisis Hotline for Teens)
1-800-999-9999

Planned Parenthood Federation of America
(212) 541-7800

Youth Crisis Hotline, National
1-800-448-4663

Teen Web Sites
Covenant House
www.covenanthouse.org

National Youth Crisis Hotline
www.allaboutcounseling.com/crisis.hotlines.html

Teen Education and Crisis Hotline (TEACH)
www.teachhotline.org

Women's Health

Menopause Hotlines
American Menopause Foundation
212-714-2398

American Society for Reproductive Medicine
205-978-5000

Menopause Web Sites
American Menopause Foundation
www.americanmenopause.org

American Society for Reproductive Medicine
www.asrm.org

International Menopause Society
www.imsociety.org

Menopause Canada
wvw.menopausecanada.com

North American Menopause Society
www.menopause.org

Power Surge: Menopause Community
www.power-surge.com

Other Women's Health Hotlines
Depression After Delivery
(908) 575-9121

Endometriosis Association
(414)355-2200

Menopause Society, North American
(440)442-7550

Planned Parenthood Federation of America
(212) 541-7800

PMS Access
1-800-222-4767

Women's Health Research, Melpomene Institute for
(651) 642-1951

Women's Health Resource Center, National (NWHRC)
(877)986-9472

Women's Sports Foundation 1-800-227-3988

Other Women's Health Web Sites
National Women's Health Information Center
www.4woman.gov

North American Menopause Society
www.menopause.org

Society for Women's Health Research
www.womens-health.org

Miscellaneous Hotlines

Abortion Federation, National
(800)772-9100

Catholic Charities USA
(703) 549-1394

Center for Interpersonal Growth
1-800-699-8206

Consumer Nutrition Hotline
1-800-366-1655

Couple to Couple League (Interpersonal Relationships)
(513) 471-2000

Dietetic Association, American (ADA)
1-800-366-1655

Displaced Homemakers
1-800-432-9168

Food and Drug Administration
1-888-894-6361

Girls and Boys Town
1-800-448-3000

Patient Information and Education, National Council on
(301) 656-8565

TOPS (Take Off Pounds Sensibly)
(414) 482-4620

U.S. Dept, of Health and Human Services, Public Health
(877) 696-6775

APPENDIX F
Informational Resources

APPROVED ABBREVIATIONS AND SYMBOLS

AB	Abortion
Abd.	Abdomen
Ac	Acute
ACEP	America/College of Emergency Physicians
ADL	Activities of Daily Living
ADR	Adverse Drug Reaction
Adv	Advised
AF	Atrial Fibrillation
Agg-	Aggravated
AIDS	Acquired Immune Deficiency Syndrome
Alt.	Altered
AM	Before noon
Amt.	Amount
Ant.	Anterior
Anticoag.	Anticoagulant
Appt.	Appointment
ASA	Aspirin
ASAP	As Soon As Possible
Asp.	Aspiration
Assoc.	Associated
ASWB	Altered State of Well Being
A-V	Arterial Venous
AVED	Age, Veracity, Emotional State, Debilitation/ Distance
BCM	Birth Control Method
BCPs	Birth Control Pills
BE	Barium Enema
BF	Breastfeeding
BID	Twice a Day
BM	Bowel Movement
BP	Blood Pressure
BRAT	Diet of Bananas, Rice, Applesauce, Toast
C	Centigrade
Ca	Caller
CA	California
CF	Cystic Fibrosis
Char.	Character
CHD	Congenital Heart Defect
Chemo	Chemotherapy
CHF	Congestive Heart Failure
Circ.	Circulation; Circulatory
Cl	Client
CNS	Central Nervous System
c/o	Complains of
Comp.	Complication
Conj.	Conjunctiva
COPD	Chronic Obstructive Pulmonary Disease
Corn.	Corneal
CPD	Cephalopelvic Disproportion

CPS	Child Protective Services
CSF	Cerebrospinal Fluid
CV	Cardiovascular
CVA	Cardiovascular Accident
D&C	Dilation and Curettage
DIC	Disseminated Intravascular Coagulation
Disp	Disposition
Dk.	Dark
DKA	Diabetic Ketoacidosis
DM	Diabetes Mellitus
DPT	Diphtheria/Pertussis/Tetanus
DTS	Dysfunctional Thoracic Syndrome
DUB	Dysfunctional Uterine Bleeding
Dx	Diagnosis
ed.	Edition
Ed.	Editor
ED	Emergency Department
EEG	Electroencephalogram
e.g.	For example
EMD	Emergency Medical Dispatcher
Emerg	Emergent
Emot	Emotional
ENA	Emergency Nurses' Association
Ep-Barr	Epstein-Barr
Epi	Epinephrine
ERT	Estrogen Replacement Therapy
Esp.	Especially
EST	Established
ETOH	Alcohol
Exp.	Exposure
Expir.	Expiration, Expiratory
F	Fahrenheit
FA	Future Appt.
Fac.	Factor
FB	Foreign Body
Fri.	Friday
FUO	Fever of Unknown Origin
Fut	Future
Fx	Fracture
GC	Gonococcus
GE	Gastroesophageal
GI	Gastrointestinal
Gtts.	Drops
GYN	Gynecological
HCG	Pregnancy Test
HIB	*Haemophilus Influenzae* Type B
HIV	Human Immunodeficiency Virus
HPV	Human Papillomavirus
Hr, hr(s) Hour(s)	
HTN	Hypertension
Hx	History (of)

IAQ	Initial Assessment Questions	Post.	Posterior
ICP	Intracranial Pressure	Post-Op	After surgery
i.e.	That is	Pot.	Potential
IM	Intramuscular	PP	Postpartum
Immz	Immunization	Preg	Pregnancy
Info	Information	Pre-Op	Before Surgery
Inj-	Injury	Prev.	Previous
Insp.	Inspiration, Inspiratory	prn	As needed
Irreg.	Irregular	Prob.	Problem
IUD	Intrauterine Device	PROM	Premature Rupture of Membrane
IUGR	Intrauterine Growth Retardation	Psych.	Psychiatric
IV	Intravenous	Pt.	Patient
L&D	Labor and Delivery	Pul.	Pulmonary
LEEP	Loop Electrosurgical Excision Procedure	q	Every
LLQ	Left Lower Quadrant	QID	Four times a day
LMP	Last Menstrual Period	qt	Quart
Loc	Location	RDS	Respiratory Distress Syndrome
Lrg-	Large	Re:	Regarding
LUQ	Left Upper Quadrant	Rec.	Rectal
MD	Doctor	Reg.	Regular
Med(s)	Medication(s)	Rel.	Relieving
MI	Myocardial Infarction	Resp.	Respiratory
min	Minute(s)	Rheum.	Rheumatism; Rheumatoid
MMR	Measles/Mumps/Rubella	Risk Fx	Risk Factor(s)
mo	Month(s)	RLQ	Right Lower Quadrant
mod.	Moderate	RN	Registered Nurse
Mon.	Monday	R/O	Rule out
Mono	Mononucleosis	ROM	Range of Motion
MRI	Magnetic Resonance Imaging	RPR	Rapid Plasma Reagent (test for syphilis)
MVA	Motor Vehicle Accident	RR	Respiratory Rate
N/A	Not Applicable; when doesn't apply	R/T	Related to
Neg	Negative	RUQ	Right Upper Quadrant
NOC	Night	Rx	Prescription Medication
NPO	Nothing by mouth	SA	Self-Assessment
NSAIDs	Nonsteroidal Anti-Inflammatory Drugs	SAB	Spontaneous Abortion
Ntg	Nitroglycerin	Sat.	Saturday
N/V	Nausea/Vomiting	SBE	Subacute Bacterial Endocarditis
Obj.	Object	SDA	Same-Day Appointment
Occ.	Occasionally	sec	Second(s)
OD	Overdose	Sev.	Severe
OM	Otitis Media	SI	Supplemental Information
OPV	Oral Polio Vaccine	Sib.	Sibling
OTC	Over the Counter	SIDS	Sudden Infant Death Syndrome
OV	Office Visit	Sm.	Small
oz	Ounce	SOB	Short of Breath
P	After (post)	SQ	Subcutaneous
Per	Through	St	States
PHN	Public Health Nurse	STI	Sexually Transmitted Infection
PID	Pelvic Inflammatory Disease	Strep	Streptococcus
PIH	Pregnancy-Induced Hypertension	Sun.	Sunday
PM	After noon	Sx	Symptom
PND	Postnasal Drip	T	Temperature
PO	By mouth	TAB	Therapeutic Abortion
Poss.	Possible	TB	Tuberculosis

Tbsp.	Tablespoon		Wed.	Wednesday
Temp.	Temperature		w/in	Within
Thurs.	Thursday		Wk, wk(s)	Week(s)
TIA	Transient Ischemic Attack		WNL	Within Normal Limits
TID	Three times a day		w/o	Without
TM	Tympanic Membrane		Wt.	Weight
TMJ	Temporomandibular Joint		x	Times
Trnspt	Transportation		Yr, yr(s)	Year(s)
Tsp.	Teaspoon		#	Number
TSS	Toxic Shock Syndrome		O	Degree(s)
Tues.	Tuesday		/	Per; Or; And/or
Tx	Treatment		+	Plus or Positive
UC	Uterine Contraction		-	Negative
UCC	Urgent Care Clinic		±	Plus or minus; with or without
Urg.	Urgent		>	Greater than; increases
URI	Upper Respiratory Infection		<	Less than; decreases
UTI	Urinary Tract Infection		≥	Greater than or equal to
Vag.	Vaginal		≤	Less than or equal to
Veg.	Vegetable		A	Negative when response is "no"
w	With		®	Rectal

Protocol-Specific References

Abdomen Problem
Briggs, J. K. (2007). *Telephone Triage Protocols for Nurses.* New York: Wolters Kluwer.

Brunicardi, F. C., Andersen, D. K., Billiar, T. R., et al. (Eds.). (2005). *Schwartz's Principles of Surgery* (8th ed.). New York: McGraw-Hill Companies, Inc.

Goldman, L,, and Ausiello, D. (Eds.). (2007). *Cecil Medicine* (23rd ed.). Philadelphia: Elsevier Inc.

Karmath, B., Holden, M.D., Hussain, N. et al. (2004, April), Chest pain: Differentiating cardiac from noncardiac causes. *Hospital Physician,* 24-28.

Lafferty, S., and Baird, M. (2001). *Telenurse: Telephone Triage Protocols.* Albany, NY: Delmar Thomson Learning.

Long, V., and McMullen, P.C. (2003). *Telephone Triage for Obstetrics and Gynecology.* New York: Lippincott Williams and Wilkins.

Marx, J. A., Hockberger, R. S., Wall, R. M., et al. (Eds.). (2006). *Rosen's Emergency Medicine: Concepts and Clinical Practice* (6th ed.). Philadelphia: Mosby Elsevier.

Porter, R. D,, Kaplan, J. D., Homeier, B. P,, et al. (Eds.). (2006). *The Merck Manual of Diagnosis and Therapy* (18th ed.). Whitehouse Station, NJ: Merck and Co., Inc.

Teichman, J. M. (2004). Clinical Practice. Acute Renal Colic from Ureteral Calculus. *New England Journal of Medicine, 350,* 684-693.

Abuse
American Medical Association. (1992). Violence: A Compendium from JAMA, American Medical News and Specialty Journals of the AMA. *JAMA.* Chicago: American Medical Association.

Briggs, J. K. (2007). *Telephone Triage Protocols for Nurses.* New York: Wolters Kluwer.

Cowell, N. A., and Burgess, A. W. (Eds.). (1996). *Understanding Violence against Women.* Washington, DC: National Academy Press.

Jezierski, M. (1999). Family violence screening: Opportunities in prehospital settings. *Journal of Emergency Nursing,* 25(3), 201-205.

Lee, D., and Anderson, L. F. (1995). *Improving Your Community Clinic's Response to Domestic Violence.* Sacramento, CA: California Department of Health Services.

Lipscomb, G. H., et al. (1992). Male victims of sexual assault. *Journal of the American Medical Association, 267(22),* 3064-3066.

Markus, K. (1999, April 19). Reporting signs of abuse. *Nurse Week,* 13.

Reece, R. M. (1994). *Child Abuse: Medical Diagnosis and Management.* Philadelphia: Lea and Febiger.

Shea, C.A., Mahoney, M., and Lacey, J. K. M. (1997). Breaking through the barriers to domestic violence intervention. *American Journal of Nursing, 97(6),* 26-33.

West, C. M. (1999). *Partner Violence in Military Families.* Durham, NH: University of New Hampshire, Family Research Laboratory.

Winfrey, M. E., and Smith, A. R. (1999). The suspiciousness factor: Critical care nursing and forensics. *Critical Care Nursing, 22(1),* 1-7.

Back Problem
Briggs, J. K. (2007). *Telephone Triage Protocols for Nurses.* New York: Wolters Kluwer.

Goldman, L., and Ausiello, D. (Eds.). (2007). *Cecil Medicine* (23rd ed.). Philadelphia: Elsevier Inc.

Karmath, B., Holden, M.D., Hussain, N. et al. (2004, April). Chest pain: Differentiating cardiac from noncardiac causes. *Hospital Physician,* 24-28.

Lafferty, S., and Baird, M. (2001). *Telenurse: Telephone Triage Protocols.* Albany, NY: Delmar Thomson Learning.

Marx, J. A., Hockberger, R. S., Wall, R. M., et al. (Eds.). (2006). *Rosen's Emergency Medicine: Concepts and Clinical Practice* (6th ed.). Philadelphia: Mosby Elsevier.

Bowel Problem
Briggs, J. K. (2007). *Telephone Triage Protocols for Nurses.* New York: Wolters Kluwer.

Goldman, L., and Ausiello, D. (Eds.). (2007). *Cecil Medicine* (23rd ed.). Philadelphia: Elsevier Inc.

Lafferty, S., and Baird, M. (2001). *Telenurse: Telephone Triage Protocols.* Albany, NY: Delmar Thomson Learning.

Marx, J. A., Hockberger, R. S., Wall, R. M., et al. (Eds.). (2006). *Rosen's Emergency Medicine: Concepts and Clinical Practice* (6th ed.). Philadelphia: Mosby Elsevier.

Porter, R. D., Kaplan, J. D., Homeier, B. P., et al. (Eds.). (2006). *The Merck Manual of Diagnosis and Therapy* (18th ed.). Whitehouse Station, NJ: Merck and Co., Inc.

Thielman, N. M., and Guerrant, R. L. (2004). Clinical practice. Acute infectious diarrhea. *New England Journal of Medicine, 350,* 38.

Chest Pain

American Heart Association. (2008). Heart disease and stroke statistics—2008 update. Retrieved July 2, 2008, from http://www.americanheart.org/presenter.jhtml?identifier=3018163.

Briggs, J. K. (2007). *Telephone Triage Protocols for Nurses.* New York: Wolters Kluwer.

Calabro, J. J. (1977). Costochondritis. *New England Journal of Medicine, 296,* 946.

Chobanian, A. V., Bakris, G. L., Black, H. R., et al. (2003). Seventh report of the Joint National Committee on Prevention, Detection, Evaluation, and Treatment of High Blood Pressure. *Hypertension, 42(12)* 6-1252.

Epstein, S. E., Gerber, L. H., and Borer, J. S. (1979). Chest wall syndrome: A common cause of unexplained cardiac pain. *Journal of the American Medical Association, 241,* 2793-2797.

Fam, A. G., and Smythe, H. A. (1985). Musculoskeletal chest wall pain. *Canadian Medical Association Journal, 133(5),* 279-289.

Grundy, S. M., Cleeman, J. I., Bairey Merz, C. N., et al. (for the Coordinating Committee of the National Cholesterol Education Program). (2004). Implications of recent clinical trials for the National Cholesterol Education Program Adult Treatment Panel III guidelines endorsed by the National Heart, Lung, and Blood Institute, American College of Cardiology Foundation, and American Heart Association. *Circulation, 110,*227-239.

Karmath, B., Holden, M.D., Hussain, N. et al. (2004, April). Chest pain: Differentiating cardiac from non-cardiac causes. *Hospital Physician,* 24-28.

Lafferty, S., and Baird, M. (2001). *Telenurse: Telephone Triage Protocols.* Albany, NY: Delmar Thomson Learning.

National Cholesterol Education Program, National Heart, Lung, and Blood Institute, National Institutes of Health. (2002, September). *Third Report of the Expert Panel on the Detection, Evaluation, and Treatment of High Blood Cholesterol in Adults (Adult Treatment Panel III) Final Report* (NIH Publication No. 02-5214, VII1 -4). Washington, DC: U.S. Department of Health and Human Services.

National Institute of Diabetes and Digestive and Kidney Diseases. (2008). *National Diabetes Statistics, 2007 Fact Sheet.* Bethesda, MD: U.S. Department of Health and Human Services, National Institutes of Health.

Schocken, D., Benjamin, E., Fonarow, G., et al. (2008). Prevention of heart failure. A scientific statement from the American Heart Association Councils on Epidemiology and Prevention, Clinical Cardiology, Cardiovascular Nursing and High Blood Pressure Research; Quality of Care and Outcomes Research Interdisciplinary Working Group; and Functional Genomics and Translational Biology Interdisciplinary Working Group. *Circulation, 117,*2544-2564.

Wolf, E., and Stern, S. (1976). Costosternal syndrome: Its frequency and importance in differential diagnosis of coronary heart disease. *Archives of Internal Medicine, 136(2),* 189-191.

Cold Exposure

Briggs, J. K. (2007). *Telephone Triage Protocols for Nurses.* New York: Wolters Kluwer.

Lafferty, S., and Baird, M. (2001). *Telenurse: Telephone Triage Protocols.* Albany, NY: Delmar Thomson Learning.

Confusion

Briggs, J. K. (2007). *Telephone Triage Protocols for Nurses.* New York: Wolters Kluwer.

Lafferty, S., and Baird, M. (2001). *Telenurse: Telephone Triage Protocols.* Albany, NY: Delmar Thomson Learning.

Selwa, L. M., Ozuna, J., Taylor, L. et al. (2002). *Neuro-Triage Telephone Advice.* Boston: Butterworth Heinemann.

CPR

Dizziness and Fainting

Briggs, J. K. (2007). *Telephone Triage Protocols for Nurses.* New York: Wolters Kluwer.

Goldman, L., and Ausiello, D. (Eds.). (2007). *Cecil Medicine* (23rd ed.). Philadelphia: Elsevier Inc.

Huff, J. S,, Decker, W. W,, Quinn, J. V., et al. (2007). Clinical policy: Critical issues in the evaluation and management of adult patients presenting to the emergency department with syncope. *Annals of Emergency Medicine, 49,4,*431-440.

Karmath, B., Holden, M.D., Hussain, N. et al. (2004, Aprilfa 10]). Chest pain: Differentiating cardiac from non-cardiac causes. *Hospital Physician,* 24-28.

Marx, J. A., Hockberger, R. S., Wall, R. M., et al. (Eds.). (2006). *Rosen's Emergency Medicine: Concepts and Clinical Practice* (6th ed.). Philadelphia: Mosby Elsevier.

Porter, R. D,, Kaplan, J. D., Homeier, B. P., et al. (Eds.). (2006). *The Merck Manual of Diagnosis and Therapy* (18th ed.). Whitehouse Station, NJ: Merck and Co., Inc.

Selwa, L. M., Ozuna,J.,Taylor, L. et al. [all](2002). *Neuro-Triage Telephone Advice.* Boston: Butterworth Heinemann.

Ear Problem
Briggs, J. K. (2007). *Telephone Triage Protocols for Nurses.* New York: Wolters Kluwer.

Goldman, L., and Ausiello, D. (Eds.). (2007). *Cecil Medicine* (23rd ed.). Philadelphia: Elsevier Inc.

Lafferty, S., and Baird, M. (2001). *Telenurse: Telephone Triage Protocols.* Albany, NY: Delmar Thomson Learning.

Marx, J. A., Hockberger, R. S., Wall, R. M., et al. (Eds.). (2006). *Rosen's Emergency Medicine: Concepts and Clinical Practice* (6th ed.). Philadelphia: Mosby Elsevier.

National Institute of Health. (2000). *Sudden Deafness* (NIH publication 00-4757, rev. 2003). Bethesda, MD. National Institute of Health.

Porter, R. D., Kaplan, J. D., Homeier, B. P., et al. (Eds.). (2006). *The Merck Manual of Diagnosis and Therapy* (18th ed.). Whitehouse Station, NJ: Merck and Co., Inc.

Emotional Problem
American Academy of Child and Adolescent Psychiatry. (1999). *Being Prepared: Knowing When to Seek Help for Your Child* (No. 24). Bethesda, MD: American Academy of Child and Adolescent Psychiatry. Retrieved April 18, 2000, from http://www.aacap.org/publications/factsfam/ whenhelp.htm.

American Psychological Association. (2000). *Warning Signs: Recognizing Violence Warning Signs in Others.* Washington DC: American Psychological Association. Retrieved April 4, 2000, from http://www.helping.apa. org/warningsigns/recognizing.html.

Arem, R. (1999). *The Thyroid Solution: A Mind-Body Program for Beating Depression and Regaining Your Emotional and Physical Health.* New York: Ballantine.

Jamison, K. R. (1997). *An Unquiet Mind.* New York: Random House.

Jamison, K. R. (1999). *Night Falls Fast, Understanding Suicide.* New York: Alfred Knopf.

Joiner, T. E. (1999). Assessment of suicidality in outpatient practice. *Professional Psychology: Research and Practice*, 30(5), 447-453.

Kleespies, P. M., Deleppo, J. D., et al. (1999). Managing suicidal emergencies. *Professional Psychology; Research and Practice*, 30(54), 454-463.

Kleiman, K. R,, and Raskin, V. R. (1994). *This Isn't What I Expected: Overcoming Postpartum Depression.* New York: Bantam.

Matsakis, A. (1996). *I Can't Get over It: A Handbook for Trauma Survivors* (2nd ed.). Oakland, CA: New Harbinger Publishers.

Meyer, E. (2000). *Suicide Prevention by Phone, Conversation with Wheeler.* San Francisco: San Francisco Suicide Prevention.

National Institute of Mental Health. (1991). *Let's Talk about Depression.* Rockville, MD: National Institute of Mental Health. Retrieved April 20, 2000, from http://www.medscape.com/govmt/NIMH/patient/depre ssion/TalkAboutDepression.html.

National Institute of Mental Health. (1993). *Understanding Panic Disorder.* Rockville, MD: National Institute of Mental Health. Retrieved April 20, 2000, from http://www.medscape.com/govmt/NIMH/patient/Panic Disorder.html.

National Institute of Mental Health. (1994-2000). *Schizophrenia.* Rockville, MD: National Institute of Mental Health. Retrieved May 10, 2000, from http://www. medscape.com/govmt/NIMH/patient/schizophrenia. html.

National Institute of Mental Health. (1995). *Bipolar Disorder.* Rockville, MD: National Institute of Mental Health. Retrieved April 20,2000, from http://www.medscape.com/ govmt/IMH/patient/depression/BipolarDisorder.html.

National Institute of Mental Health. (1996). *Obsessive-Compulsive Disorder.* Rockville, MD: National Institute of Mental Health. Retrieved May 10, 2000, from http://www.medscape.com/govmt/NIMH/patient/Anxiety Disorders/ocd.html.

National Institute of Mental Health. (2000). *Depression in Children and Adolescents.* Office of Communications and Public Liaison. Rockville, MD: National Institute of Mental Health. Retrieved April 18, 2000, from http://www.nimh.nih.gov/publicat/depchildresfact.cfm.

Schwartz, J. M,, and Beyette, B. (1998). *Brain Lock, Free Yourself from Obsessive-Compulsive Behavior: A Four-Step Self-treatment Method to Change Your Brain Chemistry.* New York: Harper.

Torrey, E. F. (1995). *Surviving Schizophrenia: A Manual for Families, Consumers and Providers* (3rd ed.). New York: Harper-Perennial Library.

West, J. W., and Ford, B. (1997). *The Betty Ford Center Book of Answers: Help for Those Struggling with Substance Abuse and for the People Who Love Them.* Las Vegas, NV: Pocket Books.

Wilson, R. R. (1996). *Don't Panic: Taking Control of Anxiety Attacks.* New York: HarperCollins.

Extremities Problem
Briggs, J. K. (2007). *Telephone Triage Protocols for Nurses.* New York: Wolters Kluwer.

Goldman, L., and Ausiello, D. (Eds.). (2007). *Cecil Medicine* (23rd ed.). Philadelphia: Elsevier Inc.

Hagen, K. B., Hilde, G., Jamtvedt, G., and Winnem, M. (2004). Bed rest for acute low-back pain and sciatica. *Cochrane Database of Systematic Reviews,* 3(CD001254).

Karmath, B., et al. (2004, April). Chest pain: Differentiating cardiac from non-cardiac causes. *Hospital Physician,* 24-28.

Lafferty, S., and Baird, M. (2001). *Telenurse: Telephone Triage Protocols.* Albany, NY: Delmar Thomson Learning.

Marx,). A., Hockberger, R. S., Wall, R. M., et al. (Eds.). (2006). *Rosen's Emergency Medicine: Concepts and Clinical Practice* (6th ed.). Philadelphia: Mosby Elsevier.

Porter, R. D., Kaplan, J. D., Homeier, B. P., et al. (Eds.). (2006). *The Merck Manual of Diagnosis and Therapy* (18th ed.). Whitehouse Station, NJ: Merck and Co., Inc.

Selwa, L. M., et al. (2002). *Neuro-Triage Telephone Advice.* Boston: Butterworth Heinemann.

Eye Problem
Briggs, J. K. (2007). *Telephone Triage Protocols for Nurses.* New York: Wolters Kluwer.

Goldman, L., and Ausiello, D. (Eds.). (2007). *Cecil Medicine* (23rd ed.). Philadelphia: Elsevier Inc.

Lafferty, S., and Baird, M. (2001). *Telenurse: Telephone Triage Protocols.* Albany, NY: Delmar Thomson Learning.

Marx, J. A., Hockberger, R. S., Wall, R. M., et al. (Eds.). (2006). *Rosen's Emergency Medicine: Concepts and Clinical Practice* (6th ed.^Philadelphia: Mosby Elsevier.

Porter, R. D., Kaplan, J. D., Homeier, B. P., et al. (Eds.). (2006). *The Merck Manual of Diagnosis and Therapy* (18th ed.). Whitehouse Station, NJ: Merck and Co., Inc.

Selwa, L. M., et al. (2002). *Neuro-Triage Telephone Advice.* Boston: Butterworth Heinemann.

Face/Jaw Problem
Bennetto, L., Patel, N. K., and Fuller, G. (2007). Trigeminal neuralgia and its management. *British Medical Journal, 334,* 201-205.

Briggs, J. K. (2007). *Telephone Triage Protocols for Nurses.* New York: Wolters Kluwer.

Gilden, D.H. (2004). Clinical practice. Bell's Palsy. *New England Journal of Medicine, 351,* 1323.

Goldman, L., and Ausiello, D. (Eds.). (2007). *Cecil Medicine* (23rd ed.). Philadelphia: Elsevier Inc.

Karmath, B,, et al. (2004, April). Chest pain: Differentiating cardiac from non-cardiac causes. *Hospital Physician,* 24-28.

Lafferty, S., and Baird, M. (2001).*Telenurse: Telephone Triage Protocols.* Albany, NY: Delmar Thomson Learning.

Marx, J. A., Hockberger, R. S., Wall, R. M,, et al. (Eds.). (2006). *Rosen's Emergency Medicine: Concepts and Clinical Practice* (6th ed.). Philadelphia: Mosby Elsevier.

Porter, R. D., Kaplan, J. D., Homeier, B. P., et al. (Eds.). (2006). *The Merck Manual of Diagnosis and Therapy* (18th ed.). Whitehouse Station, NJ: Merck and Co., Inc.

Selwa, L. M., et al. (2002). *Neuro-triage Telephone Advice.* Boston: Butterworth Heinemann

Fever
Briggs, J. K. (2007). *Telephone Triage Protocols for Nurses.* New York: Wolters Kluwer.

Goldman, L., and Ausiello, D. (Eds.). (2007). *Cecil Medicine* (23rd ed.). Philadelphia: Elsevier Inc.

Lafferty, S., and Baird, M. (2001).*Telenurse: Telephone Triage Protocols.* Albany, NY: Delmar Thomson Learning.

Mandell, G. L., Bennett, J. E., and Dolin, R, (Eds.) (2005). *Principles and Practices of Infectious Diseases* (6th ed.). Philadelphia: Elsevier Churchill Livingstone.

Marx, J. A., Hockberger, R. S., Wall, R. M., et al. (Eds.). (2006). *Rosen's Emergency Medicine: Concepts and Clinical Practice* (6th ed.). Philadelphia: Mosby Elsevier.

Porter, R. D., Kaplan, J. D., Homeier, B. P., et al. (Eds.). (2006). *The Merck Manual of Diagnosis and Therapy* (18th ed.). Whitehouse Station, NJ: Merck and Co., Inc.

Head Problem
Briggs, J. K. (2007). *Telephone Triage Protocols for Nurses.* New York: Wolters Kluwer.

Fitch, M. T., and van de Beek, D. (2007). Emergency diagnosis and treatment of adult meningitis. *Lancet Infectious Diseases, 7,*191.

Goldman, L., and Ausiello, D. (Eds.). (2007). *Cecil Medicine* (23rd ed.). Philadelphia: Elsevier Inc.

Kasper, D. L., Braunwald, E., Hauser, S., Longo, D., Jameson, J. L,, and Fauci, A. S. (Eds.). (2004). *Harrison's Principles of Internal Medicine* (16th ed.). New York: McGraw-Hill.

Lafferty, S., and Baird, M. (2001).*Telenurse: Telephone Triage Protocols.* Albany, NY: Delmar Thomson Learning.

Lipton, R. B., et al. (2004). Classification of primary headaches, *Neurology, 63,*427-435.

Marx, J. A., Hockberger, R. S., Wall, R. M., et al. (Eds.). (2006). *Rosen's Emergency Medicine: Concepts and Clinical Practice* (6th ed.). Philadelphia: Mosby Elsevier.

Porter, R. D., Kaplan, J. D,, Homeier, B. P., et al. (Eds.). (2006). *The Merck Manual of Diagnosis and Therapy* (18th ed.). Whitehouse Station, NJ: Merck and Co., Inc.

Ropper, A., and Gorson, K. C. (2007). Concussion, *New England Journal of Medicine, 356(2),* 166-172.

Selwa, L. M., et al. (2002). *Neuro-triage Telephone Advice.* Boston: Butterworth Heinemann.

Heat Exposure
Briggs, J. K. (2007). *Telephone Triage Protocols for Nurses.* New York: Wolters Kluwer.

Joint Problem
Briggs, J. K. (2007). *Telephone Triage Protocols for Nurses.* New York: Wolters Kluwer.

Lafferty, S., and Baird, M. (2001). *Telenurse: Telephone Triage Protocols.* Albany, NY: Delmar Thomson Learning.

Michota, F.A., Jr., M.D., (Eds.) (2001). *Diagnostic Procedures Handbook* (2nd ed.). Hudson, OH: Lexi-Comp, Inc.

Skinner, H.B. (Ed.) (2000). *Current Diagnosis & Treatment in Orthopedics* (2d ed.). New York: McGraw-Hill.

Lip/Mouth; Teeth/Gums; Tongue Problem
Briggs, J. K. (2007). *Telephone Triage Protocols for Nurses.* New York: Wolters Kluwer.

Goldman, L., and Ausicllo, D. (Eds.). (2007). *Cecil Medicine* (23rd ed.). Philadelphia: Elsevier Inc.

Lafferty, S., and Baird, M. (2001). *Telenurse: Telephone Triage Protocols.* Albany, NY: Delmar Thomson Learning.

Marx, J. A., Hockberger, R. S., Wall, R. M,, et al. (Eds.). (2006). *Rosen's Emergency Medicine: Concepts and Clinical Practice* (6th ed.). Philadelphia: Mosby Elsevier.

Pigman, E. C., and Scott, J. L. (1993). Angioedema in the emergency department: The impact of angiotensin-converting enzyme inhibitors. *American Journal of Emergency Medicine, Il(*4), 350-354.

Porter, R. D., Kaplan, J. D., Homeier, B. P., et al. (Eds.). (2006). *The Merck Manual of Diagnosis and Therapy* (18th ed.). Whitehouse Station, NJ: Merck and Co., Inc.

Neck Problem
Briggs, J. K. (2007). *Telephone Triage Protocols for Nurses.* New York: Wolters Kluwer.

Goldman, L., and Ausiello, D. (Eds.). (2007). *Cecil Medicine* (23rd ed.). Philadelphia: Elsevier Inc.

Karmath, B., et al. (2004, April). Chest pain: Differentiating cardiac from non-cardiac causes. *Hospital Physician,* 24-28.

Lafferty, S., and Baird, M. (2001). *Telenurse: Telephone Triage Protocols.* Albany, NY: Delmar Thomson Learning.

Marx, J. A., Hockberger, R. S., Wall, R. M., et al. (Eds.). (2006). *Rosen's Emergency Medicine: Concepts and Clinical Practice* (6th ed.). Philadelphia: Mosby Elsevier.

Porter, R. D., Kaplan, J. D,, Homeier, B. P., et al. (Eds.). (2006). *The Merck Manual of Diagnosis and Therapy* (18th ed.). Whitehouse Station, NJ: Merck and Co., Inc.

Selwa, L. M., et al. (2002). *Neuro-triage Telephone Advice.* Boston: Butterworth Heinemann.

Nose/Sinus Problem
Briggs, J. K. (2007). *Telephone Triage Protocols for Nurses.* New York: Wolters Kluwer.

Goldman, L., and Ausiello, D. (Eds.). (2007). *Cecil Medicine* (23rd ed.). Philadelphia: Elsevier Inc.

Kucik, C. J., and Clenney, T. (2005). Management of epistaxis. *American Family Physician, 71,* 305.

Lafferty, S., and Baird, M. (2001). *Telenurse: Telephone Triage Protocols.* Albany, NY: Delmar Thomson Learning.

Marx, J. A., Hockberger, R. S., Wall, R. M., et al. (Eds.). (2006). *Rosen's Emergency Medicine: Concepts and Clinical Practice* (6th ed.). Philadelphia: Mosby Elsevier.

Piccirillo, J. F. (2004, August). Acute bacterial sinusitis. *New England Journal of Medicine 351,* 902-910.

Porter, R. D., Kaplan, J. D., Homeier, B. P., et al. (Eds.). (2006). *The Merck Manual of Diagnosis and Therapy* (18th ed.). Whitehouse Station, NJ: Merck and Co., Inc.

Snow, V., et al. (2001). Position paper endorsed by the American Academy of Family Physicians, the American College of Physicians-American Society of Internal Medicine, and the Infectious Diseases Society of America. *Annals of Internal Medicine, 134,* 495.

Penile/Scrotal/Testicle Problem
Briggs, J. K. (2007). *Telephone Triage Protocols for Nurses.* New York: Wolters Kluwer.

Lafferty, S., and Baird, M. (2001). *Telenurse: Telephone Triage Protocols.* Albany, NY': Delmar Thomson Learning.

Marx, J. A., Hockberger, R. S., Wall, R. M., et al. (Eds.). (2006). *Rosen's Emergency Medicine: Concepts and Clinical Practice* (6th ed.). Philadelphia: Mosby Elsevier.

Mueller, N. M. (Ed.). (2000). *Telephone Nursing Practice in Adult Urology. A Manual for Urology Nurses.* Pitman, NJ: Society of Urologic Nurses and Associates.

Rosenstein, D., and McAninch, J. W. (2004). Urologic emergencies. *Medical Clinics of North America, 88,* 495.

Workowski, K. A., and Berman, S. M. (2006). Sexually transmitted diseases treatment guidelines. *MMWR Recommendations and Reports,* 55,1-94.

Rectal Problem
Bharucha, A., Wald, A., Enck, P., and Rao, S. (2006). Functional anorectal disorders. *Gastroenterology, 130,* 1510.

Briggs, J. K. (2007). *Telephone Triage Protocols for Nurses.* New York: Wolters Kluwer.

Brunicardi, F. C., Andersen, D. K., Billiar, T. R., et al. (Eds.). (2005). *Schwartz's Principles of Surgery* (8th ed.). New York: McGraw-Hill Companies, Inc.

Goldman, L., and Ausiello, D. (Eds.). (2007). *Cecil Medicine* (23rd ed.). Philadelphia: Elsevier Inc.

Lafferty, S., and Baird, M. (2001). *Telenurse: Telephone Triage Protocols.* Albany, NY: Delmar Thomson Learning.

Marx, J. A., Hockberger, R. S,, Wall, R. M,, et al. (Eds.). (2006). *Rosen's Emergency Medicine: Concepts and Clinical Practice* (6th ed.). Philadelphia: Mosby Elsevier.

Porter, R. D., Kaplan, J. D,, Homeier, B. P., et al. (Eds.). (2006). *The Merck Manual of Diagnosis and Therapy* (18th ed.). Whitehouse Station, NJ: Merck and Co., Inc.

Respiratory Problem
Briggs, J. K. (2007). *Telephone Triage Protocols for Nurses.* New York: Wolters Kluwer.

Karmath, B., et al. (2004, April). Chest pain: Differentiating cardiac from non-cardiac causes. *Hospital Physician,* 24-28.

Lafferty, S., and Baird, M. (2001). *Telenurse: Telephone Triage Protocols.* Albany, NY: Delmar Thomson Learning.

Shock
Briggs, J. K. (2007). *Telephone Triage Protocols for Nurses.* New York: Wolters Kluwer.

Seizures
Briggs, J. K. (2007). *Telephone Triage Protocols for Nurses.* New York: Wolters Kluwer.

Skin Problem: Bites/Stings
Briggs, J. K. (2007). *Telephone Triage Protocols for Nurses.* New York: Wolters Kluwer.

Lafferty, S., and Baird, M. (2001). *Telenurse: Telephone Triage Protocols.* Albany, NY: Delmar Thomson Learning.

Skin Problem: Burns
Briggs, J. K. (2007). *Telephone Triage Protocols for Nurses.* New York: Wolters Kluwer.

Lafferty, S., and Baird, M. (2001). *Telenurse: Telephone Triage Protocols.* Albany, NY: Delmar Thomson Learning.

Skin Problem: Discoloration
Briggs, J. K. (2007). *Telephone Triage Protocols for Nurses.* New York: Wolters Kluwer.

Lafferty, S., and Baird, M. (2001). *Telenurse: Telephone Triage Protocols.* Albany, NY: Delmar Thomson Learning.

Skin Problem: Laceration/Wound
Briggs, J. K. (2007). *Telephone Triage Protocob for Nurses.* New York: Wolters Kluwer.

Lafferty, S., and Baird, M. (2001). *Telenurse: Telephone Triage Protocob.* Albany, NY: Delmar Thomson Learning.

Skin Problem: Lesion/Lump/Swelling
Briggs, J. K. (2007). *Telephone Triage Protocols for Nurses.* New York: Wolters Kluwer.

Lafferty, S., and Baird, M. (2001). *Telenurse: Telephone Triage Protocols.* Albany, NY: Delmar Thomson Learning.

Skin Problem: Rashes
Briggs, J. K. (2007). *Telephone Triage Protocols for Nurses.* New York: Wolters Kluwer.

Lafferty, S., and Baird, M. (2001). *Telenurse: Telephone Triage Protocols.* Albany, NY: Delmar Thomson Learning.

Skin Problems: All
MRSA, Frequently Asked Questions. San Francisco Department of Public Health Communicable Disease Control and Prevention. Retrieved July 7, 2008, from http://www.sfcdcp.org/index.cfm?id=100.

Weber, D. J., Cohen, M. S., and Rutala, W. (2005). The acutely ill patient with fever and rash. In G. L. Mandell, J. E. Bennett, and R. Dolin (Eds.), *Principles and practices of infectious diseases* (6th ed.) (p. 729). Philadelphia: Elsevier Churchill Livingstone.

Zetola, N., Francis, J. S., Nuermberger, E. L., and Bishai, W. R. (2005). Community-acquired meticillin-resistant *Staphylococcus aureus:* An emerging threat. *Lancet Infectious Diseases, 5,* 275.

Substance Abuse Problem
Briggs, J. K. (2007). *Telephone Triage Protocob for Nurses.* New York: Wolters Kluwer.

Lafferty, S., and Baird, M. (2001). *Telenurse: Telephone Triage Protocols.* Albany, NY: Delmar Thomson Learning.

American Academy of Family Physicians. (2003). *Problem Drinking—How to Recognize It.* http://Familydoctor. Org/Handouts/755.Html. Retrieved July 17, 2003.

American Academy of Pediatrics. (2003). *Common Inhalants.* http://Search.Nlm.Nih.Gov/Medlineplus/Query? Disambiguation=True&Function=Search&Server2=Server2 &Server 1 =Server 1 &Parameter=Inhalants&X=21 &Y= 12. Retrieved July 17,2003.

American College of Obstetricians and Gynecologists. (2002). *Illegal Drugs and Pregnancy.* http://Www.Medem. Com/Medlb/Article-_Detaillb.Cfm?Article_Id=Zzzn0x8997c &Sub_Cat=2005. Retrieved July 17,2003.

Mayo Clinic.Com. (2001). *Date-Rape Drugs: Keep an Eye on That Drink.* http://www.Mayoclinic.Com/Invoke. Cfm?Id=Hq00507. Retrieved July 17, 2003.

National Institute on Alcohol Abuse and Alcoholism. (1998). *Alcohol Alert: Alcohol and Sleep.* http://www. Niaaa.Nih.Gov/Publications/Aa41-Text.Htm. Retrieved July 17, 2003.

National Institute on Alcohol Abuse and Alcoholism. (2002). *Alcoholism: Getting the Facts.* http://www.Niaaa. Nih.Gov/Publications/Booklet.Htm. Retrieved July 17, 2003.

National Institute on Alcohol Abuse and Alcoholism. (2002). *FAQs on Alcohol Abuse and Alcoholism.* http://www.Niaaa.Nih.Gov/Publications/Booklet.Htm. Retrieved July 17,2003.

National Institute on Drug Abuse. (2003). *Club Drugs.* http://www.Nida.Nih.Gov/Infofax/Clubdrugs.Html. Retrieved July 17, 2003.

National Institute on Drug Abuse. (2003). *Heroin.* http://www.Nida.Nih.Gov/Infofax/Heroin.Html. Retrieved July 17, 2003.

National Institute on Drug Abuse. (2003). *Research Report Series—Methamphetamine Abuse and Addiction.* http://www.Nida.Nih.Gov/Research-Reports/ Methamph/Methamph.Html. Retrieved July 17, 2003.

National Institute on Drug Abuse. (2002). *Research Report Series—Prescription Drugs: Abuse and Addiction.* http://www.Nida.Nih.Gov/Research-Reports/Prescription/ Prescritption.Html. Retrieved July 17, 2003.

Peck, P. (2003). *Senior Drinking, Drug Abuse often Missed.* UPI Science News Web site. http://www.Nlm.Nih. Gov/Medlineplus/News/Fullstory-_13395.Html. Retrieved July 17,2003.

Waldron, T. (2003). *Sniffing, Snorting Drugs May Raise Hepatitis C Risk.* Reuters Health Information Web site. http://www.Nlm.Nih.Gov/Medlineplus- News/Fullstory_13262.Html. Retrieved July 17,2003.

Urinary Problem

Fihn, S. D. (2003). Clinical practice. Acute uncomplicated urinary tract infection in women. A practical overview. *New England Journal of Medicine; 349,* 259-266.

Goldman, L., and Ausiello, D. (Eds.). (2007). *Cecil Medicine* (23rd ed.). Philadelphia: Elsevier Inc.

Lafferty, S., and Baird, M. (2001). *Telenurse: Telephone Triage Protocols.* Albany, NY: Delmar Thomson Learning.

Long, V., and McMullen, P.C. (2003). *Telephone Triage for Obstetrics and Gynecology.* New York: Lippincott Williams and Wilkins.

Marx, J. A., Hockberger, R. S., Wall, R. M., et al. (Eds.). (2006). *Rosen's Emergency Medicine: Concepts and Clinical Practice* (6th ed.). Philadelphia: Mosby Elsevier.

Mueller, N. M. (Ed.). (2000). *Telephone Nursing Practice in Adult Urology. A Manual for Urology Nurses.* Pitman, NJ: Society of Urologic Nurses and Associates.

Porter, R. D., Kaplan, J. D., Homeier, B. P., et al. (Eds.). (2006). *The Merck Manual of Diagnosis and Therapy* (18th ed.). Whitehouse Station, NJ: Merck and Co., Inc.

Vomiting/Nausea

Briggs, J. K. (2007). *Telephone Triage Protocols for Nurses.* New York: Wolters Kluwer.

Goldman, L., and Ausiello, D. (Eds.). (2007). *Cecil Medicine* (23rd ed.). Philadelphia: Elsevier Inc.

Hasler, W. L., and Chey, W. D. (2003). Nausea and vomiting. *Gastroenterology, 125,* 1860.

Karmath, B., et al. (2004, April). Chest pain: Differentiating cardiac from non-cardiac causes. *Hospital Physician,* 24-28.

Marx, J. A., Hockberger, R. S., Wall, R. M., et al. (Eds.). (2006). *Rosen's Emergency Medicine: Concepts and Clinical Practice* (6th cd.). Philadelphia: Mosby Elsevier.

Mehler, P. S. (2003). Clinical practice. Bulimia nervosa. *New England Journal of Medicine, 349,* 875.

Porter, R. D., Kaplan, J. D,, Homeier, B. P., et al. (Eds.). (2006). *The Merck Manual of Diagnosis and Therapy* (18th ed.). Whitehouse Station, NJ: Merck and Co., Inc.

Selwa, L. M., et al. (2002). *Neuro-triage Telephone Advice.* Boston: Butterworth Heinemann.

Women's Health

Birth Control Options
ACOG Practice Bulletin #69: Emergency Contraception. (2005). *Obstetrics and Gynecology, 106,* 1443.

Long, V., and McMullen, P.C. (2003). *Telephone Triage for Obstetrics and Gynecology.* New York: Lippincott Williams and Wilkins.

Petitti, D. B. (2003). Clinical practice. Combination estrogen-progestin oral contraceptives. *New England Journal of Medicine, 349,* 1443.

WHO Birth Control Summary, (n.d.). Retrieved July 9, 2008, from http://www.who.int/reproductive-health/ publications/mec/summary.html.

Breast Problem
Briggs, J. K. (2007). *Telephone Triage Protocols for Nurses.* New York: Wolters Kluwer.

Long.V., and McMullen P. C. (2003). *Telephone Triage for Obstetrics and Gynecology.* New York: Lippincott Williams & Wilkins.

Santen, R., and Mansel, R. (2005). Benign breast disorders. *New England Journal of Medicine, 353,* 275-285.

Smith, R. L., Pruthi, S., and Fitzpatrick, L. A. (2004). Evaluation and management of breast pain. *Mayo Clinic Proceedings, 79,* 353.

Breastfeeding Problem
Gartner, L. M., Morton, J., Lawrence, R. A., et al. (2005). Breastfeeding and the use of human milk *Pediatrics, 115,*496.

La Leche League. Web site, www.llli.org. 8/8/2008

Lawrence, R. A., and Lawrence R. M. (2005). *Breastfeeding: A Guide for the Medical Professions* (5 th ed.). St Louis: Mosby.

Long, V., and McMullen, P.C. (2003). *Telephone Triage for Obstetrics and Gynecology.* New York: Lippincott Williams & Wilkins.

Menopause Options
Executive summary. (2004). Hormone therapy. *Obstetrics and Gynecology, 104,* IS.

Grady, D., Herrington, D., Bittner, V., et al. (2002). Cardiovascular disease outcomes during 6.8 years of hormone therapy: Heart and Estrogen/progestin Replacement Study follow-up (HERS II). *Journal of the American Medical Association, 288,* 49.

Long.V., and McMullen, P. C. (2003). *Telephone Triage for Obstetrics and Gynecology.* New York: Lippincott Williams and Wilkins.

USPSTF guidelines for hormone replacement therapy. (2007). Retrieved July 9, 2008, from www.ahrq. gov/clinic/uspstfix.htm

Postpartum Problem
Brockington, I. (2004). Postpartum psychiatric disorders. *Lancet,* 363,303.

Cunningham, F. G., Hauth, J. C., Leveno, K. J., Gilstrap III, L., and Bloom, S. L. (Eds.). (2005). *Williams Obstetrics* (22nd ed.). New York: McGraw-Hill.

Long.V., and McMullen, P.C. (2003). *Telephone Triage for Obstetrics and Gynecology.* New York: Lippincott Williams and Wilkins.

Marx, J. A., Hockberger, R. S., Wall ,R. M., et al. (Eds.). (2006). *Rosen's Emergency Medicine: Concepts and Clinical Practice* (6th ed.). Philadelphia: Mosby Elsevier.

Pregnancy Problem
Creasy, R.K., and Resnik, R. (1999). *Maternal-Fetal Medicine.* (4th ed.). Philadelphia: W.B. Saunders.

Cunningham, F. G., Hauth, J. C., Leveno, K. J., Gilstrap III, L., and Bloom, S. L. (Eds.). (2005). *Williams Obstetrics* (22nd ed.). New York: McGraw-Hill.

Long, V., and McMullen, P. C. (2003). *Telephone Triage for Obstetrics and Gynecology.* New York: Lippincott Williams and Wilkins.

Marin County Women's Health. (1998). *Common Discomforts of Pregnancy.* San Rafael, CA: Marin County Women's Health.

Oyelese, Y., and Ananth, C. V. (2006). Placental abruption. *Obstetrics and Gynecology, 108,* 1005.

Peck, D., and Griffis, N. (1999). Preterm labor in the triage setting. *Journal of Nurse-Midwifery. 44(5),* 449-457.

Post Partum Health Alliance of Northern California. (2000). *PostPartum Depression, Psychosis, and Baby Blues.* San Jose, CA: Post Partum Health Alliance of Northern California.

Queenan, J.T., and Hobbins, J.C. (1996). *Protocols for High-Risk Pregnancies.* (3rd ed.). Cambridge, MA: Blackwell.

Sibai, B. M. (2005). Diagnosis, prevention, and management of eclampsia. *Obstetrics and Gynecology, 105,* 402.

TB Screening
American Thoracic Society (ATS) and the Centers for Disease Control and Prevention (CDC). (2000). Targeted tuberculin testing and treatment of latent tuberculosis infection (Official statement adopted by the ATS Board of Directors, July 1999). *American Journal of Respiratory Critical Care Medicine, 161,* S221.

American Thoracic Society and the Centers for Disease Control and Prevention. (2000). Diagnostic standards and classification of tuberculosis in adults and children (Official statement adopted by the ATS Board of Directors, July 1999). *American Journal of Respiratory Critical Care Medicine, 161,* 1376.

Screening for tuberculosis and tuberculosis infection in high-risk populations. Recommendations of the Advisory Council for the Elimination of Tuberculosis. (1995). *MMWR—Morbidity and Mortality Weekly Report, 44,* 19.

Vaginal Bleeding
Daniels, R., and McCuskey, C. (2003). Abnormal vaginal bleeding in the nonpregnant patient. *Emergency Medicine Clinics of North America, 21,* 45.

Lafferty, S., and Baird, M. (2001). *Telenurse: Telephone Triage Protocols.* Albany, NY: Delmar Thomson Learning.

Long, V., and McMullen, P. C. (2003). *Telephone Triage for Obstetrics and Gynecology.* New York: Lippincott Williams and Wilkins.

Marx, J. A., Hockberger, R. S., Wall, R. M., et al. (Eds.). (2006). *Rosen's Emergency Medicine: Concepts and Clinical Practice* (6th ed.). Philadelphia: Mosby Elsevier.

Pitkin, J. (2007, May). Dysfunctional uterine bleeding, *British Medical Journal, 334(7603),* 1110-1111.

Vaginal Problem: OB/Gyn Procedures
ACOG Practice Bulletin. (2006, May). Clinical management guidelines for obstetrician-gynecologists (No. 72): Vaginitis. *Obstetrics and Gynecology, 107(5),* 1195-1206.

Anderson, M. R., Klink, K., and Cohrssen, A. (2004). Evaluation of vaginal complaints. *Journal of the American Medical Association, 291,*1368.

Long, V., and McMullen, P. C. (2003). *Telephone Triage for Obstetrics and Gynecology.* NewYork: Lippincott Williams and Wilkins.

Workowski, K. A., and Berman, S. M. (2006). Sexually transmitted diseases treatment guidelines. *MMWR Recommendations and Reports, 55,* 1.

RESOURCE LIST

American Pain Society. (1999-2001). Pain: The fifth vital sign, www.ampainsoc.org

Benner, P. (1984). *From Novice to Expert: Excellence and Power in Clinical Nursing Practice.* Menlo Park, CA: Addison-Wesley.

Briggs JK. (2007). *Telephone Triage Protocols for Nurses.* New York: Wolters Kluwer.

Brillman, J., Wachter, D. A., et al. (1999). Pediatric telephone triage protocols: Standardized decision making or false sense of security? *Annals of Emergency Medicine, 33(4),* 368-394.

Brocklehurst, J. C., Tallis, R. C., and Fillit, H. M. (1992). *Textbook of Geriatric Medicine and Gerontology* (4th ed.). London: Churchill Livingstone.

Clawson, J. J., and Dernocoeur, K. B. (1998). *Principles of Emergency Medical Dispatch* (2nd ed.). Salt Lake City: Priority Press.

Daugird, A. J., and Spencer, D. C. (1989). Characteristics of patients who highly utilize telephone medical care in a private practice. *The Journal of Family Practice, 27,* 420-421.

Edmonds, E. (1997, January). Telephone triage: 5 years' experience. *Accident and Emergency Nurse, 5(1),* 8-13.

Edwards, B. (1998, January). Seeing is believing—picture building: A key component of telephone triage. *Journal of Advanced Nursing, 7(1),* 51 -57.

Edwards, B. (1994, April). Telephone triage: How experienced RNs reach decisions. *Journal of Advanced Nursing, 19(4),* 717-724.

Farand, L., Lepcohon, J., Kalina, M., et al. (1995, September). The role of protocols and professional judgment in emergency medical dispatching. *European Journal of Emergency Medicine, 2(3),* 136-148.

Fifield, M. (1995). Telephone triage: Protocols for an unacknowledged practice. *Australian Journal of Advanced Nursing, 13(2),* 5-9.

Fillit, H,, and Capello, C. (1994). Making geriatric assessment an asset to your primary care practice. *Geriatrics, 49(1),* 27-50.

Finley, R. (1995). *Polypharmacy and the Elderly.* Presented at the Contemporary Forums Conference, Telephone Triage: Essential for Expert Practice, Dublin, CA.

Fischer, P. M., and Smith, S. R. (1979). The nature and management of telephone utilization in a family practice setting. *Journal of Family Practice, 8,*321-327.

Fletcher, K. (1995). *Polypharmacy in the elderly.* Presented at the Contemporary Forums Conference, Telephone Triage: Essential for Expert Practice, Dublin, CA.

Goldman, L., and Ausiello, D. (Eds.). (2007). *Cecil Medicine* (23rd ed.). Philadelphia: Elsevier Inc.

Guy, D. H. (1995). Telephone care for elders. *Journal of Gerontological Nursing, 12,* 27-34.

Helliker, K., and Burton, T. M. (2003). Knowledge gap: Medical ignorance contributes to toll from aortic illness. *Wall Street Journal,* Tuesday, November 4, Vol. CCXLII No 89, p. 1.

Hickey M, Newton S, et al. (2005) *Telephone Triage for Oncology Nurses.* Pittsburgh: Oncology Nursing Society;.

Horan, M. A. (1992). Introduction: Presentation of disease in old age. In: J. C. Brocklehurst, R. C. Tallis and H. M. Fillit (Eds.), *Textbook of Geriatric Medicine and Gerontology*. New York: Churchill Livingstone, pp. 145-149.

Joint Commission on Accreditation of Healthcare Organizations (JCAHO). (Oct 14, 2008). Pain standards for 2001. www.jcaho.org/standard/pm.html.

Kennedy, K., Aghababian, R.V., Gans, L., et al. (1996). Triage: Techniques and applications in decision making. *Annals of Emergency Medicine, 28(2),* 136-144.

Lafferty S, and Baird M. (2001) *Telenurse: Telephone Triage Protocols*. Albany, NY: Delmar Thomson Learning;.

Landau, T. P., Ledley, R. S., Campion, H. R., et al. (1982). Decision theory model of the emergency medical triage process. *Computers in Biology and Medicine, 12(1),* 27-42.

Langewiesche, W. (1998, March). The lessons of Valujet 592. *The Atlantic Monthly,* 81-98.

Leape, L. L. (1994, December). Error in medicine. *Journal of American Medical Association, 272(23),* 1851-1857.

Lephrohon, J., and Patel, V. L. (1995, July-September). Decision-making strategies for telephone triage in emergency medical services. *Medical Decision Making, 15(3),* 240-253.

Long V and McMullen PC. (2003) *Telephone Triage for Obstetrics and Gynecology.* New York: Lippincott Williams and Wilkins;.

Marx, J. A., Hockberger, R. S., Wall, R. M., et al. (Eds.). (2006). *Rosen's Emergency Medicine: Concepts and Clinical Practice* (6th ed.). Philadelphia: Mosby Elsevier.

Nobles-Knight, D. (1995). *Polypharmacy in the Elderly.* Lecture presented at the Contemporary Forums Conference, Telephone Triage: Essential for Expert Practice, Dublin, CA.

Osgood, N. J. (1985). *Suicide in the Elderly.* Richmond, VA: Aspen.

Porter, R. D., Kaplan,). D,, Homeier, B. P., et al. (Eds.). (2006). *The Merck Manual of Diagnosis and Therapy* (18th ed.). Whitehouse Station, NJ: Merck and Co., Inc.

Selwa LM, et al. (2002) *Neuro-Triage Telephone Advice.* Boston: Butterworth Heinemann.

Tanner, C. A. (1998). *Clinical Judgment and Evidence-Based Practice: Conclusions and Controversies.* Portland, OR: Oregon Health Sciences University.

Todd, C. (1998). Pain in the elderly, Part I: Assessing a complex population. *NurseWeek.* Feb. 9, 12-13.

Wheeler, S. Q. (2003). *Telephone Triage Protocols for Adult and Pediatric Populations.* San Anselmo, CA: Tele-Triage Systems (www.teletriage.com)

Wheeler SQ. *Telephone Triage Protocols for Infants and Children (Birth to Six Years).* San Anselmo, CA: Tele-Triage Systems; 2003 (www.teletriage.com).

Wheeler SQ. (2003) *Telephone Triage Protocols for School Age Children Age Six to 18.* San Anselmo, CA: TeleTriage Systems; (www.teletriage.com). Accessed Jan 2008.

Wheeler, S. Q. (1993). *Telephone Triage: Theory, Practice and Protocol Development.* San Anselmo, CA: TeleTriage Systems (www.teletriage.com). Accessed Jun 2008

Wheeler, S. Q. (1993). *Telephone Triage: Theory, Practice and Protocol Development.* Albany, NY: Delmar.

Wheeler, S. Q. (1998). *Time Bind/flying Blind: Decision Making under Conditions of Uncertainty and Urgency.* Presented at the Contemporary Forums Conference, Telephone Triage: Essential for Expert Practice, Dublin, CA.

Williams, D. O. (2004). Treatment delayed is treatment denied. *Circulation,* 109,-1806-1808.

Winfrey, M. E., and Smith, A. R. (1999). The suspiciousness factor: Critical care nursing and forensics. *Critical Care Nursing,* 22(1), 1-7, Gaithersburg, MD: Aspen.

Audio Scripts adapted from the following Legal Cases
1998   Burnett vs. Hacker, Hople, Wenzke, Medical Group
1999   Stallings vs. Kaiser Foundation Health Plan of the Mid Atlantic States
2000   Fuentes vs. Thomas-Davis Medical Center
2000 Entwhistle vs. Kaiser Foundation Health Plan of the Mid Atlantic States
2006 Geyer vs Pediatric Resource Medical Group, Inc., et al.

Task Force Biographies

TASK FORCE LEADER

Sheila Quilter Wheeler, RN, MS, has practiced nursing for over 30 years, primarily in the critical care, ED, and clinic settings. She is an accomplished writer, educator, and researcher. Since 1984, Ms Wheeler has pioneered the field of telephone triage. Ms Wheeler is the author of *Telephone Triage: Theory, Practice, and Protocol Development,* has written for the *Journal of Emergency Nursing;* and lectures nationally. She is the founder of the annual national conference "Telephone Triage: Essentials for Expert Practice." In addition to an MA in film, Ms Wheeler holds an MS degree in community health nursing from the University of California, San Francisco.

2009 Contributing Authors/Medical Reviewers

Expert Reviewers

Elsa Tsutaoka, MD, has practiced family medicine in the San Francisco area since 1998. She has a primary care practice in an urban underserved area in San Francisco. Dr. Tsutaoka also serves as assistant clinical professor in the Department of Family and Community Medicine, University of California at San Francisco. She also works in Urgent Care in various locations in the San Francisco bay area, from urban to suburban settings, and has a practice as a student health center physician at City College of San Francisco.

Dr. Tsutaoka's interests include chronic disease care, community involvement, and self-management. She also works in Urgent Care and Student Health Centers. She graduated from UC, San Diego.

Cindy Lamendola, MSN, ANP, is an adult nurse practitioner and clinical research coordinator at the Stanford University in Stanford, California. Ms. Lamendola has a specialized practice in cardiovascular nursing. She currently researches and practices in the areas of insulin resistance, Type 2 diabetes, and cardiovascular disease.

Ms. Lamendola has an extensive background in cardiac rehabilitation and risk factor management. She has lectured nationally and published articles on insulin resistance and CVD risk factors. She is a founding member and past president of the Preventive Cardiovascular Nurses Association and a fellow of the American Heart Association.

Adult/Geriatric Physician Medical Reviewers

Russ J. Kino, MD, is currently director of emergency services at St. John's Hospital and Health Center, Santa Monica, California. He is also assistant clinical professor of medicine at UCLA Medical Center in Los Angeles as well as director of ER on Call, a telephone triage program at St. John's. Dr. Kino has broad experience in emergency medicine both in the United States and in Western Australia, where he did internship and residency rotations at the Royal Perth Hospital. Awards for achievement include the Jack Bercove Memorial Prize in general practice, best scientific paper, National Conference of the Australian College for Emergency Medicine, and Buchanan Prize for top score in National Examination for Fellow of Australian College for Emergency Medicine. Dr. Kino has given numerous presentations on a wide range of topics internationally. His research articles have appeared in peer-reviewed publications.

Edwin Cary Pigman, MD, has served as the medical director of World Access Group, an international travel and medical assistance service organization. Dr. Pigman is assistant professor of Emergency Medicine at George Washington University Medical Center, Washington, DC, and has received awards for excellence in teaching and research. In addition to numerous presentations, Dr. Pigman is a frequent contributor to the *American Journal of Emergency Medicine, Annals of Emergency Medicine,* and others. Dr. Pigman graduated from the Ohio University College of Medicine and received a B. of S. from Edgecliff College of Xavier University, Cincinnati, Ohio.

Pediatric Physician Medical Reviewer

Robert H. Pantell, MD, is chief of the General Pediatrics Division and professor of pediatrics at the University of California, San Francisco. Past positions include chief of adolescent medicine and associate professor of pediatrics, family medicine, and biometry at Medical University of South Carolina; assistant coordinator of ambulatory pediatrics at Stanford University Medical Center; and pediatrician at a community health program in rural Idaho. Since 1974, Dr. Pantell has received numerous awards for his writing and research. He is winner of the American Medical Writers Association award, Robert Wood Johnson Foundation grant, David and Lucille Packard grant, Agency for Health Care Policy and Research grant award, and many others. Dr. Pantell has served as contributor and author for numerous articles and books and is a frequent presenter at regional and national forums. The major focuses of his creative activities are Doctor-Patient Communications, Common Clinical Problems, Health Care Provider Behavior and Modification by Education. Dr. Pantell received his MD from Boston University in 1969, completed his pediatrics residency at North Carolina Memorial Hospital in Chapel Hill in 1972, and a fellowship as a Robert Wood Johnson clinical scholar at Stanford University in 1977.

Adult/Geriatric Nurse Task Force Members

Jeff Howell, RN, CEN, has practiced emergency and trauma nursing for 10 years. He has practiced in New York City and San Francisco. He currently resides and practices in Sonoma County, California. He has also worked as an MICN, paramedic clinical preceptor, telephone triage RN, drug/AIDS counselor at San Francisco General Hospital, and emergency flight transport nurse in the Bahamas. Mr. Howell is currently at work on his MA at San Francisco State University.

Jean Berg Meddaugh, RN, began working for the East Valley Clinic in 1968 when she converted a small room in the Alexian Brothers Hospital into a satellite clinic for the Santa Clara Valley Medical Center. Over the years, she has managed the clinic, which has expanded to become an important community resource, committed to providing care to seniors and the medically underserved on the east side of San Jose. In 1993, Ms. Meddaugh coordinated the development of an Urgent Care Center that offers pediatric and adult medical services seven days a week.

Bertha A. Ruiz, DNSc, RN, GNP, CS, has been a nurse for 15 years, primarily in the areas of medical-surgical nursing and as a gerontological nurse practitioner. Her research and written work has focused on patient health care outcomes and cost effectiveness of nursing interventions. Dr. Ruiz's current research project addresses hip fracture recovery in older persons. She has been active locally, statewide, and nationally on issues regarding education of ethnic populations, specifically those of Latinos. Dr. Ruiz is the founder and immediate past president of the San Francisco Bay Area Chapter of the National Association of Hispanic Nurses and a key member of the California Nursing Coalition for the Emerging Majority. She holds a DNSc degree from the University of California, San Francisco. Dr. Ruiz has held various nursing positions in Oregon, Idaho, Utah, and California.

Adult/OB/GYN Nurse Task Force Members

Laura Wachter Alexander, RN, BSN, IBCLC, has a broad background in nursing as a clinical instructor and patient educator. Ms. Alexander currently works as a lactation consultant and prenatal instructor to California Pacific Medical Center, San Francisco. In the past she has worked for the National Center for Education in Maternal and Child Health, Washington, DC. Ms. Alexander graduated from Northern Illinois University School of Nursing and has practiced nursing since 1979.

Stacy Bischoff, RN, NP, has practiced for more than 19 yr as a women's health care nurse practitioner. She has practiced most recently with Women's Medical Associates, a private OB/GYN practice in Greenbrae, California. Ms. Bischoff has worked extensively for the last 10 years in the areas of family planning and planned parenthood, specializing in infertility, patient education, and adoption counseling. Most recently, Ms. Bischoff has worked in integrative medicine and women's health. Ms. Bischoff received her diploma from Norton Medical Infirmary and nurse practitioner training at Harbor-UCLA Medical Center.

Joan Marks, BSN, NP, has been in a private OB/GYN practice for the last 20 yr in Marin County with Richard H. Printz, MD. Women's health is her primary interest. Ms. Marks received her Nurse Practitioner Certificate from University of California at San Francisco in 1977. She is a graduate of the University of Colorado School of Nursing, 1969.

Suellen Miller, RN, CNM, MHA, PhD, is currently a postdoctoral research fellow at the Institute for Health Policy Studies at the University of California, San Francisco, School of Medicine. Dr. Miller has practiced as a certified nurse-midwife since 1977. She has worked with international organizations as a researcher, educator, and technical advisor in the Philippines, West Indies, and Thailand. Dr. Miller has authored numerous articles and books and is a regular presenter on women's issues. Dr. Miller received her PhD at UCSF, MHA at Antioch University West, San Francisco, and nurse-midwifery at Meharry Medical School in Nashville, Tennessee.

Pediatric Nurse Task Force Members

Jeff Howell, RN, CEN (See Adult/Geriatric Nurse Task Force Members.).

Elizabeth San Luis, MSN, PNP, has practiced nursing since 1972, primarily in the areas of intensive care, dialysis, and pediatrics. Currently Ms. San Luis practices at the Ambulatory Care Center at the University of California Medical Center, where she services low-income, high-risk pediatric patients. Ms. San Luis developed the Clinic for Children of Teen Parents to provide primary care. She provides breastfeeding consultation to patients and providers. Ms. San Luis also provides primary care in a unique family-oriented clinic for children with HIV or AIDS. Ms. San Luis received a MS and a degree as a pediatric nurse practitioner at the University of California, San Francisco.

Susan Valeriote, RN, CPNP, MS, has worked as a pediatric nurse practitioner since 1984. Ms. Valeriote worked for seven years in the Pulmonary Center at Children's Hospital in Oakland, caring for a predominantly Medi-Cal population—single young mothers of minority, lower socioeconomic status with children. As a pediatric nurse practitioner, she was responsible for all telephone triage at the center. Her publications include a tracheotomy care booklet and teaching videos for tracheotomy care and bronchodilator therapy. Most recently she was a clinical professor at the University of California, San Francisco, in the Pediatric Nurse Practitioner program. She holds a BS in nursing from USF, a BSB from Santa Clara University, and an MS from UCSF.

Expert Reviewers

Patricia A. Crane, MSN, RNC, NP, has practiced nursing for 25 yr. Ms. Crane attended the University of Texas Health Science Center at Dallas' Women's Health Care

Nurse Practitioner program and obtained her MSN degree from the University of California, San Francisco, in 1991. As an educator and practitioner, Ms. Crane has provided reproductive health care in a variety of settings and coordinated and lectured in the education program Associate Women's Health Care Nurse Practitioner program for 5 years. As a forensic nurse consultant, she has spoken at national and international conferences on medical-legal issues, specifically interpersonal violence and the cultural practice of female genital mutilation.

Eve R. Meyer, MSW, MSHA, has been executive director of San Francisco Suicide Prevention for 12 yr. She has specialized in training staff members of small community organizations to be part of the larger mental health system. Prior to working in Suicide Prevention, she was marketing director for a group of for-profit health care facilities. She worked at California Pacific Medical in marketing, and for SMP Health Care Architects in system design. She received a masters in social work at the University of Chicago and an MSHA at the University of Michigan.

Adrienne Plasse, MPH, CNM, has been a certified nurse-midwife since 1978, when she graduated from Johns Hopkins School of Public Health's Nurse-Midwifery program. She has worked primarily in underserved communities, Planned Parenthood, and in Central America. She has served in faculty positions at Case Western Reserve University, The Frontier School of Midwifery in Kentucky, and currently at the University of California, San Francisco, in both the School of Medicine and the Nurse-Midwifery Education Program. Ms. Plasse has extensive and current experience in protocol design for OB/GYN, NP, and CNM practice. At present, she works in a community-based women's health clinic and attends births at Marin General Hospital, in Marin County, California.

Donna M. Vincent, RN, BSN, MA, has practiced nursing for 28 yr. She began her career in the neonatal intensive care unit of a large academic center and then went on to develop and teach a perinatal outreach education program for the Robert Wood Johnson Foundation Rural Infant Care Project. Ms. Vincent acted as the director of the Perinatal Advisory Council for Los Angeles communities, which published guidelines for perinatal and neonatal care. She has served as director of four major telephone triage programs across the United States, including those at Boston Children's Hospital at Harvard and Stanford Medical Centers. Ms. Vincent has published numerous articles in the areas of perinatal/ neonatal care and telehealth and has presented lectures at several natural conferences.

Lindsay Wheeler, DC, has been a practitioner of chiropractic since 1982. She has a private practice in Berkeley, California. She lectures frequently on back injury prevention and rehabilitation. She has published numerous articles in chiropractic journals. She has a longstanding interest in self-care and education in the treatment of back pain.

AFTERWORD

"We don't look for patterns of our recurrent mistakes or devise and refine potential solutions for them. But we could, and that is the ultimate point". Gawande, 2009

Any mistake or failure in the diagnostic process can lead to a diagnosis that is wrong, missed or delayed. Inpatient diagnostic errors tend to be more lethal, however more diagnostic errors occur in ambulatory settings". Groszkruger,

It has been my life's work to devise solutions for patterns of error in practice and systems. In 1993, I authored the first "how to" training manual in telephone triage. Two years later, I led a Task Force of 25+ expert nurses, nurse practitioners and physicians to complete the first three-volume set of age-specific, 5-Level Triage adult and pediatric guidelines. Our goal was to create a decision support tool that met the needs of clinicians.

Twenty Years Later

Evidence-based practice Since 1995, research and standards have validated the guideline structure, process and system (training, guidelines, documentation, standards). For example,

- Research on patient safety and error (Institute of Medicine) has emphasized the use of a system-based approach. The guidelines are one part of a system.
- The Joint Commission has pointed out root causes of error (inadequacies of assessment, communications, cognitive error, informed consent, and continuity) -- which these guidelines and system reduce through improved nursing process, force functions and checklists.
- Clinical Call center standards have emerged (URAC), as have practice standards (American Academy of Ambulatory Care Nursing) – both supported by the structure and process of the guideline and system.
- The guidelines improve communications through refined and clarified triage nomenclature developed by American College of Emergency Physicians.
- Finally, Emergency Medicine Standards have been published that emphasize the use of pattern recognition, context and identification of high-risk populations.

In the light of these developments, I felt the guidelines needed to be revised and updated, because these differences constitute significant change.

Health Information Technology Also during the same 20-year period technology literally exploded -- Internet, Healthcare Informational Technology, the electronic medical record (EMR) and electronic guidelines known as Computerized Decision Support Systems (CDSS). In 2011, the global telemedicine market was $11.6 billion in 2011 and is expected to triple to $27.3 billion in 2016, according to a BCC report (http://www.bccresearch.com/pressroom/hlc/global-telemedicine-market-reach-$27.3-billion-2016). Professionally, however, the field lagged behind technology.

"All learned occupations have a definition of professionalism, a code of conduct. It is where they spell out their ideals and duties. They all have at least three

*common elements: expectation of selflessness; of skill; and of trustworthiness.
Aviators have a fourth expectation -- discipline".*   *(Gawande, 2010)*

Malpractice in Telephone Triage Since 1995, I have served as an expert witness related
to telephone triage malpractice -- reviewing and analyzing between 30-35 cases. In the
majority of cases, malpractice was related to recurrent patterns of error -- inadequate
assessments, incomplete documentation, poor communication, and cognitive bias and as
well as inadequate systems.

Many malpractice cases are related to *Delay in Care.* Telephone triage is a risk-prone
clinical subspecialty due to challenges of assessing the symptoms of invisible patients.
The propensity for cognitive bias is worsened due to ambiguity, decision fatigue and a
time-driven work atmosphere that stresses efficiency over proficiency.

By virtue of its difficulty, telephone triage -- of all clinical specialties -- requires a high
degree of professionalism. Early on in the guideline development process, I was
informed that patient patterns of distress are predictable (for example, potential for sepsis
and dehydration in pediatric populations). The information leads us to develop guidelines
to *routinely* investigate and try to rule out these patterns. Our goal was to develop tools
that would anticipate problems, resulting in timely referrals. However, over that 20-year
span, I found that in 30-40% of malpractice cases on which I consulted the outcome were
sepsis – *problems that other guidelines had failed to anticipate and address.*

Research: Current Decision Maker Safety In 2015 I performed a narrative review of the
literature (2002-2012), to evaluate the status of Decision maker Safety in telephone
triage. Despite the small number of substantive studies I found an adequate number upon
which to base the review. Not surprisingly, we found nurses to be as proficient and safer
than physicians; nurses appear to be the best match of clinician to the task of telephone
triage. This prospective conclusion may be due to:

- more *complete* systems
- use of pattern recognition and context in decision-making
- right strategy: estimation of symptom urgency rather than differential
  diagnosis

It is important to note that after decades of practicing *telephone medicine*, physicians still
have no formal telephone triage system, and their documentation is inconsistent. It
appears that physicians are largely unfamiliar how nurses perform the task -- urgency
estimation, pattern recognition, context, the nursing process (for telephone triage). Yet,
since the mid-90's, physicians have developed electronic guidelines (CDSS) that nurses
are required to use.

Despite the introduction of physician-developed CDSS -- presumably designed to make
the process safer – mistriage and delays in care persist. In my opinion, nurses best
utilized as guideline developers, and physicians as reviewers.

Current CDSS Approach to Decision Making

Differential Diagnosis vs Urgency Estimation To date, no independent research has demonstrated the validity and reliability of a given CDSS (Marklund, Randell). In fact, researchers have found that savvy nurses resist using software as intended, instead developing "workaround approaches" (Greatbatch, Holmstrom).

Many current CDSS developers use algorithms. It may be overly deterministic -- aimed at a differential diagnosis. Whereas, medical diagnoses are based on face-to-face encounters and one or more of the following processes http://omerad.msu.edu/ebm/Diagnosis/Diagnosis2.html With the exception of pattern recognition (modified for phone encounters) these diagnostic approaches appear to break down in telephone triage for the reasons described in Box 1.

BOX 1: Medical Diagnostic Processes

Diagnosis may be defined as the "process of using the history, physical examination, laboratory, imaging studies, and other tests to identify the disease responsible for the patient's complaint. Diagnoses help clinicians make informed decision about treatment and prognosis. Physicians use several types of reasoning during the diagnostic process:

- *Pattern-recognition -- "instant recognition" of a disease commonly used for diagnosis of common conditions such as urinary tract infection or sinusitis.*
- *Algorithmic -- using flowcharts and algorithms, this approach is useful for conditions where patient information is discrete and accurate, such as diagnosis of anemia or an abnormal liver function test. Decision trees of individual symptoms are dependent upon automated reasoning, with little or no pattern elicitation, or working hypothesis. Automated reasoning is deterministic (diagnostic; establish a cause) it requires accurate, complete information.*
- *Exhaustive -- gathering every possible piece of data. Used for unusual presentations where other modes of decision-making have failed and after patients have already received a basic evaluation. However, it is generally inefficient in the primary care setting for an initial evaluation.*
- *Hypothetic deductive -- generating and rejecting hypotheses as more data are collected. involves proposing a differential diagnosis, asking a question, using the answer to refine the differential diagnosis, asking another question, again refining the differential, and so on".*

ADAPTED AND MODIFIED FROM
http://omerad.msu.edu/ebm/Diagnosis/Diagnosis2.html

Telephone triage is time-limited, and is not face-to-face. Unlike office or ED visits, there is no immediate access to lab results, x-rays or other resources. The best approach appears to be to use a solid operating procedure – the nursing process -- including thorough assessments, pattern recognition, and urgency estimation.

The algorithmic approach (currently employed in CDSS) appears to be the wrong match of tool to task because it requires accurate information and uses "automated reasoning". In addition, the exhaustive, or hypothetico-deductive approaches are both extremely time-consuming and impractical. Thus, pattern recognition with urgency estimation appear to be the best match of tools to task.

However, in order for pattern recognition to be effective, clinicians must follow the nursing process, perform comprehensive assessments, communicate effectively, provide informed consent, ensure continuity and avoid cognitive bias. These elements are built into the design for the guidelines and system we have developed. We integrated standards and components in order to achieve safety and quality.

They differ from other guidelines in several ways. Some electronic software appear to function like *decision-making* systems (CDMS) and are devoid of clinical training programs or professional standards. These guidelines are *decision support* tools and include an integrated form for documentation as well as standards with optional training. The structure and processes supporting guidelines are robust, reliable and used consistently – in other words, a strong system and professional discipline.

Design Standards for Guidelines

In 2011 the Institute of Medicine recommended that developers set forth design standards for the assumptions, analytic methods, and rationales used in any guideline development. In Clinical Practice Guidelines We Can Trust (2011), IOM sets forth seven criteria required for appraising Guidelines (p 213, Appendix C). While such design standards apply to all telephone triage guidelines, no developer has produced evidence that their guidelines meet such standards. Our goal has always been to meet and surpass these standards, and to make the guidelines as evidence-based as possible.

These guidelines are based on evidence (Goodman & Perrin, 1978; Patel, 1995) related to a clinical pattern recognition strategy (by nurses and nurse practitioners) in telephone triage. They are also derived from categories and descriptions established by ACEP. Finally, they are based on a 5-Tier Triage approach supported by ENA. They were specifically designed to meet and/or exceed the following IOM criteria:

Validity – if guidelines are followed, it will lead to expected outcomes — one of 5 Level dispositions

Reliability/reproducibility – given the same data and using the guidelines, another set of nurses would produce the same results or expected outcomes — safe, timely 5-Tier dispositions

Clinical applicability – explicitly states the populations to which they apply

Flexibility – identifies exceptions to their recommendations

Clarity & Transparency – unambiguous language, precisely defined terms, easy to follow mode of presentation

1) *Validity and Reliability/Reproducibility*

If followed, it will lead to expected outcomes. Reliable: given the same data, another set of nurses using these guidelines would produce the same outcomes. Validity and reproducibility are feasible only if qualified nurses — with adequate clinical training — operate them.

2) *Clinical applicability*

Guidelines were designed to explicitly address three distinct populations: Adults (Age 18+), School Age (Age 6-18), and Infant Child age groups (Birth to Six years) of all risk levels, socioeconomic status and literacy levels.

3) *Flexibility*

The Users Guide identifies exceptions to guideline recommendations, rules or provisions for situations, which do not fall into typical presentations. Some examples include:

- When dealing with high-risk patients, atypical symptoms or situations
- When in doubt about what is the right decision
- When the nurse wishes to upgrade or downgrade
- A robust Standardized Guideline, used as a "go to" or "fall back" guideline for situations where no specific guideline seems to apply.

4) *Clarity*

The authors of the protocols made every attempt to achieve the goal of clarity. As recommended by the Manchester Triage Group (2016), we worked tirelessly to create a product with unambiguous language, precisely defined terms, clear operating instructions and a consistent and user-friendly presentation.

We used 5th – 8th grade level language, so information could be *read directly* to the caller, rather than risk introducing error by having to "retranslate" it from medical jargon or college to 8th grade level.

We simplified the format to streamline the process and to direct the eye through the guideline. Table of Contents are Site-based for ease of locating the correct title.

Guideline dispositions are based on the 5-Tier Triage model, which provides complete instructions for when, where, and why patients should be seen for each of five levels of acuity. The guidelines have been 5-Level since 1995 — when first published in 1993.

5) *Transparency*

By their very nature, books are transparent. Similar to the classic Merck Manual reference, which describes a broad array of symptom patterns, these guidelines are also a reference book format. In addition, the User's Guide has full instructions. The reader can easily understand how the manuals operate.

Changes to 2017 Edition

Since 1995, several experts have reviewed and contributed content revisions to the first editions of Infant-Child, School Age and Adult versions in 2003, 2005 and 2009 respectively. The structure and process are further bolstered by the aforementioned research and standards. We have reframed several key features of the Guidelines -- Checklists (Gawande, Wachter), Force Functions (Wachter) and 5-Tier Triage (Emergency Severity Index, Manchester Triage Group). In the light of new research and standards, these updates can enhance safety and quality.

Built-In Standards to avoid Error

*T*elephone triage interactions represent "virtual visits", not unlike an ED visit. Early research emphasized thorough assessment, contextual and pattern recognition leading to decisions (Perrin, Patel). One method is the use of checklists -- *a key feature of these guidelines.*

Checklists

In the 1995 versions of the guidelines, we developed four Assessment Checklists to use with the guidelines: SAVED, SCHOLAR, RAMP, and ADL. Those checklists remain intact with minor modifications and additions (DEMERIT and SEPSIS). The new approach is to rely heavily on these checklists.

Atul Gawande, MD, set out to improve safety in the surgical process by developing a checklist that would prevent clinicians from forgetting key steps. Dr. Gawande based his book on checklists used by very risk averse industries -- the airline and the building industries. Pilots use the aviation industry checklist before taking off in order to prevent plane crashes. Building contractors consult detailed lists for constructing high-rise buildings – to prevent them from falling down. The World Health Organization noted that as numbers of surgeries increased worldwide, so were complications and deaths. WHO asked Gawande to develop a checklist to make surgery safer.

Gawande saw that two lists were necessary – a detailed list for critical steps to be taken (process); and a list of required communications (assessment). In 1993, I developed checklists to improve communications by avoiding cursory assessments assess symptoms, using the nursing process to insure consistent communication, informed consent and (patient flow) continuity. All of these are consistently built into the process

- Assessment Checklists (SAVED, RAMP, SCHOLAR, ADL, ADEMERIT)
  - Identify high risk populations by age, chronic illness, communication problems, immunodeficiency and other risk factors
  - Identify and rule out certain high risk symptoms
  - Rule out sepsis and dehydration -- more common in high-risk populations

(elderly, debilitated, disabled and pediatric populations).

Force Functions or Safety Features

Guidelines have built-in safety features to avoid errors related to:

- *Assessment to support adequate assessments related to symptoms, patient history, and identifying high risk symptoms and patients.*
- *Communication* to ensure clear, accurate instructions throughout the process. Promote improved oral, written, electronic communications, among staff, with physicians, patient or family.
- *Continuity* to strengthen and promote safe, timely access, correct sites for care, and continuity of care.
- *Human Error* to improve decision-making, reduce decision fatigue, distraction, complacency
- *Patient Rights* elements to ensure informed consent, participation in care, pain management

5-Tier Triage Approach to Dispositions

Telephone Triage Task Force worked tirelessly to simplify – in a reasonable, prudent way -- what can be a mentally arduous and labor-intensive process – that of eliciting, recognizing and sorting symptoms (triage). This approach, now known as "5-Tier Triage" is a current trend (ENA). Early telephone triage research (Perrin, Lephrohon,1985) hypothesized that pattern recognition was the cognitive skill shown to aid decision making without the benefit of visualization or guidelines.

- *2015 ENA Policy Statement (see Appendix B) outlines a policy to develop a 5-level urgency approach for face-to-face triage **and** telephone triage. Our approach has been based on 5-Level Urgency Triage since 1995. It includes flexible time frames and sites for further evaluation that apply 24/7/365, rather than limited to Office Hours.*

Disposition Clarity and Transparency

A "body of knowledge" for triage requires agreed-upon triage terminology (Manchester Triage Group, 2015)

- nomenclature (Classifications: 5-Tier)
- definitions (Definitions for emergent, urgent, etc)
- teaching (Medical and legal tradition, Joint Commission, evidence-based)
- methodology (Nursing Process)
- audit (QA based on AAACN standards)

Our five-level approach builds upon nomenclature based upon ACEP and Manchester Triage Group standards, dividing symptom patterns into five categories of Urgency as follows:

- Life Threatening

- Emergent
- Urgent
- Acute
- Non-Acute

Each level has a time frame and access sites to be further evaluated -- as appropriate -- depending upon the time and day of the week. Each urgency level is intended as a flexible *time frame **and*** a flexible *access venue* for the nurse to determine what is safe, timely and prudent. Nurses have a professional responsibility to use good judgment. A common rule of thumb to apply being "when in doubt, err on the side of caution, and bring patients in sooner rather than later".

Life threatening symptoms always require paramedic transport to ED within minutes. They must be kept NPO. Remain on the line with the caller. Whenever possible, institute a three-way conference call with both parties (patient and EMS services, Suicide Prevention, Rape Crisis or Poison center, for example) as directed by your policies.

Emergent level symptoms always require ED services. Some must be kept NPO. Some patients will require paramedic transport; some may be brought by car by a person who can safely bring them in within the appropriate time frame (0-1 hour). Always notify Labor and Delivery or Emergency Department of pending arrivals of any patient coming via car.

Urgent symptoms typically require evaluation within 1-8 hours (same-day appointment). Some may require evaluation within the hour and are instructed by guideline to "Come in now". Depending upon the time of day and day of the week, some patients may be directed, as appropriate, to Emergency Department, Urgent Care, or office settings for further evaluation.

Some patients in Urgent category may also require paramedic transport due to transportation problems. Some may require other reliable, timely transport as is practical, i.e. Uber, Lyft or Taxi etc. if there is no readily available car or if relatives are too anxious to drive them in. Always notify Labor and Delivery or Emergency Department of pending arrivals any patient arriving via car.

Acute Symptoms typically require evaluation within an 8-24 hour time frame, or a next day appointment. Depending upon the time of day and day of the week, some patients may be directed, as appropriate, to Emergency Department, Urgent Care, or office settings for further evaluation. Always notify Labor and Delivery Department, Emergency Department or Psychiatric Emergency of any pending arrivals of patient being transported via car.

Non-Acute Symptoms may require evaluation within a 24+ time frames or future appointment or advice only. Depending upon the time of day and day of the week (available access), these patients may be directed to Emergency Department, Urgent Care, or office settings for further evaluation, as appropriate.

CONTINUING EDUCATION OPTIONS

PLEASE NOTE: *The Preceptor Workbook (details below) is only available with one of the following CE training packages from teletriage.com in CE section:*

"The Update Package" for Telephone Triage: 18 CE Order online at teletriage.com *(CE is available to a single individual only) Provides an update to recent trends in safety, regulations and legal issues in telephone triage.*

- *Risk Management 1 In Telepractice (2005, 2014) (3 CE)*
- *Risk Management 2 In Telepractice (2005, 2014) (3 CE)*
- *Risk Management 3 in Telepractice (2014) (1 CE)*
- *Safety of Decision makers in Telephone Triage (2015) (6 CE)*
- *Protocol Competency (2012) (5 CE)* Includes one volume of Adult or Pediatric Guidelines
- *Audiolinks to* 10 case studies (2009)
- Preceptor Workbook Download 200 pages (Free)
- Standards Manual Download 80 pages (Free)

Guideline Competency: 5 CE Course may be ordered online at teletriage.com.

- A single volume of Adult, Infant-Child or School-Age Guidelines
- Audio links to 10 case studies (2009)
- Preceptor Workbook Download 200 pages (Free)
- Standards Manual Download 80 pages (Free)

PRECEPTOR WORKBOOK

Telephone Triage: Essentials for Expert Clinical Practice

Description: 200-page workbook with Answer Key serves as an update to the 1993 training manual. It focuses on the essential elements the Role, Risks, Rules of Thumb, Red Flags, Red Herrings, Right Assessment, Right Disposition, and the clinical decision-making process. It also emphasizes methods to reduce errors related to inadequacies in assessment, communication, continuity and human error. The goal of the training manual is to teach participants to get patients to the right place, at the right time, for the right reason.

This training program and tools, processes and strategies utilized in it (for Assessment, Documentation, and Decision Making) represent best practices grounded in an evidence- and standards- based, complete, comprehensive *system* (training program, standards, guidelines, documentation form).

Workbook with Exercises utilizes the methodologies of reading, workbook exercises, and analysis and critique and triage practicum with case studies. Includes 50 Adult and Pediatric written case studies, End of Chapter Exercises and Answer Key. Participants may practice triage skills with Adult and Pediatric written case studies, using a Master

(Generic) Guideline and QA score sheet. Participants will be able to coach less experienced nurses to an adequate level of competency in these areas:

- How to avoid five root causes of error related to telephone triage
- How to utilize Rules of Thumb, Red Flags to make better decisions
- How to utilize five assessment Check Lists and purpose of each
- Improved clinical decision-making process (nursing process), with an emphasis on assessment and communications
- Consistently select safe, timely dispositions from 5-Tier System using 50 Adult and Pediatric case studies

The content contained in this workbook is based on recent research and an article from the American Society of Risk Managers (Groszkruger, D. (2014) Diagnostic Error: Untapped Potential For Improving Patient Safety? Journal of Healthcare Risk Management, Vol 34, No 1, P 38-41), wherein the author stresses the current lack of knowledge about the extent of diagnostic error, and uncertainty about error characteristics and variations in definitions. He recommends remedies such as evidence-based guidelines, remedial education, organizational efforts to reduce human error, improved decision support systems, triggers to identify high risk populations, simulations, post mortem examinations, audits and patient involvement.

Table of Contents

Chapter 1: *Overview*
Chapter 2: *Risk Management Legal Issues & Malpractice*
Chapter 3: *Rules Of Thumb as Decision Support Tools*
Chapter 4: *Assessment Tools & Strategies*
Chapter 5: *Clinical Decision Making Process*
Chapter 6: *Intro to Master Guideline*
Chapter 7: *Communication Strategies*
Chapter 8: *The Documentation Tool*
Chapter 9: *Avoidable Human Errors*
Chapter 10: *Assessment By Proxy*
Chapter 11: *Crisis Calls & "War Stories"*

Made in the USA
Monee, IL
11 September 2022

13771682R00256